In Pursuit of Health Equity

STUDIES IN SOCIAL MEDICINE

Allan M. Brandt, Larry R. Churchill, and Jonathan Oberlander, *editors*

This series publishes books at the intersection of medicine, health, and society that further our understanding of how medicine and society shape one another historically, politically, and ethically. The series is grounded in the convictions that medicine is a social science, that medicine is humanistic and cultural as well as biological, and that it should be studied as a social, political, ethical, and economic force.

A complete list of books published in Studies in Social Medicine is available at https://uncpress.org/series/studies-social-medicine.

ERIC D. CARTER

In Pursuit of Health Equity

A History of Latin American Social Medicine

The University of North Carolina Press *Chapel Hill*

This book was published with the support of the Macalester College Dewitt Wallace Library Open Access Fund.

© 2023 The University of North Carolina Press
All rights reserved
Set in Arno Pro by Westchester Publishing Services
Manufactured in the United States of America

Complete Library of Congress Cataloging-in-Publication data for this title is available from the Library of Congress at https://lccn.loc.gov/2023004208.

ISBN 978-1-4696-7444-5 (cloth: alk. paper)
ISBN 978-1-4696-7445-2 (pbk.: alk. paper)
ISBN 978-1-4696-7446-9 (ebook)

Cover illustration: Pill bottles by paitoonpati/stock.adobe.com.

To Neela, with deep appreciation for your love, patience, and great ideas

Contents

Acknowledgments

I would like to acknowledge the support and advice I have received over the five-plus years that have gone into conceptualizing, researching, and writing this book.

This project was supported by generous funding from Macalester College, the American Council of Learned Societies (ACLS), and the US Fulbright Scholar Program. Chapter 2 of the book was published, in slightly modified form, in the journal *Global Public Health*, and I thank the publisher Taylor and Francis for permission to use it here.

I have a group of longtime supporters who have encouraged my research into the history of medicine and public health, since the time of my dissertation research on malaria control in Argentina, even when that path led me away from some of the central theories and approaches of my home discipline, geography. They include Karina Ramacciotti, Daniel Campi, Marcos Cueto, Andrew Sluyter, Kent Mathewson, Christian Brannstrom, Karl Zimmerer, Susan Craddock, Diego Armus, Carlos Reboratti, Hilda Sábato, Maria Julia Dantur Juri, and Paul Robbins.

This research would not have been possible without the help of colleagues and collaborators abroad, and at other universities in the United States: Jonathan Ablard, Margarita Abraham, Graciela Agnese, Claudia Agostoni, Abel Agüero, Annabelle Alfaro, Marcela Belardo, Enrique Beldarraín Chaple, Carolina Biernat, Anne-Emanuelle Birn, Iris Borowy, Ana Maria Botey, Eve Buckley, José Buschini, Pablo Camus, André Felipe Cândido da Silva, Andrés Carbonetti, Yuri Carvajal, Romina Casali, Horacio Chamizo, Jahi Chappell, Laura Cordero, Maria José Correa, Andrea del Campo, Carlos Dimas, Juan Carlos Eslava, Norberto Ferreras, Federico Ferretti, Cynthia Folquer, Nicolás Fuster Sánchez, Chris Gaffney, Diego Galeano, Raquel Gil Montero, Christopher Hartmann, César Hermida, Patricio Herrera Gonzalez, Jennifer Gunn, Gilberto Hochman, Teresa Huhle, Bob Huish, Verónica Ibarra García, Nora Jarma, Brian Johnson, Ana Kapelusz-Poppi, Jó Klanovicz, Simone Kropf, Nadia Ledesma Prietto, Juan Martín Librandi, Maria Silvia Di Liscia, Renzo Llorente, Fernando Longhi, Gabriel Lopes, Marcelo López Campillay, Ana Paulina Malavassi, Juliana Martinez Franzoni, Kendra McSweeney, Ivan Molina, Mario Morera, Abby Neely, Susana Nuccetelli, Pedro Ottonello, Jairnilson Silva

Paim, Carlos Henrique Paiva, Lara Paixão, Patricia Palma, Steven Palmer, Pablo Paolasso, Marcelo Perez, Jadwiga Pieper-Mooney, Fernando Pires-Alves, Stefan Pohl Valero, Pablo Roberto Possé, Federico Rayez, Karin Rosemblatt, Tobias Ruprecht, Dominchi Miranda de Sá, Marcelo Sánchez Delgado, Pablo Scharagrodsky, Hugo Spinelli, Edna Suárez-Díaz, Mario Testa, Chris Vaughn, Marcela Vignoli, Francisco Viola, Howard Waitzkin, Rob Wallace, Mario Zaidenberg, and María Soledad Zárate.

I benefited tremendously from sharing my research with audiences at conferences in the United States and abroad, including the ALAMES meeting in La Paz, Bolivia, in October 2018. Particular gratitude for the opportunity to present my work at two themed workshops, "Socialist International Health" (Exeter, UK, 2018), organized by Dora Vargha, and "Global Histories of Social Medicine" (Rosendal, Norway, 2022), led by Anne Kveim Lie, Jeremy Greene, and Warwick Anderson. Sebastian Fonseca Chaparro has been a valuable interlocutor. His dissertation, "Latin American Social Medicine: The Making of a Thought Style," was completed when this book project was in its final stages. So, I cite it sparingly here, confident that publications flowing from his dissertation will offer a new and fuller perspective on the Latin American Social Medicine collective since the 1970s.

I am grateful to my research assistants, who helped me locate documents during my time abroad and after I returned to the United States: Diego Labra, Alejandra Raffo, and Enzo Videla. Thanks also to students at Macalester College for their assistance, particularly Anna Bebbington for her transcribing work, and Caroline Duncombe, Finn Odum, Suzanne Rubinstein, Luiza Montesanti, Miranda Harris, and Jordy Marin Urbina for other research and editorial assistance.

Thanks to all the archivists and librarians who helped me gather information, including at the US National Library of Medicine (Stephen Greenberg); the Health Sciences Library at the University of Minnesota (Nicole Theis-Mahon); El Ágora in Buenos Aires (Julia Gago and Mario Rovere); Facultad de Medicina, University of Buenos Aires; the archives of the Biblioteca Nacional in Buenos Aires (Nicolás Del Sotto and Natalia González Tomassini); Biblioteca Nacional in Santiago, Chile; Biblioteca de Museo Enrique Laval (Andrés Diaz) in Santiago; Juan Dalma Archive in Tucumán; Instituto Superior de Estudios Sociales in Tucumán (César Canseco); Archivo Nacional Costa Rica; BINASSS Costa Rica (Irene Ramirez Chavez); Biblioteca Nacional Costa Rica; Biblioteca Luis Demetrio Tinoco at the Universidad de Costa Rica. Special thanks to the interlibrary loan department at Macalester College (Connie Karlen).

Thanks to all the individuals who agreed to be interviewed for this project, who are listed in the bibliography. I did not interview Jairnilson Silva Paim, but I appreciate his willingness to answer many questions via email. I am also grateful for the ALAMES members who spoke with me informally at the 2018 La Paz meeting.

I appreciate the support of all my colleagues in the geography department at Macalester College: Laura Smith, Holly Barcus, Bill Moseley, Dan Trudeau, I-Chun Catherine Chang, Ashley Nepp, Dave Lanegran, Kelsey McDonald, Xavier Haro-Carrión, and Laura Kigin. Thanks also to other colleagues and friends in Saint Paul and elsewhere: Zsolt Nagy, Karla Nagy, Elizabeth Prevost, Mike Guenther, Pablo Silva, Jessemy Jungman, Robert Jungman, Denny Hansen, Julie Lindholm, Ernie Capello, Jess Pearson, Ron Barrett, Devavani Chatterjea, Olga Gonzalez, Erica Busse, Jesse Zarley, Roopali Phadke, Chris Wells, Karine Moe, Paul Overvoorde, and David Van Riper.

The team at the University of North Carolina Press offered indispensable guidance on the writing of this book. Thanks especially to Elaine Maisner, who gave the book much-needed attention (and many opportunities for revision) during her final years as editor for the Latin America collection, María García, and Andreína Fernández.

Last but not least, a deep appreciation to my family who has supported and valued my education throughout my life: my father, Dale, who passed away in 2019; my mother, Virginia; and my sisters, Nicole and Susan; along with my whole extended family. And of course, I could not have done this without my wife, Neela, and daughters, Nalini and Bianca. Thank you for everything.

Abbreviations

AABEMS	Asociación Argentina de Biotipología, Eugenesia y Medicina Social (Argentine Association for Biotypology, Eugenics, and Social Medicine)
ABRASCO	Associação Brasileira de Saúde Coletiva (Brazilian Association for Collective Health)
AFP	Alliance for Progress
ALAMES	Asociación Latinoamericana de Medicina Social (Latin American Social Medicine Association)
AMECH	Asociación Médica de Chile (Chilean Medical Association)
ANEC	Asociación Nacional de Estudiantes Católicos (National Association of Catholic Students, Chile)
APHA	American Public Health Association
APRA	Alianza Popular Revolucionaria Americana (American Popular Revolutionary Alliance, Peru)
BMC	*Boletín Médico de Chile*
CCSS	Caja Costarricence de Seguridad Social (Costa Rican Social Security Fund)
CEBES	Centro Brasileiro de Estudos de Saude (Brazilian Center for Health Studies)
CELADE	Centro Latinoamericano y Caribeño de Demografía (Latin American and Caribbean Demographic Center)
CEPAL	Comisión Económica para América Latina y el Caribe (United Nations Economic Commission for Latin America and the Caribbean)
CESS	Centro de Estudios Sanitarios y Sociales (Center for Health and Social Research, Rosario, Argentina)
CM	Colegio Médico (College of Physicians, Chile)
COMRA	Confederación Médica de la República Argentina (Medical Federation of Argentina)

CSO	Caja del Seguro Obrero Obligatorio (Chile) (Obligatory Workers' Insurance Fund)
CTAL	Confederación de Trabajadores de América Latina (Confederation of Latin American Workers)
DNH	Departamento Nacional de Higiene (Argentina) (National Department of Hygiene)
FAO	Food and Agriculture Organization (of the UN)
FECh	Federación de Estudiantes de Chile (Chilean Students' Federation)
FLACSO	Facultad Latinoamericana de Ciencias Sociales (Latin American School of Social Sciences)
FP	Frente Popular (Popular Front coalition, Chile)
IHB	International Health Board (of the Rockefeller Foundation)
IIPI	Instituto Internacional Americano de Protección de la Infancia (International American Institute for the Protection of Childhood)
ILO	International Labor Organization or Office
IMF	International Monetary Fund.
IOPAA	Integración Operacional de Abajo hacia Arriba (Operational Integration from Below to Above, Colombia)
ISAPRE	Institución de Salud Previsional (Health Insurance Institution, Chile)
IWW	International Workers of the World
LASM	Latin American social medicine
LN	League of Nations
LNHO	League of Nations Health Organization
LRMSC	*La realidad médico-social chilena*
MAB	Movimento de Amigos de Bairros (Neighborhood Friends Movement, Brazil)
MAPU	Movimiento de Acción Popular Unitaria (Popular Unitary Action Movement, Chile)
MOPS	Movimento Popular em Saúde (Popular Health Movement, Brazil)

NAP	National AIDS Program (Brazil)
OIT	Organización (Oficina) Internacional del Trabajo
OPS	Organización Panamericana Sanitaria or de la Salud
OPS/ CENDES	Organización Panamericana Sanitaria/Centro de Estudios del Desarrollo (Pan American Health Organization/Center for Development Studies)
PAHO	Pan American Health Organization
PASB	Pan American Sanitary Bureau
PESES	Programa de Estudos Socioeconômicos em Saúde (Program for Socioeconomic Research in Health, Brazil)
PHC	Primary Health Care
PHM	People's Health Movement
RF	Rockefeller Foundation
SAFCI	Salud Familiar Comunitaria Intercultural (Family Community Intercultural Health, Bolivia)
SNS	Servicio Nacional de Salud (National Health Service, Chile)
SUS	Sistema Único de Saúde (Unified Health System, Brazil)
UERJ	Universidade do Estado do Rio de Janeiro (State University of Rio de Janeiro)
UHC	Universal Health Coverage
UNICEF	United Nations International Children's Emergency Fund
UP	Unidad Popular (Popular Unity coalition, Chile)
USAID	United States Agency for International Development
WHO	World Health Organization

In Pursuit of Health Equity

Introduction

The Pursuit of Health Equity

In March of 1986, more than four thousand people gathered in the national indoor sports stadium for Brazil's National Health Conference. Although this was the eighth time such a conference had been convened since the 1930s, it was unprecedented in its form and focus. Emerging from two decades of authoritarian rule, Brazilian society in the 1980s experienced a dizzying surge of democratic activity, with new spaces for citizen participation in shaping the direction of national life. The 1986 Brasilia conference was one of those spaces: while previous meetings had involved only representatives from the health sector, this time the doors were opened to the public, with delegates from trade unions, grassroots neighborhood associations, nongovernmental organizations, churches, and other civil society groups. Collectively, they planned to lay the foundations for a new national health system, one responsive to the needs and demands of the impoverished masses that had been excluded from Brazil's celebrated "economic miracle" of the previous decades.

Sérgio Arouca, the president of the organizing committee, opened the proceedings with a nationally televised speech. With passion and precision, Arouca explained that the assembly had to decide whether every Brazilian—and indeed, every human being—should be guaranteed a right to health. If so, who was the guarantor of this right? Who would control and regulate the system to make health services available to all Brazilians? And how would a new system be financed? In his speech, Arouca articulated his concept of a right to health, which transcended a mere absence of disease. Instead, Arouca's vision of health encompassed rights to all the resources necessary for human thriving: adequate housing, a formal education, freedom from violence, freedom of expression, and an ability to participate as a citizen in democratic decision making. At a time when Latin America was experiencing an exciting yet fragile transition from dictatorship to democracy, now was the moment to invite full public participation in a complete rethinking of the Brazilian health system, as part of the larger task of reinventing Brazilian society under genuine egalitarian principles.

Arouca's "Democracy and Health" speech sparked four days of intense discussion that yielded a plan for a new Brazilian health system. After several more years of debate and deliberation, including a convention to write a new national constitution, this plan became the Sistema Único de Saúde (SUS), the country's unified health system. For Arouca and his peers, this moment had been building for a long time. As a physician, Marxist academic, and political activist, he belonged to a field known as *saúde coletiva*, or collective health, which in the early 1970s began to formulate a more equitable, just, and effective approach to health in a society marked by extreme division, inequality, and repression. This small group of scholars, political activists, and health system technocrats was, in turn, nurtured and stimulated by connections to a wider movement known as *medicina social*, or social medicine.

Participants in the Latin American social medicine network seldom made their impact as dramatically as Arouca did at the 1986 conference. Mostly they worked out of the limelight, in medical schools, hospitals, community health projects, international health bureaucracies, research centers, universities, and ministries of health, nudging the health field bit by bit toward equity, openness, and new ways of thinking about social determinants of health and disease. Some carried these values into the political arena, as elected legislators and high-ranking health officials. And during times of intense political repression, as in Chile in the 1970s, many in the social medicine group lost their livelihoods, went into exile, or even gave their lives to the cause of promoting health justice. The goal of this book is to tell these stories, in order to make sense of Latin American social medicine, how it responds to and shapes a dynamic political environment, and how lessons from this movement might lead to new ways of thinking about how to achieve health equity in the twenty-first century.

Latin American Social Medicine: The Need for a New History

Social medicine is a field that helped produce broad-based public health improvements across Latin America in the twentieth century, and continues to do so today. However, the deep historical roots, institutional bases, political influence, and public health achievements of Latin American social medicine (LASM) have received scant attention, even with rising interest in the subject among scholars and public health practitioners.[1] Moreover, despite the concurrent rise of social medicine in various countries of Latin America, no one has comprehensively pieced together the institutional, interpersonal, and intellectual connections that made social medicine an international movement. This book, then, attempts to offer the first comprehensive treatment of the history of social medicine in Latin America, with potential lessons for understanding how to promote health equity under challenging political and economic conditions. In short, I seek to offer an intellectual and political history of this influential yet often fragmented movement.

How do we define social medicine? Unfortunately, there is no widely agreed-upon meaning; it has been classified as a philosophy, a field of study, a social movement, or a political stance. Despite the efforts of its most ardent proponents, social medicine has never been universally formalized as a specialty in the way of pediatrics, pathology, or epidemiology (although, as we will see, social medicine has been in a productive dialogue with these fields and many others). Over the course of time, the thematic domain of social medicine also shifts dynamically, despite persistent analytical, ethical, and political threads. In seeking a definition, we confront another issue: not everything that qualifies as "social medicine" was actually labeled as such, perhaps instead filed under "social epidemiology," "community health," "preventive medicine," "collective health," or "critical epidemiology."[2] For all these reasons, it is not easy to construct a definition of social medicine that is consistently valid across time.

Nevertheless, as I define it, social medicine is an academic field that principally focuses on structural determinants of health and illness. Encompassing diverse disciplinary perspectives, social medicine consistently takes a critical stance toward mainstream ideas and practices in medicine and health policy. Social medicine is also typified by a commitment to achieving health equity through political action, meaning that the lines separating medical practitioner, scholar, and activist are fuzzy, if they exist at all. This definition is intended to be broad enough to encompass a complex and heterogeneous field, and one that changes considerably over time.

We should also distinguish "social medicine" and "socialized medicine." Social medicine is an academic field that hinges on an integrative, biosocial perspective on the root causes of illness, whereas socialized medicine is a policy model for organizing the health system. Even though there is good reason to maintain this analytical distinction, the concepts of "social medicine" and "socialized medicine" have often been conflated, not just by academic researchers but also by those involved in the social medicine movement.[3] The two concepts are clearly different but a formal distinction does not do justice to the slippage between them in actual practice. While the domain of academic social medicine extends far beyond analysis of health systems and their defects, social medicine advocacy is often directed toward reforming health systems, with a strong policy preference for socialized medicine. Even today, the main Latin American social medicine organization, Asociación

Latinoamericana de Medicina Social (ALAMES), holds fast to support for universal, state-run health care—that is, socialized medicine. In a recurring pattern, progressive doctors and other health workers often "fall back" to a position of improving the health-care system from within—as a system they can more easily shape, and in which they have authority and expertise—when broader political projects lose momentum.

Difficult to even define or classify, social medicine has been an elusive subject in the historiography of public health and health politics in Latin America. While scholars have written many interesting national case studies—for example, on Chile, which was a hotbed for social medicine starting in the 1920s—we lack a synthesis of these national-scale stories and a tracing of international expert networks within a single narrative across the region. Another shortcoming of much of the historiography on social medicine in Latin America is that its intellectual roots are almost invariably traced back to Europe and its left-wing political and labor movements. As I will argue throughout the book, European influences on Latin American social medicine are overstated. LASM has been a homegrown response to health problems within the specific political-economic context of an "underdeveloped" region. And just as the big questions of Latin American development have invited diverse ideologies and approaches, so too social medicine cannot be reduced to a project solely of the Latin American left.

Thus, one goal of this book is to trace the history of the concept of social medicine in Latin America and how ideas from social medicine are transformed into policies, lasting institutions, and discursive formations that continue to shape perspectives on public health and health systems in Latin American countries. At the same, this book is about people: mostly leftist-progressive doctors, health workers, technocrats, and academics who engage the dynamic political conditions around them, at local, national, and international scales. Some, like Arouca in Brazil or Salvador Allende in Chile, are already renowned for their political skill and leadership. Others are well-known to those familiar with the LASM community, such as Nila Heredia of Bolivia, Asa Cristina Laurell of Mexico, and María Isabel Rodríguez in El Salvador. But we will also hear the stories of lesser-known figures, like Juan Gandulfo, Juan Lazarte, Mario Testa, Clara Fassler, and Francisco de Assis Machado, who all made important contributions in the development of social medicine in the region.

Social medicine also needs to be understood in relation to the larger community of medical practitioners and health professionals. In much of Latin America, physicians were politically active and, especially in the first half of the twentieth century, often members of tight-knit circles of social elites. The interests of their social class, their profession, and the nation as a whole were often in tension. I will argue that social medicine originally thrived in those places where the medical profession had high status and where health technology and infrastructure had reached a sufficiently sophisticated level, but where doctors saw their own power as being under threat. In early social medicine, progressive doctors tended to promote a vision of society where the state would guarantee collective well-being, but under the leadership of scientific experts such as themselves. Early social medicine sought to introduce or accentuate principles of rational management of society; even as many of its proponents pursued public office, they disdained the normal aspects of electoral politics: partisanship, dealmaking, short-term thinking, clientelism, and corruption. Their interventions into the lives of others, well-meaning and supported increasingly by international norms, rarely involved the participation of those being managed.[4]

Thus early social medicine tended to be marked by the same paternalism as medicine more generally, and formations of political alliances with working-class groups (like labor unions) were interesting but exceptional episodes. Only with the revival of social medicine in the 1970s—what I call "second wave" social medicine—did the field begin to take seriously the question of broader participation in the health sector while also developing a critique of the medical profession's (sometimes) self-serving politics. How doctors, especially, understand and advocate politically for their professional interests, often in ways that conflict with the aspirations of social medicine, is a recurring theme in this book.

I also seek to address why some societies are able to lay the foundations for promotion of public health and well-being, while others do not make it a priority. One common answer to this health policy puzzle centers on the notion of "political will," meaning that through deliberative and (usually) democratic processes, some nations have made, as Anne-Emanuelle Birn puts it, a "historical commitment to health as a social goal."[5] Such an emphasis on using the political process to construct lasting health systems is seen as a vital corrective for defects in twenty-first-century global health practice, which tends to favor technology-heavy interventions against specific diseases, often funded by private philanthropies. But where does such "political will" for a commitment to public health come from?[6] It would be gratifying to believe that political pressure for generous welfare states and effective health-care systems comes "from below," generated by grassroots activism within expanding democratic structures. However, as the political scientist James

McGuire points out, the reality is often different: some of the most "progressive" health policies in Latin American countries are actually generated by insulated technocrats, while the political pressure of groups like organized labor often ends up creating fragmented health systems with uneven benefits.[7] In this book, I argue that social medicine has exerted outsized influence in the realm of Latin American health politics; to be even more precise, politically engaged doctors, other health workers, and academics have constructed institutions that function as think tanks, forums for discussion, and pressure groups to steer health policy in more progressive and egalitarian directions. But it would be wrong to call social medicine a grassroots movement, although more recent iterations of social medicine have prioritized democratizing the health sector and forming strategic coalitions with other social movements.

Another major goal of this book is to highlight, and even promote, perspectives from the Global South on health and development questions. In the discourse of global health today, developing countries are often portrayed as sources of problems and bastions of infectious disease rather than as intellectual inspirations or policy models. Even in more critical academic fields, such as medical anthropology or health geography, there is a tendency to take theoretical frameworks native to the Anglo-American academy and impose them on case studies from the Global South.[8] However, in much of Latin America there is a rich scholarly conversation and animated public discourse on health policy questions. Put simply, there is a different way of looking at things. To give one example, Latin American scholars have developed a concept of social *determination* of health, focused on political-economic processes that produce health inequality, in contrast to the concept of social *determinants*, which is viewed as politically neutral and therefore more widely acceptable to the World Health Organization (WHO) and other players in international development.[9] To some, Latin American social medicine exemplifies what Boaventura de Sousa Santos has called "epistemologies of the south" (meaning the Global South), to rival the rigid, unimaginative, and destructive modes of thought that characterize Western modernity.[10] As a US-based academic with an interest in questions of health equity and justice, I am drawn to Latin American social medicine's counterhegemonic tendencies, which push against the grain of both biomedicine (as individualistic, commercialized, and apolitical) and global health policy (with its emphasis on narrow, technical interventions and problematic geopolitical imaginaries).[11]

Social medicine may or may not have the emancipatory potential claimed by some of its most ardent theoreticians, like Jaime Breilh or Edmundo

Granda. But it does matter that this work comes *from* the Global South, based on experiences of health in conditions of underdevelopment and nurtured by networks of solidarity across Latin America and into other areas of the Global South.[12] The theoretical tool kit of LASM is expansive, and includes the structuralist Marxist perspectives that have long characterized Latin American social sciences, along with feminist, post-structural, and Indigenous approaches. Many universities in the region now have full-fledged programs in social medicine or collective health. Even though biomedicine continues to hold more prestige, social medicine has visibility, status, and influence in many Latin American countries, while the field is extremely marginalized in US academia, even in schools of public health.

As alluded to above, social medicine may go by other names. In the Latin American academy, the term "collective health"—a field whose Brazilian origins and broader achievements are described in more detail in chapter 6— is perhaps overtaking "social medicine." Sometimes, in Spanish usage, the terms are used in conjunction, abbreviated as "ms-sc" (*medicina social-salud colectiva*). However, I have decided to use the simpler term "social medicine" throughout the book, except in situations where disambiguation and finer distinctions between fields of study are necessary to do justice to the subject.

The Contested Historiography of Social Medicine

Social medicine has been a somewhat slippery subject in the historiography of public health and medicine in Latin America. In historicizing their field, most prominent scholars in LASM lean on a narrative that emphasizes its European origins and its later diffusion to the Americas, as well as the relatively recent (post-1960s) consolidation of social medicine in Latin America. It is important, therefore, to say a bit about the conventional narrative of social medicine's origins, how this story spread, and why it is due for reconsideration.

The idea of social medicine is frequently traced back to Rudolph Virchow, a pioneering pathologist, and Frederick Engels, the famed critic of capitalism. Born just a year apart in different regions of what would become Germany, they came of age in an era of political revolution. In 1848, while Engels was writing *The Communist Manifesto* with Karl Marx, Virchow reported on a typhus epidemic in Upper Silesia, the causes of which he traced not so much to biological factors, but to social problems, such as poverty, unemployment, and poor housing.[13] Just a few years before, in his report "The Condition of the Working Class in England," Engels, who was not a physician, demonstrated the physical, life-shortening toll of factory work and urban squalor in the early stages of the Industrial Revolution. Virchow, an excellent lab scientist, made prolific contributions to fields such as cell biology, pathology, forensic medicine, and oncology. But his "visions of the social origins of illness pointed out the wide scope of the medical task: the study of social conditions as part of clinical research and health workers' engagement in political action."[14] Virchow's name is often invoked as a symbol of social medicine's transformative potential and revolutionary credentials, as in a 2021 *New York Times* commentary by the epidemiologist Jay S. Kaufman.[15]

The standard history of social medicine, with origins in the revolutionary year of 1848, was first crafted by a group of European and US historians in the 1930s and 1940s, and this narrative lent support to a particular vision for health policy and the medical profession's role in it. Henry Sigerist, George Rosen, and Erwin Acknerknecht, in particular, first constructed the image of Virchow as the founder of social medicine, over and above his long-recognized contributions as a pioneer in cellular pathology.[16] Beyond their writings on social medicine, these scholars transformed the history of medicine in general; by introducing an analytical framework based in historical materialism, Sigerist and his disciples situated the development of medicine and public health in dynamically changing societies under capitalist political economies and moved the field away from triumphalist narratives of scientific progress.[17]

Thus, Sigerist, based at Johns Hopkins University, was never just narrating the history of social medicine; he was also crafting important analytical tools for contemporary scholars and engaging in political advocacy, especially at a time—the Great Depression, followed by World War II and the liberal internationalist hopes of the early postwar period—when the continued growth of the welfare state seemed desirable and perhaps inevitable. Sigerist was also a consultant of sorts in the development of the universal health-care system for the province of Saskatchewan, under the leadership of Tommy Douglas, which was the model for Canada's national health system.[18] Later, Sigerist's sociopolitical histories of medicine inspired the cutting analyses of a vocal, international, leftist-progressive front against business as usual in the health field, including Milton Roemer, Milton Terris, Vicente Navarro, Gustavo Molina, Howard Waitzkin, Elizabeth Fee, Nancy Krieger, and Paul Farmer.

As an academic field, social medicine's first peak, in the Atlantic world, happened just after the end of World War II.[19] At that time, there were professorial chairs or institutes of social medicine at Johns Hopkins, Yale University, Columbia University, the New York Academy of Medicine, Oxford University,

Cambridge University, and the University of Edinburgh. The field attracted support from such philanthropic organizations as the Milbank Memorial Fund in the United States and the Nuffield Trust in the United Kingdom.[20] Social medicine seemed in sync with the humanitarian liberal internationalism of the early postwar period, evident in the elevation of the Canadian Brock Chisholm to the role of first director-general of the new World Health Organization.[21] As the proceedings of a 1947 New York conference on social medicine attest, there was optimism about the postwar order, as a triumph of liberalism and the best aspects of modernism, with encouraging signs of further expansion of welfare state institutions in the victorious Western nations.[22] (Notably, the so-called Beveridge Report of 1942 laid the foundations for the British National Health Service, established in 1948.[23])

But in these same proceedings, one can also see characteristic aspects of the field that would lead to its decline, or at least its temporary eclipse: unfashionable holism, eclectic philosophical influences, incoherence as a scholarly field, and the lack of a research agenda. John Ryle, of Great Britain, promoted social medicine as "an expression of scientific humanism" and hoped to turn "clinical medicine into a new discipline of holistic socio-biology of health and disease." Yet as Dorothy Porter noted, "Ryle's holistic conception of social medicine did not survive him."[24] Medical education—whether in the formation of clinicians or medical researchers—became even more reductionist and oriented toward biomedicine, under the hegemony of the ideas of Abraham Flexner and his reforms of medical education in the United States, starting at Johns Hopkins (giving us the term "Flexnerian," applied, usually pejoratively, in many later social medicine texts). Meanwhile, social medicine gave way to social epidemiology, "highly quantitative and, by contrast to Ryle's holism . . . methodologically reductive and positivistic" (although other commentators, like Nancy Krieger, see no intrinsic antagonism between the social justice-oriented values of social medicine, a quantitative methodological approach, and rigorous theory building).[25] Meanwhile, in response to geopolitical pressures and following the technocratic development logic of the Cold War, the WHO turned its back on rights-based, horizontal approaches that required comprehensive, critical analysis of social inequalities. A sort of "medical McCarthyism"—starting in the United States, but spreading widely through international health circles—also discouraged anything vaguely socialist in health politics.[26] Thus began the long postwar hiatus of social medicine.[27]

As a coherent Latin American social medicine movement began to take shape in the early 1970s, some of its key actors developed an origin story for

LASM that leaned heavily on the accounts of Sigerist and colleagues. This narrative of the movement's history implied a rebirth of social medicine after decades of nonactivity, and an ideological base in leftist political thought. The genealogical connections of LASM to the founding-father figure of Rudolf Virchow were seemingly solidified with the historical writing of the US sociologist-physician Howard Waitzkin, who contended that Virchow's student, Max Westenhöfer, became a mentor to a young Salvador Allende in Chile. In this way, social medicine ideals were ostensibly handed down from one generation to the next, into the contemporary era. As I have argued elsewhere (with Marcelo Sánchez Delgado), this narrative, though popular, lacks empirical support and presents a distorted vision of early Chilean social medicine. During social medicine's first wave in Latin America, before historians like Sigerist began to revive his memory, Virchow was considered a trailblazing biomedical researcher but was not influential in social medicine thought. The association between Westenhöfer and Allende is tenuous, if it existed at all, and they did not align ideologically, given that Westenhöfer supported the Third Reich and Allende was a steadfast anti-fascist.[28]

Since the late 1990s, there has been rising interest in the history of LASM, motivated partly by an effort to show the "deep roots" of progressive, social-justice-oriented health policy. Other charismatic figures, like the leftist icon Che Guevara or the colonial-era doctor Eugenio Espejo, have been added into the historical pantheon of LASM.[29] The new historiography of LASM suggests that a social justice orientation is deeply rooted in Latin American health systems, and the invocation of such a tradition helps in the struggle to protect and expand hard-won gains and to resist the incursion of neoliberalism and US-inspired models of health care.[30]

In Latin America, the historiography of second-wave LASM is often dominated by what Carlos Henrique Paiva and Luiz Antonio Teixeira call "actor-authors," that is, veterans of social medicine writing the history of the movement as they experienced it.[31] These accounts are richly detailed but the narratives tend to start no earlier than the 1960s, ignoring affinities and continuities between the different waves of Latin American social medicine.[32] Meanwhile, Latin American historians of health and medicine who focus on the 1930s and 1940s, particularly, tend to treat social medicine as a tendency that arises abruptly in episodes of health systems reform or welfare state expansion, quite bounded by national historiographical contexts, rather than recognizing international connections.[33]

In this book, I build on this recent historiography while seeking to develop a historical narrative of social medicine in Latin America that is less dependent on European origin stories, transnational in scope, ideologically plural-istic, and concerned with the translation of ideas into policies and lasting institutions. Many accounts of social medicine's history in Latin America, written by committed members of the movement today, skip over inconve-niently non-leftist figures of social medicine's first wave in the early twentieth century (such as Carlos Paz Soldán in Peru, Eduardo Cruz-Coke in Chile, or Ramón Carrillo in Argentina), erase vibrant debates within the movement, and neglect the reasons for social medicine's mid-century ebb before its re-vival around 1970. Rather than creating movement idols, historical research should connect the dots to explain why social medicine becomes prominent in some places rather than others, how its concerns change over time, how institutional and interpersonal networks sustain an interest in social medi-cine, and how it gains influence in the realms of health and social policy. By exploring the contributions of a range of actors, taking seriously the geneal-ogy of ideas and ideology, and being attentive to broader political and geopo-litical contexts, I present a new perspective on the development of LASM.

Method and Approach

At the outset of this project, my goal was to combine a history of ideas, a his-tory of expert networks, and a history of policy. That is, I aimed to examine the intellectual roots of social medicine and its development as a scholarly field, the expert networks and institutions that sustained or advanced social medicine ideas, and how these ideas translated into policy. Here, I explain my analytical approach and why I made certain choices in my research.

Using a broadly Foucauldian approach, I consider the history of social medicine as a story of the construction of disciplinary knowledge, and how a discipline becomes formalized, professionalized, and institutionalized. Ricardo Salvatore, in his history of US academics constructing knowledge of South America in the early twentieth century, writes: "I consider disciplinary knowledge itself to be imperial. Disciplinary knowledge can only increase its scope, consolidate its domain, and build comparative inquiries by extending its reach to incorporate the territory of the Other."[34] While this is typically true, the story of social medicine is almost the opposite of what Salvatore suggests. Social medicine has always been something of an underdog, strug-gling for recognition and respect against mainstream medicine, hegemonic models in international development, and adverse geopolitical conditions. Yet, as Margarita Fajardo writes in her study of Latin American economists and other social scientists at the Comisión Económica para América Latina y el Caribe (CEPAL), an "overbearing focus on and the presence of Northern institutions in the region" may obscure the success of Latin American intellectuals and activists.[35] Put another way, a position in the global scientific, geopolitical, and economic periphery is not simply, or mainly, an obstacle for social medicine; rather, these same conditions may be a source of critique, creative inspiration, and movement solidarity. International health has been a "dynamic arena" where "local [Latin American] actors ... national politicians, researchers and policy specialists, transnational professionals, and international agencies interact and mold one another."[36] How social medicine experts navigate uneven power relations in many domains (academia, medical science and practice, international development, geopolitics) is one motif throughout the book's narrative. The larger point is that the formation of a field like social medicine cannot be understood in a vacuum, outside of larger academic and political contexts.

Given the importance of how scientific fields define boundaries around themselves, I have also found a need to reconstruct the history of the health-related social sciences in Latin America. Only recently have scholars like Salvatore, Fajardo, and Joanne Rappaport started to uncover the history of the social sciences in Latin America.[37] LASM scholarship itself, especially the writings of Juan César García and Everardo Duarte Nunes, is useful for constructing the history of the social sciences as applied to health in the region.[38] Simplifying a bit here, the protagonists of first-wave social medicine were mostly doctors with eclectic intellectual inspirations at a time when the academic social sciences were in their infancy in Latin America. Second-wave LASM, by contrast, took social theory very seriously, with harsh criticism of dominant paradigms in the health field (behaviorialism, functionalism, positivism), in favor of critical, neo-Marxist approaches, along with nascent post-structural analyses, such as Foucault's influential work on power/knowledge in the field of medicine.

The persistence and development of social medicine in Latin America have depended on the growth and maintenance of networks that connect individuals and institutions, in a common endeavor but with spaces for debate and disagreement, as well as linkages to other networks (for example, in the international health and development bureaucracies) not explicitly devoted to the cause of social medicine. Most scholars would appreciate the importance of networks in knowledge production; academic life is made up of associative spaces, such as conferences, scholarly associations, academic journals, groups of collaborators, university faculty, classrooms, and so forth; we expend uneven amounts of effort on the development and maintenance of these associative spaces, given our personal and professional priorities, scholarly interests, and assessments of influence; and these institutions transcend us as individuals—they have momentum of their own.

Initially, one of my research objectives was an effort at *historical reconstruction* of networks: to actually reassemble, formally and systematically, nodes (individuals and institutions) and linkages or relationships between the nodes (e.g., as collaborators, colleagues, mentors and students, etc.). Newer computer software applications facilitate what could be a tedious and complex task. While I did use network visualizations to organize my thoughts, I decided not to let my analysis rest on such formal, quantitative network analysis methods, since the archival record that is vital to "abstracting relational information from sources" is too fragmentary for this field (especially in the early twentieth century), and so much qualitative interpretation is necessary to determine what constitutes important and substantive relationships.[39] Instead, I use a "life trajectory" approach, which was suggested by an article that happens to be about a pivotal figure in second-wave LASM, Juan César García (whom I discuss in more depth in chapter 6).[40] This approach emphasizes the role played by significant individuals (like García, in this instance) moving through trajectories in time and space, some well-planned and others more serendipitous, that help produce and congeal networks that carry out collective intellectual and political work. At the same time, I adhere to the same general approach rising in Latin American historiography, tracing the international networks in areas like natural science, social sciences, health, and labor organizing that work to transcend conventionally insular national case study approaches.[41] This approach is explained in more detail in chapter 2, where I analyze international influences on first-wave LASM.

In 2015–2016, I conducted archival and interview-based research in Argentina, Chile, and Costa Rica, thanks to funding from the Fulbright US Scholar Program and an American Council of Learned Societies fellowship. I selected these countries because of their often-cited public health achievements, diverse political-economic circumstances, and centrality in international networks in social medicine and health policy. Key primary sources include medical journals, newspapers, correspondence, conference proceedings, and government documents, with a focus on the fields of public health and social medicine. For the latter period under study (essentially, from the 1960s onward), I make use of long and wide-ranging interviews I conducted with key players in social medicine and public health policy. These conversations are especially useful for reconstructing expert networks and understanding the political challenges faced by left-leaning social medicine advocates; many of the medical professionals I spoke to were exiled from Argentina or Chile during the military dictatorships there. I later spent some time in Brazil to establish connections that helped me understand the collective health movement, and I participated in the 2018 ALAMES meeting in La Paz, Bolivia, where I shared a preliminary outline of the book project and spoke to ALAMES members (although I am not a member of the association). Since the book covers a lot of ground, both chronologically and spatially, I also take full advantage of the growing and conceptually rich secondary literature on social medicine, public health, health systems, social development, and the welfare state in Latin America. I have benefited tremendously from the open, accessible culture of academic publishing in Latin America.

As I assembled the pieces of this new history of Latin American social medicine, I also contemplated the temporal and spatial boundaries of the narrative. The story begins around the end of World War I, due to several coinciding factors: rising frequency of use of the term "social medicine" in the region, for example, in medical and public health journals; the apogee of the medical profession's influence on national politics through the related hygiene movement; and the shifting political environment favorable to new welfare state institutions (at least in welfare state "pioneers" like Argentina, Uruguay, and Chile). The story ends around the early 2000s, as social medicine gained renewed prominence in the health policy planning of so-called Pink Tide governments of the region. Given my choice to take the long historical view on Latin American social medicine, what follows is not primarily an institutional history of ALAMES (founded in 1984) or the Brazilian national collective health organization, Associação Brasileira de Saúde Coletiva (ABRASCO; founded in 1979), which have received fuller treatments elsewhere.[42]

In terms of spatial extent, it is impossible to cover every part of Latin America with the same amount of depth, so I have centered the narrative selectively on prominent nodes of research and activism in social medicine, especially Chile, Argentina, and Brazil. Some countries that might seem logical to include because of their famously effective universal health systems, like Costa Rica and Cuba, are largely left out of the story (as I explain in chapter 7). Without a doubt, the country most conspicuous in its (near) absence is Mexico. Historians have examined rural health projects connected to the process of agrarian reform in the postrevolutionary period, along with other innovative public health programs under the presidency of Lázaro Cárdenas.[43] Such endeavors could rightly be seen to epitomize a social medicine approach, and they coincide with the most energetic period of first-wave social medicine in the 1930s. However, it was a challenge to treat the country's public health politics with the same level of detail and nuance I devote to Chile and Argentina. Given that Mexican actors and institutions appear in the context of rural health projects (chapter 1), international labor organizing (chapter 2), new academic spaces for social medicine (chapter 6), and the translation of social medicine theory into health policy (chapter 7), one could envision an alternate history of Latin American social medicine anchored in Mexico. And I think there is much more to be said about progressive health movements in Ecuador, Venezuela, and Peru. Again, the goals of comprehensive coverage and narrative coherence were sometimes at odds, but the *Latin Americanness* of social medicine, as a question of movement identity, is hard to dispute.

It is also important to say a bit about my identity as a researcher and how it influences my work on this project. I am a geographer, but engaged with debates in fields like the history of science, history of public health, and history of international development.[44] Reflecting my affiliation with the subfield of medical or health geography, I have always been interested in theories of "the social" in the health field; that is, how to conceptualize the ways individuals interact with the natural, social, and built environment around them, in ways that can produce health-promoting outcomes—or not. For many health geographers, this concern is the core of the field, which accommodates a wide range of epistemological positions, influenced to varying degrees by structural, post-structural, and humanist approaches. And, with my background in political ecology and development studies, I am especially mindful of the power of hegemonic discourses in the international development field and how some voices (from the political left, usually, but also from grassroots, Indigenous, and other subaltern social movements) are silenced or marginalized. As a geographer, I also believe it is crucial to connect global- and local-scale processes through the workings of institutions, discourses, and networks. Much of the failure of development planning (whether specifically in the health field or in other domains) comes from a lack of careful historicizing of local social, political, and environmental contexts. That is why, throughout this book, I try to develop textured historical narratives to explain how social medicine emerged from experiences in specific times and places.

Outline of the Book

Chapter 1 begins with a political-intellectual history of the origins of social medicine in the Latin American context. I offer an alternative history that disputes the notion that social medicine diffused from Europe to Latin America as a coherent leftist ideological project. In the region, social medicine emerged as one response to what was termed the "social question," a coming to grips with the social consequences of modernization and urbanization. With the academic social sciences still in their infancy, the pioneers of social medicine, such as Paz Soldán, used an eclectic analytical tool kit that adapted ideas from the natural sciences about organisms, systems, harmony, growth, and decay and applied them to understand the workings of society. Social medicine was also strongly tied (and at times hard to distinguish from) other streams of scientific-reformist thought, including eugenics (and "race science," more generally), scientific hygiene, and puericulture. Special attention is paid to the ideological foundations of different strands of social medicine, including socialist ideas, Catholic social doctrine, and anarchism.

Chapter 2 examines the international networks that influenced ideas and policy in social medicine in the 1930s and 1940s in Latin America, focusing on institutional networks shaped by the League of Nations Health Organization (LNHO), the International Labor Office (ILO), the Rockefeller Foundation (RF), and the Pan American Sanitary Bureau (PASB, the predecessor of the Pan American Health Organization, PAHO). After examining the architecture of these networks, this chapter traces their influence on the policy domain of social insurance, or social security, a cornerstone of the welfare state. Closer scrutiny of a series of international conferences and local media accounts of them reveals that international networks were not just "conveyor belts" for policy ideas from the industrialized countries of the United States and Europe into Latin America; rather, there was often contentious debate over the relevance and appropriateness of health and social policy models in the Latin American context. Furthermore, the weakness of these international institutions, as compared to postwar health and development organizations, meant that Latin American countries had more latitude for policy experiments based in progressive social medicine concepts. In parallel, an international network of Latin American socialists grew, but I argue that their influence on contemporary social medicine was subtle, indirect, and delayed.

Chapters 3 and 4 center on two countries where social medicine made a difference in the construction of health and social policy, Chile and Argentina, in the 1930s and 1940s. While these countries are often recognized as welfare-state "pioneers" in Latin America, the influence of actors and institutions of social medicine on the development of the welfare state is not well understood. In Chile, social medicine was a fluid field of policy experiment, where participants drew inspiration from a hodgepodge of internationally available health policy options and worked to adapt them to their diagnosis of Chilean realities. The political engagement of progressive physicians led eventually to the creation of the Chilean National Health Service, a major landmark in the development of comprehensive health systems in Latin America. Chapter 4 focuses on the development of the social medicine milieu and its political consequences in Argentina, with special attention on the "classic" Perón era from 1945 to 1955. It is easy to portray Peronist health reforms as having been undermined by outside conservative forces, but in this chapter I argue that the move toward an ambitious universal health-care system was stymied in large part by competing interests within the Peronist governing coalition. In addition, the medical profession organized to offer either active or passive resistance to many of the gestures toward centralization of health services of the Perón government. As a result, even today Argentina's health system is marked by fragmentation and stratification.

In chapter 5, I argue that social medicine receded in the face of increasingly technocratic modes of health policymaking in the early Cold War era. In part, social medicine was a victim of its own success, as much of its agenda became institutionalized in national health systems planning. With the guidance of international organizations such as PAHO, the WHO, and CEPAL, the cultivation of health systems professionals became more formalized, and with expertise developed in modern social sciences with roots in behavioralism, functionalism, and positivism. The postwar international development apparatus performed a function of ideological discipline, driving out radical proposals for health equity and democratic participation in health planning. The career of the Chilean Abraham Horwitz, who maintained a kind of political neutrality despite Cold War tensions, serves as an archetype of trajectories in mainstream international health. I also examine the life of Josué de Castro of Brazil as Horwitz's ideological opposite; Castro's expansive worldview and politically charged analyses of the roots of hunger and disease were, in a way, ahead of their time. Tracking the hiatus of social medicine in the 1950s and 1960s helps clarify the meaning and focus of the field and sets the stage for a revival of LASM in the 1970s, which was led by disaffected health technocrats inspired by new kinds of social theory and political critique.

Chapters 6 and 7 describe this second wave of social medicine in Latin America. Starting in the early 1970s, new theoretical currents from the social sciences reinvigorated social medicine thought. During an era of right-wing authoritarian governments across the region, these ideas were often too radical for open discussion in universities, academic journals, or the media. The political climate of the time, marked by the Cuban Revolution, new student movements in Mexico and elsewhere, and the violent overthrow of Allende's government in 1973, added urgency to social medicine debates, and many left-leaning health professionals from Argentina and Chile were forced into exile by military regimes. New ideas in social medicine (or in Brazil, *saúde coletiva*) flourished in key nodes across the region. From a privileged position in the PAHO, the Argentinean Juan César García coordinated, sometimes covertly, the research and activism of these nodes, eventually coalescing in the formation of ALAMES, an international association of professionals in social medicine.

In chapter 7, I analyze LASM from the 1980s to the early 2000s, a turbulent period marked by both a restoration of democracy in much of the region and the rise in neoliberal or free-market-oriented policy prescriptions, often imposed by the World Bank or International Monetary Fund. LASM, as a left-leaning academic-activist field, thrived in the new openings created by democratization, as demonstrated by the successful health reform movement in Brazil. At the same time, second-wave social medicine resisted neoliberal schemes to transform the health sector, by investigating the transnational financial interests behind privatization, by analyzing the life-threatening consequences of the disintegration of the welfare state, and by directly influencing and guiding health policy under leftist-populist regimes in the early 2000s. In this chapter, I also discuss the cases of two countries, Cuba and Costa Rica, that have been largely disconnected from second-wave social medicine networks, despite their renowned egalitarian health policies, and I sketch the lines of research that sustain social medicine and collective health as a critical academic field, into the present.

In sum, Latin American social medicine is a movement and an idea that, though it might not heal the world, deserves broader consideration. At this time of great uncertainty, I hope that this book demonstrates the power of ideas and the value of political activism by doctors, academics, and others dissatisfied with the status quo—not only in health policy but also in the organization of society, the international geopolitical order, and even the way we understand our bodies and our well-being.

CHAPTER ONE

Roots

The Origins of Social Medicine in Latin America

This chapter and chapter 2 focus on the formative period of social medicine's first wave in Latin America, from around 1900 to the early 1930s. The main goal of this chapter is to offer an intellectual history that sorts out the often-subtle differences between social medicine and other, overlapping schools of thought that were dominant among reform-minded groups in the medical profession. Chapter 2 analyzes how international networks and institutions linked to Europe and North America shaped the development of social medicine in Latin America. As discussed in the book's introduction, conventional narratives portray social medicine as a field that originated in Europe and imported into Latin American scientific circles by way of notable figures. However, such narratives should be approached with caution, due to a lack of supporting evidence for specific chains of diffusion and because diffusionist narratives overemphasize the role of Europe as a source for innovation in the social medicine field.[1] A related misconception is that social medicine bloomed suddenly in the 1930s, as the worldwide economic depression reversed progress in population health conditions, threw a capitalist economic model into crisis, and opened up new political possibilities—not least, a channeling of popular demands into the structure of modern welfare states.[2] This periodization also aligns with interpretations that classify social medicine as mainly a project of the political left.

In this chapter, I argue that we do not need to look to Europe to understand the origins of social medicine in Latin America and that social medicine thought germinated in the region well before the 1930s. I trace the origins of social medicine to the so-called social question, which, in many Latin American countries, was a coming to grips with the consequences of capitalist modernization. As in contemporary Europe, the social question centered on how to design political institutions to manage rapid social and economic change. Situated between traditional, conservative elites, on the one hand, and the more radical proposals of movements like anarchism, anarcho-syndicalism, and socialism, on the other, the positivist intellectuals who addressed the social question settled largely for a middle way that entailed slow political reforms to channel the demands of the working class along with social policies meant to improve living standards and buffer the worst excesses of capitalist development.

As I see it, social medicine was born in this broad, reformist middle ground. Under the sway of Comtean positivism, health reformers saw society as malleable and manageable through the application of scientific knowledge. Reformers also drew, to a lesser degree, on the notion of "social justice" from Catholic social doctrine, which was essentially the church's doctrinal reckoning with the social question. The major ideological formations of the era—socialism, anarchism, and liberalism—do not map neatly onto different types of social medicine. Rather, we find that social medicine eclectically borrowed ideas that may not at first seem ideologically compatible. As Dorothy Porter and Roy Porter aptly put it, "The history of ideas about social medicine brings to light many competing—often contradictory—systems of belief."[3]

It is not really possible to understand social medicine of the time without recognizing that its advocates were fully immersed in the tenets of *higienismo*, the hygiene movement. In a way, social medicine was a stronger expression of the hygiene movement's conviction that society's ills could be managed with the analytical tools of medical science backed by strong states. To contend that social medicine drew inspiration from the social sciences in this early period has it exactly backward; rather, hygienists projected the frame of the natural sciences onto the workings of society. Here, I concur with Foucault's interpretation of the "birth of social medicine": it was not an "anti-medicine" but rather signified an intensification of medicalization as developmental states became concerned with the productivity of human capital and the environmental conditions of cities.[4]

Again, this chapter is intended as a history of ideas. In this analysis, I try to be attentive to how historical actors in the early 1900s actually employed the term "social medicine," while also recognizing the indefinite boundaries (and complex connections) between it and other fields or epistemes, such as hygiene, eugenics, puericulture, and anarchism. My analytical strategy here is inspired by Foucault's "genealogical" approach. One of the most lucid explanations of this approach comes from an article on the history of the concept of "disaster medicine" by Cécile Stephanie Stehrenberger and Svenja Goltermann. "Analyzing the history of disaster medicine by using a genealogical method," they write, "means that we can neither pinpoint a single origin of disaster medicine nor discern any linear progressive history leading toward its perfection."[5] The same could be said of social medicine. With the genealogical approach, I try to avoid the error of teleology, which would be a reading backward from the "endpoint" or current conceptualization of social medicine in a search for its origins. Since "genealogy is as much interested in ruptures and discontinuities as it is in conti-nuities," I also make a point of discussing movements that were truncated, such as an anarchist tendency of social medicine.[6] So the genealogical approach is also concerned with what "might have been" under different historical circum-stances. This approach also differs from overly simplistic genealogical frame-works where ideas, ideologies, and values seemingly get "passed down" from mentor to disciple, one generation after another.

The chapter first explores how liberal elites of the early 1900s in Latin America constructed the social question as a public health crisis. Miserable health conditions were a manifestation of poverty and stark social divisions that could spark radical political movements. Imbued with positivist ideas of progress through science, reformers offered a program of state-led improve-ments in sanitation and hygiene to ameliorate the worst consequences of capitalism and to incorporate urban workers, in particular, into a project of national development. Next, I turn to the hygiene movement and its rela-tionship with social medicine. Here I use the writings of a renowned hygien-ist, Carlos Paz Soldán, of Peru, to construct a "syllabus" for social medicine of that era, which encompassed the higienistas' narrower fields of concern, like puericulture, sexual hygiene, occupational medicine, and rural medicine. The subsequent section explores the disconcerting association between social medicine and eugenics, wherein prominent ideas from race science evoked a biopolitical emergency of racial degeneration, lending urgency to the project of social medicine. My survey of social medicine's early history closes with a discussion of anarchist versions of social medicine. Although it was never that prominent, the anarchist alternative can be held up as a mirror to clarify some essential philosophical issues in social medicine, especially with respect to the relationship between individuals, society, and the state, and the capac-ity for small-scale, grassroots, and cooperative organizations to liberate and empower the working class.

Health Crisis and the Social Question in Latin America

As in Europe, social medicine emerged as a scientific project to confront the "social question" of the late 1800s and early 1900s. In essence, the social ques-tion was a reckoning with the effects of capitalist industrial development: the rupturing of traditional patterns of production, the increasing divisions be-tween social classes, rampant poverty, and mass migration from the country to the city.[7] In Latin America's largest cities, the degradation of environmental and public health conditions gave the social question a visceral urgency.[8]

The social question prompted examination of the proper role and reach of the state in regulating the economy and ameliorating social crises. How could pressures for political participation, voice, and recognition of civil and social rights be accommodated in a stable political system while avoiding a revolution from below? To the liberal elites who posed and debated the social question, such concerns were vivid and real. In Chile, for example, the national state aligned with capitalist interests to violently repress organized labor. The terror of state violence was dramatically on display in the Santa Maria School massacre in 1907, where hundreds of miners and their family members were killed in a confrontation between strikers and the Chilean army in Iquique.[9]

Meanwhile, there was a palpable shift in the nature and character of public health crises across the region. Starting around 1900, biomedicine, sanitary engineering, and the interests of international commerce converged to reduce the threat of the big epidemic diseases (smallpox, plague, cholera, and yellow fever) by way of specific interventions: vaccines, development of potable water systems in major Latin American cities, regulation of maritime trade, and port sanitation. The first international sanitary conferences and institutions (the Pan American Sanitary Bureau, which eventually grew into the PAHO), focused narrowly on tackling infectious disease epidemics to avoid interruptions of international commerce.

As these dramatic epidemics became less frequent, the persistent health problems of the impoverished masses emerged from the background into sharper focus. Infant mortality, a sensitive measure of overall population health, was astonishingly high. In Santiago, Chile, the infant mortality rate averaged over 290 per 1,000 during a five-year period in the 1920s.[10] An international survey in 1930 found national infant mortality rates of 110 per 1,000 in Argentina and around double that in Chile, ranging from 217 per 1,000 in one neighborhood of Santiago to 268 per 1,000 in one small town in central Chile.[11] Around the same time, Mexico reported an infant mortality rate of 131 per 1,000, and Costa Rica, about 193 per 1,000.[12] In other words, all across the region, something like one or two in ten children did not make it past their first birthday. Building the capacity even to gather such statistical data on the population was an integral part of the scientific answer to the social question and reflected another concern, fears of dwindling populations in many Latin American states.[13]

Reform-minded doctors tended to reframe the social question as a national health crisis. As in Europe or the United States around the same time, overcrowding, poor sanitation, and frequent disease epidemics were the corporeal manifestations of the poverty and inequality resulting from the rapid growth of cities. The response of some liberals to the social question was to design a reformist program for the state that would preempt these revolutionary tendencies. In Chile, the first exegesis of "the social question," an 1884 essay with that title, was written by a physician, Augusto Orrego Luco, who recognized the need for broader economic reforms to address problems like malnutrition and child mortality.[14] Though well-positioned in Chile's national oligarchy, Orrego Luco made little headway in enacting public health reforms. In neighboring Argentina, however, a vibrant hygiene movement took off around the same time.

A segment of social elites applied the tenets of a hegemonic epistemology of their time, positivism, to analytically dissect the workings (and dysfunctions) of modern society, which was understood in organic terms. As Marcos Cueto and Steven Palmer put it, "The basic positivist metaphor of society as an organism was reinforced by the spectacular triumphs of medical bacteriology and immunology between 1870 and 1900." They go on to say that "instead of revolutions, the positivist's notion of social 'order and progress' (appearing as the motto on Brazil's late-nineteenth-century republican flag) was consonant with the elite's aim that modernization should be led by professional, technocratic, and business elites that guided the rest of society."[15] For the Chilean historian Maria Angélica Illanes, social policy strategies in the early 1900s marked a shift in the way of doing politics. As she explains, the people—"el pueblo"—became a new "field of social action"; professionals worked on intervening on the *pueblo*, and in the lives of the poor more specifically, to meet multiple objectives: reducing social conflict via the reformist rather than the revolutionary route, guaranteeing social reproduction, and incorporating all members of society into the project of national economic development.[16] These professionals worked on the "body and blood" of the pueblo, understood literally in a nationalist metaphysics: the nation was a superorganism whose maladies could be studied, diagnosed, and cured through tools of modern science.[17]

This kind of political discourse was widespread and prefigured the developmentalist approach of modernizers throughout the twentieth century. As Eduardo Zimmermann argues, the framing of the social question by Argentine intellectuals anticipated a reformist "middle way" between state socialism and laissez-faire individualism. The rising disciplines of sociology and economics, as taught in Argentine universities in the first few decades of the 1900s, embarked on a program of "scientific social reform," inspired by "reformist intellectuals" who sparked the Progressive movement in the United States, and by promoters of working-class "cooperativism" and "mutualism," such as the French economist Charles Gide, whose ideas, in turn, led to the International Labor Organization (ILO) (as discussed in more depth in chapter 2).[18] The creation of a national Department of Labor in Argentina, studies of the conditions of the working classes in the country, and a new slew of labor laws were all concrete results of this reformist spirit. Of course, this new class of professionals, asserting a practice of scientific statecraft, did not always get their way. They had to negotiate conflicts with traditional political elites, the working class, and political parties that mobilized working-class interests by other means.

Catholic social doctrine also influenced debates on the social question. This doctrine can be dated with some precision, originating with the papal encyclical, *Rerum Novarum* ("of new things"), issued in 1891. Pope Leo XIII sensed that the church could not remain silent on matters of social and economic development, which had been mostly ceded to the secular political realm since the early modern period, especially with the rise of revolutionary—and mostly atheistic—anti-capitalist movements. The *Rerum Novarum* outlined the respective obligations of capital and labor and questioned laissez-faire economic principles, asserting instead that good Catholics should participate politically to influence governments to guarantee "social justice" for the poor.[19] In Catholic countries of Europe, such as Spain and Italy, the *Rerum Novarum* legitimated early gestures toward a welfare state and its principle of the state as arbiter of peaceful relations between labor and capital, a key rationale for the creation of the ILO in 1919.[20]

The *Rerum Novarum* had a mixed reception among the Latin American clergy, yet it nevertheless stimulated the development of social medicine. Catholic social doctrine was too progressive for many in the local church hierarchy, and deeper church involvement in social policy seemed to run against the rationalist foundations of political liberalism, positivism, anarchism, and socialism, not to mention the economic interests of national oligarchies.[21] Yet, while the effect of the *Rerum Novarum* was delayed, it provided the notion of "social justice," which became, according to Patricio Silva, an "idée-force in Chilean politics at the beginning of the twentieth century, as the so-called 'social question' became Chile's most pressing national problem."[22] In Chile, as chapter 3 explores in more depth, Catholic social doctrine provided a broadly acceptable rationale for new state protections for labor and a guiding set of principles for a group of "Social Catholic" doctors. Based at the medical school of the Universidad Católica in Santiago, they presented their own social medicine agenda in the 1930s, moved forward by Eduardo Cruz-Coke, an influential minister of health.[23] The concept of "social justice" was undoubtedly a cornerstone of *justicialismo*, the doctrine of Perón's government in Argentina, which institutionalized the demands of labor into a welfare state with relatively equitable access to health care. Catholic social doctrine was also foundational to centrist Christian Democratic parties in Latin America, like that of Eduardo Frei Montalva in mid-century Chile. While the Social Catholics may have been stifled by more conservative elements in the church, subsequent papal encyclicals—notably, the *Quadragesimo Anno* of 1931, issued in the midst of global economic depression—reiterated its core message. In the long run, Catholic social doctrine would be renewed in the 1960s and 1970s, now under the rubric of Catholic social teaching and liberation theology, whose philosophy of service to the poor has inspired some modern-day proponents of social medicine, like the American physician Paul Farmer.[24]

Carlos Paz Soldán and a Syllabus for Social Medicine

The higienistas shaped health policy in the late 1800s into the 1930s, across Latin America. As a group, higienistas were politically well connected, often serving in government offices and representing liberal tendencies of ruling oligarchies. Emboldened by the transformational impact of the bacteriological revolution on the control of infectious diseases, hygienists increasingly labeled their field "social medicine" as they extended their expert reach into solving a broad array of societal problems.

To understand how higienismo became social medicine and what kinds of problems it sought to address, I focus on a leading figure in that field, Carlos Enrique Paz Soldán. A prominent doctor in his native Peru and an energetic networker with a continental reach, Paz Soldán also attempted to define and organize the field of social medicine.[25] One of the earliest published uses of the term "medicina social" in the region is found in the title of a book by Paz Soldán, from 1916. Originally intended for use in an extension course at the University of San Marcos in Lima for working-class people, the book offered a "systematic" curriculum for the subject.[26] Much later, it was cited approvingly by the Belgian reformer René Sand in his tome, *The Advance to Social Medicine*.[27] I use Paz Soldan's curriculum as a point of departure in a "syllabus" for social medicine in the era, which encompassed other fields focused on more specific issue domains: puericulture, sexual hygiene, occupational medicine, and rural medicine.

While he bestowed the name *La Reforma Médica* on his widely distributed medical journal as an homage to Rudolph Virchow, Paz Soldán was neither a leftist nor a great scientific researcher. Pursuing eclectic endeavors that led one historian to label him "the poet and philosopher of Latin American health," he was a tireless promoter of increasing state investments in medical science and public health.[28] Borrowing from the definition of Giuseppe Tropeano—an influential advocate of socially oriented strategies of malaria control in Italy—Paz Soldán defined social medicine as "a discipline on a path towards synthesizing and popularizing the practical and scientific results of diverse biological and social doctrines" in order to "reduce morbidity and mortality, prolong the average lifespan of the poor classes, and improve the species."[29] Effective social medicine would serve to increase and cultivate the "human capital" of a country, those physical and intellectual resources that constituted the basis for economic progress.[30]

In all, Paz Soldán and his fellow hygienists across Latin America advanced an *ecological* analysis of the social determinants of health. Paz Soldán likened the urban system to a biological organism with a dynamic metabolism, with the essential functions of "feeding, eliminating, breathing, circulating, [and] connecting."[31] Hygiene dovetailed with modern urbanism, especially the construction of sanitary infrastructure (running water, sewage lines, and garbage collection); relocation of cemeteries, slaughterhouses, and other noxious land uses to the outskirts of cities; wider streets with building setbacks to allow for the penetration of sunlight; restrictions on manure-producing work animals (horses and donkeys); and development of parks, tree plantings along boulevards, fountains, and other public goods for recreation and beautification.[32] In his own writings, Paz Soldán traced the whole history of Peruvian urban planning, back through pre-Columbian times, to establish a tradition of urban modernization to promote public health—and probably to convince civic leaders of the wisdom of continuing such efforts. This kind of ecological thinking, marked by understanding dynamic interconnections in the parts of a system, and the conflation of social and biological dynamics, was commonplace in contemporary urbanism, economics, public health, and medical holism.[33]

This mode of thinking extended beyond the city, into understanding the composition of nations, which Paz Soldán treated essentially as superorganisms. Paz Soldán, as someone current in the explanatory frameworks of early twentieth-century race science, eugenics, and demography, understood nations to be engaged in a geopolitical contest where growing populations demonstrated collective vitality and the ability to control national territory.[34] As was often the case with the eugenics-inspired hygienists, Paz Soldán tended toward the "soft" eugenics line, wherein education and public health measures would gradually produce a more civilized mass culture.[35] His ideas gelled harmoniously with the nationalist political discourse of the Peruvian president Augusto B. Leguía (in his second term in office, from 1919 to 1930), who sought to quell the idea that Indigenous blood could be replaced by streams of European immigration (following the model of countries like the United States or Argentina), instead promoting public health policies for the "defense of the [Peruvian] race," which was coming to be understood, though certainly not by everyone, as a unique fusion of Indigenous and European elements.[36] Leguía sponsored the creation of Paz Soldán's Institute of Social Medicine (funded in part by a tax on soft drinks), but the institute's work stagnated after the demise of its political patron.[37]

Hygienists like Paz Soldán fixated on the extension of modern scientific discoveries into the practice of clinical medicine along with the conduct of everyday life, from cradle to grave. Paz Soldán's "social medicine" curriculum adopted this life-stage framework, applying innovations from bacteriology and physiology, particularly, to promote healthy pregnancy, infancy, childhood, working life, and so on, into old age. Improving population health meant the somewhat slow and gradual work of *inculcation* of healthy, modern habits: a change of culture and outlook, via patient-doctor conversations, public lectures, school lessons, films, newspapers, and later radio and television. This strategy clearly had a moral dimension, as hygienists despaired, in thinly veiled language, of the ignorance and vices—alcohol consumption and excessive sexuality, among others—of the urban working classes and the peasantry.

In what follows, I highlight four elements of Paz Soldán's curriculum for social medicine: puericulture, sexual hygiene, occupational medicine, and rural health. My intent is not to summarize, or much less to replicate, Paz Soldan's complete vision for social medicine; rather, I aim to show that social medicine's influence was felt in the narrower policy spheres framed by these subfields. In addition, these concerns developed in distinct institutional networks, sustained by associations, dedicated journals, conferences, and external funding, but not always under the label of "social medicine."

Puericulture

Closely allied with hygiene, the puericulture movement began in France in the 1890s, under the leadership of Dr. Adolphe Pinard, to promote scientific child-rearing. According to Nancy Leys Stepan, puericulture had an enthusiastic reception in many Latin American countries. As a variant on eugenics, it placed hope for social change and national progress not so much in restricting reproduction of undesirables, but rather in educating mothers and applying scientific insights in gynecology, obstetrics, pediatrics, nutrition, and psychiatry. Occasionally called "mothercraft" in English, puericulture was highly interventionist, as scientific experts infringed on an intimate, private realm. But, as Stepan puts it, given that children "were thought of as biological-political resources of the nation," it followed that "the state was regarded as having an obligation to regulate their health."[38] Among Latin American puericulturists, the focus of attention was the *binomio madre y niño*, the "mother-child dyad," a single "unit" that was the "special site of medical attention."[39] In Chile, the "pairing of mothers and children in an indivisible mother-child unit became the dominant reference to women."[40] The family was "the fundamental and undisputed cell of social life," according to the Uruguayan Roberto Berro; he and his fellow puericulturists "thought of mothers and children as forming a kind of reproductive, collective political economy whose health was vital to the nation."[41] In Uruguay, the field of puericulture was institutionalized as part of an advanced welfare state; leaders of this national effort, such as Berro, Julio Bauzá, and Luis Morquio, fostered an international community of puericulturists in the Americas who promoted strategies like the Gotas de Leche (milk dispensaries), regulation of *nodrizas* (wet nurses), and education on breastfeeding and nutrition.[42]

The rise of puericulture aligned with social medicine, as it reflected the extension of scientific knowledge into the traditionally private and culture-bound realm of parenting, and, concomitantly, the displacement of traditional nongovernmental institutions—for example, orphanages and hospitals run by churches or the Sociedades de Beneficencia—by centralized, scientific agencies of the state.[43] This shift was also gendered, as a mostly male cadre of physician-bureaucrats replaced the women-led Sociedades, even as imparting the lessons of puericulture was left mainly to an all-female corps of social workers, known in Chile as *visitadoras sociales*.[44] Puericulture found international institutional expression in the Instituto Interamericano de la Protección a la Infancia (IIPI), led by Morquio of Uruguay and his Argentine counterpart, the leading hygienist Gregorio Aráoz Alfaro. Along with the regular Pan American Child Congresses, the *Boletín* of the IIPI, which ran until the 1950s, was a major forum for policy ideas in puericulture, and it featured more prominent female participation than was perhaps typical in other areas of hygiene and medicine.

Sexual Hygiene

Puericulture was related to another field of study and policy action, "sexual hygiene," which grew in the interwar period. Specialists in sexual hygiene focused mainly on the control of sexually transmitted infections (to use today's terminology), particularly syphilis. To avoid explicit mention of sex, euphemisms like "social hygiene" or "social prophylaxis" were employed as labels for the field, so the field can be easily confused with hygiene or social medicine more broadly. As in those fields, sexual hygiene explanations and prescriptions alternated between biological reductionism and sociomedical holism. Insofar as salvarsan (or arsphenamine) had become more widely accessible in the 1910s—with the antibiotic penicillin arriving a few decades later—the solution to syphilis was, in part, pharmacological.

However, discussions of the social regulation of sexual behavior were inevitable. Most of the doctors and other professionals in this field saw the desires, habits, and proclivities of the working class—their vices, in other words—in need of reform. One historian evocatively categorizes sexual hygiene in Latin America as a discourse on "the bad life," with "prejudices disguised as science."[45] The problem of sexually transmitted diseases was often lumped together with other maladies that seemed endemic to the working class, the so-called social diseases. One British medical journal spoke of the "three great social evils of alcoholism, tuberculosis, and venereal disease"; similarly, Leopold Bard, a doctor who served in the Argentine Congress in the 1920s, focused on this same triad of diseases, under the rubric of "the social diseases," amenable to control through education, construction of high-quality housing, and other means to improve the "environment" for the poor.[46] Hygienists, other elites, and the labor movement converged in idealizing the single-family home, in the expanding suburban barrios of Buenos Aires, as an alternative to the morally hazardous and disease-producing *conventillos*, the notorious and decaying tenement buildings closer to the city center.[47]

This simultaneously moralizing and ecological discourse on sexual health was also infused with eugenic concerns. Nicolás Greco—in a 1935 speech to the Liga Argentina de Profilaxis Social, marking "Anti-Venereal Day," observed annually on September 7—lamented that syphilis, whose effects could be passed from one generation to the next, created a mass of "lazy, disloyal, insolent, avaricious, shameless" people.[48] Bard proposed a government agency dedicated to social hygiene, in "defense of the race," to prevent its "degeneration."[49] The leader of the Peruvian Liga Nacional de Higiene y Profilaxis Social, Carlos Bambarén, called for "preventing the procreation of undesirables, via the control of conception, sterilization, or the current knowledge of natural sterility that presents itself during the menstrual cycle," that is, the rhythm method; but in the same 1934 address, he identified education as the key to controlling reproduction and the need to fight against "socioeconomic factors that conspire against marriage," thus evincing the hygienists' concern with high (and in some countries, rising) rates of illegitimacy.[50]

Paulina Luisi, a Uruguayan doctor who was active in puericulture and sexual hygiene groups, was an early and avid proponent of a "hard" eugenics, supporting eugenic sterilization and abortion—after the example of US states like Indiana—to prevent the reproduction of degenerative elements in society.[51] At the same time, however, Luisi and other feminist social reformers (Alicia Justo de Moreau of Argentina, for example) also sought to empower women with knowledge about their sexual health. Luisi's thinking merged the eugenicist concern over scientific control of reproduction, a candid and matter-of-fact attitude about sexual education, and strict ethical standards of personal sexual conduct.[52] Similarly, anarcho-feminists in Argentina, Uruguay, and Brazil sought an end to the "sexual double standard" between men and women.[53] Luisi, for her part, led a decades-long campaign against "white slavery" and prostitution more generally.[54] Despite her connections with eugenics, Luisi was, in many ways, ahead of her time: as Asunción Lavrín writes, "No other Southern Cone feminist devoted so much time and energy to the problems of gender relationships and sexuality, and none developed a fuller set of ideas."[55]

Occupational Medicine

The field of occupational medicine was another product of the hygiene movement. In concert with industrial hygiene, it was principally concerned with workplace hazards that threatened the health of laborers. Some were specific to particular industries, and the discovery of industrial diseases was a new frontier of medical research by the late 1800s. The medical knowledge that white phosphorous (used in the manufacture of matchsticks and munitions) produced a condition called "phossy jaw" (a necrosis of the jawbone) led to the first international convention banning the use of a toxin in manufacturing, in 1906. Contemporaneously, a survey of hazardous working conditions in Argentina led by Juan Bialet Massé in 1904 resulted in the creation of the national Department of Labor, which imposed stricter regulations on industry and created a system to compensate workers for injuries, diseases, and disabilities that could be traced to working conditions.[56] Increasingly, occupational medicine took an interest in fatigue, which increased the risk of on-the-job injuries. Many new regulations dictating limits on working hours and break times, now seen as fundamental rights of labor, came from initiatives of occupational medicine.

The concern over fatigue opened up new spaces of intervention for occupational medicine, extending the hygienic gaze into the domestic lives of workers. A disease like tuberculosis occupied a liminal space since, unlike phossy jaw or silicosis, it could not be exclusively attributed to conditions in the workplace or in the home, but rather came from a patient's total environment. Thus, hygienists who had never set foot in a factory or a mine could still see themselves as guardians of worker health and productivity, offering recommendations on diet and nutrition, rest, exercise and leisure activities, proper clothing, bathing and personal hygiene, and alcohol consumption. According to René Sand—for whom, it is said, "social medicine was more or less synonymous with occupational medicine"—modern industrial relations recognized, by 1925, that "the quantity, quality, economy, and continuity of production rest on *health*, which guarantees the *power* to produce; *general and professional education*, which develops the *talent* to produce; and *contentment*, which encourages the *willingness* to produce."[57]

Sand's attitude was embodied in the ideology of the ILO. Initially created in 1919 to enforce regulation of white phosphorous and other hazardous industrial materials and workplace conditions, it promoted labor peace and industrial democracy by developing regulatory blueprints on working conditions, preventive medicine, nutrition, and social insurance. As discussed in chapter 2, the ILO had increasing influence on Latin American labor policies in the interwar period and served as a forum for the development and influence of social medicine.[58]

The labor movement's perspective on occupational medicine was ambivalent. The rising authority of hygiene led to the "medicalization" of working class life, a form of biopower exerted to discipline and control workers and their families, with the potential to defuse the radical militancy of labor.[59] Taylorist discourses on human capital and productivity tended to treat workers' bodies as "machines" absorbed into the larger mechanisms of industrial capitalism, a dehumanizing discourse that, among medical professionals, only some anarchist-leaning doctors objected to, as I explain further on. Thus, the demands of labor did not always coincide with what occupational medicine had to offer. But labor, at a political disadvantage, often welcomed the proposals of politically connected hygienists to strengthen regulation of workplace conditions. Even so, many of the occupational hygiene bills proposed by Argentine legislators like Alfredo Palacios or Leopoldo Bard never made it out of the Congress, due to recalcitrant conservative interests. When granted political power, unions demanded better working conditions and protections; in Chile, miners' unions eventually pushed the government of the Frente Popular (FP), in the late 1930s, to put regulations to prevent silicosis into practical effect.[60] And, in Chile and elsewhere, the institution of social insurance provided a mechanism to guarantee protection against or compensation for work-related illnesses and injuries, a foundational element of welfare state policies that would occupy social medicine in the 1930s and 1940s.

Rural Health

What role did social medicine play in shaping the discourse of health problems in rural areas? By the early 1930s, in Europe the League of Nations Health Organization (LNHO) took stronger interest in the underlying social and economic determinants of rural health and proposed community-led committees to support health programs in the countryside.[61] The LNHO's interest in this area was driven, in large part, by the perseverance and charismatic leadership of Andrija Stampar, whose planning for a Yugoslavian health system in the interwar period stressed the need for comprehensive reform of rural society.[62] In Latin American countries, the record of social medicine in rural health questions is mixed, with sporadic engagements rather than a consistent, studied focus of the particularities of the rural milieu and its relationship to health problems.

Rural health problems were mostly ignored because early Latin American social medicine shared the same urban bias as the hygiene movement. Hygienists treated the city as a laboratory for modernization, applying diverse tactics of sanitary engineering, control of public spaces, public health campaigns, and inculcation of hygiene into popular education for densely populated masses. For all their paternalistic rhetoric, hygienists conceded that urban working-class people were modern subjects nonetheless: interested in change, malleable and impressionable through the emerging tools of the mass media.

By contrast, rural populations were often construed as beyond the pale, living in a state of darkness, ignorance, and isolation that was so complete, they could hardly be considered as fully functioning citizens who played a role in the nation's political culture. Hygienists plumbed the depths of their lexicon to describe the wretchedness of rural folk and their habitats. In the early 1930s, Paz Soldán, through his Instituto de Medicina Social, established a malaria control project in the valley of Carabayllo, which today lies on the edge of the Lima metropolis, but was then an agricultural area distant from the city center. He wrote:

> The inspections that we have carried out, throughout the entire valley, have given us a vision of Dantesque scenes, a total contrast to a fertile

countryside abundant with rich grains. Rather than human habitations, we would call them caverns: lacking in sunlight; no flooring other than damp earth; with roofs of poorly laid out reeds, a refuge for mosquitoes; without furniture or with what could be cobbled together from tree trunks ... decorated by cobwebs that indicate how many years have passed without the simplest cleaning implements; and in this over-crowded concubinage full of hens, ducks, guinea pigs and dogs, if not pigs and sheep, these pigsties constitute the worst affront to human biology.[63]

Bear in mind that this description came from someone who was *concerned* about the health of people in rural areas; most in the medical profession would have taken no interest at all. Paz Soldán's account of conditions in the valley of Carabayllo was typical in that the objects of his interest, the rural folk, had no voice at all in these depictions. This state of passivity and objec-tification was enhanced by the opacity of provincial politics in most countries, where the votes of peasants, farmworkers, and other rural folk were routinely repressed or controlled by conservative landowning or agro-industrial elites. Indigenous groups in many countries were scarcely incorporated at all into the national political space and were treated as nonentities, even in the accounts of the most sympathetic doctors.[64]

To some extent, rural health problems differed in kind from those of the cit-ies. Rural areas across the vast region were seen as afflicted by vector-borne and infectious diseases and nutritional deficiencies that drained the life force and capabilities of people who lived in such places. When Paz Soldán wrote of the causes of malaria in rural areas, he employed a socioecological vision in which disease emerged from "geo-cosmic-social environments" or from a "rural drama" marked by the tragic motifs of ignorance, poverty, and a malevolent environ-ment.[65] Malaria, to Paz Soldán, had multiple and interlocking causes, like poor housing, lack of medical care, challenging working conditions, illiteracy, and poorly managed irrigation.[66] This socioecological perspective, which considered "interrelated, systemic causes of underdevelopment, and saw ma-laria as a multi-faceted problem that demanded multi-faceted solutions," was prominent internationally before World War II.[67]

In contrast to the holism of social medicine, in the more reductionist lens of tropical medicine these rural places functioned as field research sites and proving grounds for advances in fields like medical entomology, bacteriology, and parasitology. Across Latin America, these efforts were often spearheaded by the Rockefeller Foundation and its International Health Board (IHB). In those countries where it was especially active in public health work—such as

Brazil, Peru, and Costa Rica—the RF focused on controlling or eradicating diseases like hookworm, malaria, Chagas disease, and yellow fever while paying much less attention to local social, economic, and political conditions. Ignoring context was partly a matter of political expediency, but it also represented a philosophical orientation: that disease undermined development, and, as a corollary, that scientific research would lead to disease control and serve as a driver of economic progress.[68]

However, it would be a mistake to treat this perspective as one that the RF imposed on unwilling subjects in poorer countries. Clearly, the RF's approach dovetailed with the work of public health experts like Carlos Chagas in Brazil or Salvador Mazza in Argentina, who wanted to develop scientific excellence in their peripheral countries and use it to shoot down, one by one, old scourges like malaria or leprosy, or newly discovered ones, like Chagas disease, that hindered national progress. Thus, in Brazil the RF's work complemented the ongoing development of a network of rural health posts administered by the federal government, while in Costa Rica, the RF's health stations became the nucleus of government-run rural health services.[69] A productive collaboration between the RF's Louis Schapiro and Solón Núñez, Costa Rica's first minister of public health, as Steven Palmer writes, created "an eclectic social medicine ensemble that brought together under one roof public health nursing, home visiting, maternity and infant health, school health, and treatment and prevention of endemic and epidemic disease."[70]

Another early case of political commitment to rural health was Mexico. Rural health projects based on principles of social justice were the legacy of a political revolution in which the peasantry figured as key protagonists. This movement started in the 1920s with an active nucleus of radical physicians, the so-called Nicolaitas, who were graduates of the Colegio de San Nicolás in Morelia, Michoacán. After the left-populist governor of Michoacán, Lázaro Cárdenas, became president of Mexico in 1934, the Nicolaitas became his advisers on health policy and they developed comprehensive medical services at the level of the *ejido*, the basic territorial unit of Mexico's agrarian reform.[71] To an extent, the Cárdenas-era projects presented a challenge to the RF's ongoing work in Mexico, with their "integrated approach to medicine and public health," contrasting with the RF's commitment to biomedical and technical interventions; after Cárdenas's term ended in 1940, the process of land redistribution slowed and the ejido-level health units "began to shed their social roles and focus more narrowly on disease control, much like the RF units."[72] Notably, the Cárdenas government also established the rural service obligation for medical school graduates, a legacy that did help to improve the quality of rural medical care in the long run. As I discuss much later in the book, Cuba also made dramatic strides in rural health programs after its revolution of 1959. Otherwise, barring the pressure and restructuring of power relations brought on by major revolutions, rural health projects were a low priority for government health ministries in Latin America during this period.

Nevertheless, rural society figured in a romantic imaginary of social medicine, an idealized vision of the relationship between country doctors and their needy patients. Many doctors who worked in rural areas crafted an image of self-abnegation, sacrificing earnings, career advancement, and even their own health to work on behalf of the rural poor. Mazza, who died from complications of Chagas disease, the disease he studied most closely, after years of working in isolation in northern Argentina, epitomized this type, although few would associate him with social medicine, per se.[73] In Argentina, during the early part of the twentieth century, the memoirs of rural doctors such as Esteban Laureano Maradona constituted a mini-genre.[74] The Spanish émigré physician José María Bengoa, in a 1939 treatise on social medicine based on his work as a doctor in Sanare, a small town in northwestern Venezuela, wrote: "The rural doctor, positioned at the lowest level of the medical profession, represents a decisive factor in the social evolution of nations, which has perhaps not been recognized for its true value. He is the soldier on the front lines. There, in the vanguard, he alone is left [to act] against the enemies he has to defeat."[75]

Possibly, these doctors presented a view of social medicine that was more palatable to the public and their professional colleagues, as it placed emphasis on the "natural" vocation of medicine as serving the needs of the poor, a vision of medicine that was disconnected, mostly, from more concerted political action (such as the agrarian reform process in Mexico). Near the end of his long life, Maradona was lauded by the popular Argentine lifestyle magazine *Gente* as "one who belonged to that tiny army of enlightened ones who give their souls, lives, flesh and blood for those who suffer, the forgotten ones, those neglected people of this earth."[76] Without diminishing the value of his work in any way, we can say that this "sentimental" vision of the rural doctor was apolitical and, to the extent it equated progress with the heroic acts of exceptional individuals, quite at odds with the agenda of social medicine.

Eugenics and Social Medicine

How eugenics contributed to Latin American social medicine thought is a complex issue that cannot be avoided—and the preceding discussion suggests that racialized ideas permeated discourses on health, disease, sexuality, motherhood, work, and rural life. While historians have traced the Latin American eugenics movement in depth over the past few decades, the considerable overlap between social medicine and eugenics has hardly been recognized. Yet famous Latin American eugenicists, like Renato Kehl of Brazil, wrote about social medicine; Argentina's major eugenics association of the 1930s was known as the Argentine Association of Biotypology, Eugenics, *and* Social Medicine.[77] Many of the figures associated with social medicine's first wave in Latin America—people such as Salvador Allende, Ramón Carrillo, Juan Lazarte, Alfredo Palacios, Paulina Luisi, Carlos Bambaren, and Carlos Paz Soldán—also engaged, to varying degrees, in associations and networks linked to eugenics and regularly used the language of eugenics that was commonplace in medical discourses of the era.[78]

At first blush, it may seem puzzling that the same people could promote progressive (social medicine) and retrograde (eugenics) ideas simultaneously. But such normative evaluations on a twenty-first century ideological spectrum are anachronistic. A hundred years ago, a framing of national progress in the terms of race science provided the justification for the extension of medical knowledge and practice into other realms of social life; these were the terms of a biopolitical emergency of racial degeneration that only medical science was equipped to solve. Yet invasive tools for state control of human reproduction, like forced sterilization, were seldom employed in Latin America; rather, eugenics provided additional impetus for the use of environmental and social interventions associated with hygiene, puericulture, and social medicine.

Ideas from race science of the early twentieth century were foundational to an organicist nationalism that, in turn, was central to how Latin American social medicine understood the structure and functioning of society—and, more importantly, how a society malfunctioned, degenerated, or declined. This was the view of a national society-as-organism, one organized according to biological principles. As one Chilean doctor wrote in 1935, "Formed by living beings, society itself, to be understood, should be considered as a living organism."[79] The historian Diego Armus elaborates on this notion: "Eugenics stood at the intersection of biology and politics and was, undoubtedly, an idea of its time. It was not a pseudoscience but rather, a rationalized manifestation of the need and desire to control and dominate a population—a priority for the many modern ways of thinking that emerged at the end of the nineteenth century and the first half of the twentieth. It was largely a way of talking about social problems in biological terms."[80] Eugenics, in a sense, turned the "social question" into a "racial question" in the early 1900s, as unhealthy populations impeded national development plans.[81] Concerns over racial degeneration were spurred not only by the presence of disease and mortality but also by fears of criminality and social disorder. Under the influence of the Italian criminologist Cesare Lombroso, elite scientific and legal professionals believed in the heritability of criminal dispositions. Eugenics was mobilized not just biopolitically but geopolitically: in a competition among industrializing nations, power derived from economic strength, which in turn derived from the biological vigor and vitality of a growing population.[82]

What did Latin American eugenicists mean when they talked about race? This is a challenging question. Eugenics sometimes tended to justify and harden macro-level racial hierarchies. This was undoubtedly the case in the United States: eugenics was a handmaiden to white supremacy and its fears of the "contamination" of a national Anglo-Saxon racial stock with East Asian, African, and even other (Eastern) European elements.[83] In Latin American countries, eugenicists also grappled with the question of racial purity and mixture, framing the national racial "stock" of most countries to be a combination of European, African, and Indigenous elements. But, in the words of the anthropologist Peter Wade, while many of the Latin American eugenicists "agreed with the Anglo-American science of the early twentieth century, which held that race mixture generally brought degeneration and weakness, too close an agreement with such a view could only condemn Latin American nations to perpetual inferiority."[84]

As a result, eugenics also supported national identity construction projects based on a "constructive miscegenation" verging on "mestizophilia" in some countries, like Mexico.[85] In Chile, the discourse of a distinctive national racial type—the outcome of a distinctive, historical fusion of races—had become hegemonic by the early twentieth century, glossed as "el roto chileno," a sort of noble commoner, rough around the edges, but amenable to being civilized through education and hygiene.[86] Juan Lazarte, the Argentine anarchist doctor, remarked on his visit to Chile, "The mass of the population is homogenous, of an unmistakable Chilean type," thus painting a contrast, implicitly, with an Argentina where recent streams of European migrants had created unamalgamated ethnic communities assorted across the Argentine national space—a condition he viewed with concern.[87] These quotations suggest that eugenics offered a language of sameness and difference, in biological terms, to construct and consolidate national identities.[88]

The scientific elites affiliated with eugenics developed a distinctive vocabulary for understanding sameness and difference that relied less and less on old racial categories. In many countries of the region, long-standing racial identifiers like "Negro," "indio," or "trigueño" were eliminated from official records.[89] Eugenics, according to Wade, "focused on the 'fitness' of individuals and populations, and it targeted the working classes as much or more than people defined in terms of race."[90] This new vocabulary came, in part, from the Italian field of biotypology, "which held that there were no constant relations between constitutional biotypes and races."[91] This sense of biotype and its connection to social medicine is invoked in the words of Roberto Berro (the Uruguayan pediatrician and leader of international "puericulture" discussed above), in an essay titled "Social Medicine during Infancy": "The social importance of the role of medicine is unquestionable, to improve the living conditions that produce the three representative classes of a population: the small intellectual, physical and moral elite; the great mass of people, nine-tenths, of regular quality; and the one-tenth of *dysgenics* or *cacogenics*, who constitute the group of anti-socials, along with the insane, degenerates, epileptics, alcoholics, vagabonds, etc."[92] As Berro's statement suggests, eugenics created new categories of subjects amenable to the specific interventions of pediatrics, psychiatry, criminology, and other rising scientific disciplines.

The most severe eugenic strategies involved direct state interventions into sexual reproduction. However, measures such as forced sterilization of mentally ill or disabled people, legalization of abortion for eugenic purposes, requirement of prenuptial certificates, and criminalization of transmission of venereal diseases, despite having passionate and influential advocates, were seldom put into practice in Latin American countries. As Armus argues, the discourse of eugenics was widespread and seemed to insinuate itself into discussions of all sorts of social issues, but it seldom delivered on its goals of regulating sexual reproduction or creating durable systems of biological classification (biotypology). The failure to institute state controls over reproduction stemmed, in part, from the opposition of the Catholic Church, which "never had a good relationship" with eugenics.[93]

The distinction Nancy Leys Stepan made between "hard" Anglo-Saxon eugenics, reliant on reproductive control measures, and the "soft" Latin eugenics of Spain, France, and the Latin American countries, continues to be mostly valid. The latter variety of eugenics was founded on a "neo-Lamarckian" concept of evolution, which, in contrast to Mendelian genetics, held that diseases, vices, bad habits, lack of education, and so forth left an imprint on minds and bodies that could be passed on to the next generation. In Colombia, for example, it was widely held that "la raza entra por la boca"—race enters through the mouth—that is, by what a person eats or drinks. According to the historian Stefan Pohl-Valero, "nutrition was identified as a key element for a social engineering aimed at regulating the body-machine in order to improve national productivity; it was simultaneously related to the eugenic idea of producing better generations of workers."[94] That is why hygiene and related fields like puericulture were seen as vital to preventing further race degeneration. More recent research suggests that the structure and composition of international expert networks, for example, coming together at conferences, helped shape these different styles of eugenics.[95] These associational spaces, extending from eugenics into medicine and public health more generally, helped form a sense of community among Latin America's scientific elite—a sense of working, under challenging conditions, at the geopolitical periphery.

This raises another question: was eugenics conservative or progressive? Such a question is easily dismissed as anachronistic; still, eugenicists' self-image, at the time, was that of "defenders of progress and the new ideals of modernity who were opposed to the old customs of conservative and religious thought."[96] Wade contends, convincingly, that "during the heyday of eugenics [between 1912 and 1932] ... it was a progressivist movement driven by medics and reformers who focused as much on social 'hygiene' (i.e., an improved environment, especially for children) as on measures such as sterilization and prenuptial medical examination, which would regulate sexual reproduction and thus directly impact germ plasm."[97] Eugenics had adherents in socialists like Salvador Allende or liberal hygienists like Gregorio Aráoz Alfaro. Some radical, transformative projects—such as the "conscious procreation" movement of anarcho-feminists, discussed further below—were linked to advocacy for the "hard" eugenic measures, such as sterilization and legalized abortion.

Lastly, eugenics also offered a kind of common ground that lent ideological support to projects of national "reinvention" and the new social contract behind expanding welfare states. In the words of the Chilean historian Javiera Letelier Carvajal, "Eugenics utilized the depoliticization of the masses, so as to advocate for the unity of society under the common objective of improving the race."[98] This kind of national unity and sense of collective purpose, even if based partly on dubious reasoning about national racial origins, was essential to the development and sustainability of modern welfare states in some Latin American countries.[99] Nationalism was often dangerous but it could also be harnessed to encourage a public sentiment of solidarity that created opportunities to construct progressive social policies.

Thus, early social medicine and eugenics overlapped in discomfiting ways. More than anything, they converged in a discourse that legitimated interventions of medical science into all sorts of social realms, offered a seemingly apolitical route to managing social and public health problems, painted a grim specter of degeneration and decline as a consequence of failure to solve those problems, and constructed a national collective in racialized terms.

The Anarchist Moment

In early twentieth-century Latin America, anarchists were never numerous but they had an outsized political influence. Their militant tactics, such as general strikes, caused interruption and chaos sufficient to prompt both hard-line state repression and, as in Argentina, an opening of the political arena to organized labor.[100] Cut from the fabric of this larger movement, a small group of anarchist doctors left an imprint on early social medicine. Their contribution has been relatively neglected, overshadowed by the accomplishments of better-organized and more successful leftist groups. Deeper analysis of the agenda of anarchist doctors helps sharpen our understanding of ideas in social medicine, by showing us a road *not* taken. Anarchist notions of the state, grassroots action, and gender relations and sexuality were much *too* radical for social medicine as it gained traction and began to exert political influence. Put another way, anarchism—which inherently rejected "state medicine"— was definitely *not* on the syllabus for mainstream hygienists like Paz Soldán.

Juan Gandulfo epitomized the anarchist doctor in Chile. Now a mostly forgotten figure, in the early interwar period Gandulfo was seemingly ubiquitous in the radical political atmosphere of the classrooms, cafés, and streets of Santiago. According to the historian Raymond Craib, Gandulfo represented the "early left" of Chile: "the libertarian left" or *socialismo libertario*.[101] He was born and raised in the port city of Valparaíso, a hotbed of anarchist organizing thanks in part to the Pacific-coast organizing of stevedores by the International Workers of the World (IWW, also known as the Wobblies).[102] As a medical student at the University of Chile, along with his brother Pedro, a law student, Gandulfo became a militant member of the Federación de Estudiantes de Chile (FECh), the main student political organization, which helped lead antigovernment protests of July 1920 in Santiago. For a while, the Gandulfo name was "synonymous with revolution," in the words of another member of his youthful cohort.[103] His untimely death in a traffic accident at the age of thirty-six, in 1931, may account for his relative obscurity.

As a result of their subversive political activities, both Gandulfo brothers were jailed, during which time Juan took up the cause of prisoners' rights.[104] While he admired Peter Kropotkin and Errico Malatesta, noted European anarchist thinkers who were widely influential in Latin American circles, his intellectual interests were wide-ranging and he militated for freedom of thought and expression. His friend Pablo Neruda, a fellow *porteño*, dedicated his first book of poetry, *Crepusculario* (1923), to Gandulfo, who in turn provided the woodcut illustrations that accompanied the verses. Some of Neruda's early poems were published in *Claridad*, a literary journal that Gandulfo cofounded.[105]

Gandulfo helped start up the Policlínico Obrero of the IWW in the working-class Barrio Latino, just south of Santiago's city center, in 1923. Inspired by his experience in the Asamblea Obrera de Alimentación Nacional during medical school, the Policlínico was also testimony to the IWW's capacity for establishing collective institutions for workers to help themselves; these included *sociedades mutualistas* or mutual-aid societies, which sponsored disability, medical, and burial insurance benefits for members.[106] Gandulfo worked nights as an attending physician and offered occasional lectures on "social and biological topics," but the management of the clinic was a cooperative effort, independent from any state supervision or funding.[107]

The guiding principle behind the work of the Policlínico was *autogestión*, which roughly translates to "self-help"—or better still, "self-management." Under the ethos of autogestión, workers should manage their own organizations, like the polyclinic, autonomously. When, in 1925, Gandulfo called on workers to pitch in to fund the clinic, he declared, "We count on your help, since we cannot ask anything of the State, or the Church, given that we are fighting to destroy them."[108] But autogestión also placed demands on workers to simultaneously manage their own bodies, habits, and domestic spaces, a practice of self-care, or "autogestión del cuerpo" as Nicolás Fuster calls it.[109] This concept reflected Gandulfo's anarchist view of the relationship between the individual and the collective: as one of Gandulfo's friends eulogized him, he "fought in every way for the perfection of the individual as the instrument of collective perfection."[110]

This philosophy was revealed in the *Hoja Sanitaria*, a newspaper published monthly from 1924 to 1927 by the Policlínico. This publication can be seen as both typical and uncommon for that era: it was part of the genre of labor newspapers—*la prensa obrera*—that proliferated in the early 1900s to "feed the intellect of the masses," yet within this genre the *Hoja Sanitaria* was unique in its dedication to promoting health and hygiene.[111] Thus, close reading of this newspaper offers unique insights into anarchist framings of health questions.[112] The *Hoja Sanitaria* typically offered practical advice for workers on maintaining personal health and household hygiene, imparting lessons on anatomy, nutrition, physical exercise, mental health, cleanliness, and so forth. Fabián Pávez, a Chilean physician and historian of medicine, has lauded the "advanced concepts of integrated health" proposed by the *Hoja*

Sanitaria.[113] Yet these were didactic lessons offered by medical doctors (including Gandulfo) for uneducated workers, and in that sense were consistent with the hygiene movement.

The *Hoja Sanitaria* emphasized the capacity of *individuals* to care for themselves and control their own destinies by gaining knowledge and building self-discipline. For this reason, the *Hoja Sanitaria* railed against alcoholism, since no popular habit did more to create servile and disorganized subjects, easily bewildered and ruled by elites. Thus, self-control of alcohol consumption and other bad habits, which hygienists tended to cast in moralistic language with barely concealed fear of the working class, was for anarchists the key to working-class *emancipation.* The editors of the *Hoja Sanitaria* took a matter-of-fact approach to human sexuality, with diagrams and descriptions of sexual organs, sex acts, and the nature of sexual desire that were frank and insistently "scientific," but devoid of moralizing and thus exceptional in Chilean society of the 1920s. Gandulfo evinced a similarly knowing attitude toward sex in his advocacy for conjugal visits in prison, and liberal attitudes toward sexuality characterized the thought of other anarchist doctors. According to Víctor Muñoz Cortés, a historian of anarchism in Chile, these attitudes toward alcohol and sex were manifestations of a holistic philosophy of living in harmony with a natural order, which also led to an anarchist interest in vegetarianism, alternative medicine, and sports. However, Muñoz doubts that these kinds of values and habits were actually widespread among rank-and-file workers in the IWW and other unions.[114]

The *Hoja Sanitaria*, with its emphasis on individual reasoning, action, and self-control, assiduously avoided discussion of structural causes of poverty. For example, a Dr. Uribe y Troncoso wrote in 1924, "During a strike, a poor woman spent her last ten cents on lettuce to feed her family, who were hungry. If she had bought beans instead, she could have obtained 70 times the amount of nutrition with the same amount of money."[115] He paid no attention to the circumstances of the strike or the causes of the family's misery. Such a neglect of structural causes of poverty and health inequality in social medicine thought may seem paradoxical, given the anarchists' radical critique of capitalism, but the anarchist doctors and their IWW comrades were strong believers in direct and practical action, outside the purview of the state and the realm of electoral politics. Perhaps for this reason, the *Hoja Sanitaria* rarely alluded to national public health institutions or the news of Chilean politics.

Anarchist social medicine never had a clear program and there was little consistency in thought between doctors of anarchist persuasion. In Argentina, Juan Lazarte, whose medical labor organizing is discussed in more detail in chapter 4, was also part of an international movement of "conscious pro-creation" connected to anarcho-feminism.[116] With a similarly open attitude about sexuality, Lazarte advocated for the end of the sexual double standard between men and women, and viewed the patriarchal family structure as the base of oppressive and hierarchical social institutions. But Lazarte's ideas about reproduction were also informed by the eugenics movement, as he was sometimes preoccupied with the "improvement of the race," tended to think of many problems (like alcoholism) as heritable, and advocated for eugenic sterilization.[117] Much of his activism in social medicine was channeled into *gremialismo*, or labor union activity; however, rather than forge relationships with working-class unions in the style of Gandulfo, Lazarte worked to build a strong medical union to preserve professional autonomy as the Argentine government increasingly took charge of the health system.

What happened to anarchism and its small-scale, decentralized approach to improving workers' health and welfare? Craib, drawing on the work of Victor Muñoz, contends that in Chile, "it was less the repeated repressions— and there were many—that doomed the IWW and anarcho-syndicalism than the growing response on the part of the state to intervene favorably in labor relations, as a result of anarchist and anarcho-syndicalist agitation."[118] As Muñoz himself writes, "When the state began to intervene, to identify itself as an entity 'defending' the laboring mass, libertarian discourse lost its effectiveness among the thousands of workers who preferred to struggle under the wing of the state, rather than taking the more difficult path of organizing at its margins."[119] The incorporation of labor interests into the state apparatus was a general trend, not just in Chile but in other Latin American countries where anarchism had its political moment.[120] As Alan Knight puts it, anarchism's "rejectionist stance toward the state seemed anachronistic at a time when the state came bearing gifts, however modest."[121] Similarly, social medicine drifted away from anarchism and increasingly focused on marshaling the power and resources of the state to solve persistent health inequalities. Grassroots, nongovernmental, and collectively organized clinics, like that of the IWW, became passé and untenable. As I explain in chapter 3, socialists like Salvador Allende—although inspired by the militancy and ethical clarity of men like Gandulfo—would tend to proffer a version of social medicine that reproduced the conservative gender ideology of the labor mainstream, a notion of a healthy workforce as "human capital" for national development, and a paternalistic state with top-down technocratic practices.

Another theory about the demise of anarchism comes from the Argentine historians Leandro Gutierrez and Luis A. Romero: for working-class urbanites, anarchism's demanding codes of personal conduct made its vision of an ideal new society impractical. Leftist politics began to change: "Gone were the Utopian proposals associated with the anarchist principle of the turn of the century. The new social literature highlighted concrete problems and the search for possible and rational solutions."[122] This "new idea of social justice was not incompatible with social ascent, but rather complementary to it."[123] Anarchism was out of step with the culture of "barrio life," which included collective or cooperative action at the neighborhood level; the embrace of leisure activities, such as sports, music, dancing, and social clubs; café life and a dramatic increase in reading; and engagement in a consumer culture that promoted ideals of personal health, beauty, and achievement.

What Social Medicine Meant

During the early part of the twentieth century, social medicine meant taking the tools of medical science and directing them not just at individuals but at society at large. In ontological terms, society was construed as a national superorganism, a biopolitical entity that grew and thrived, or deteriorated and declined, in accordance with the health and vigor of its individual components. The scientific elites comprising the epistemic communities of social medicine, hygiene, and related fields did not advance a theory of society as autonomous from biological or natural laws—everything was mixed together. As a result, their analytical toolkit generally came not from Marxist theory (which made categorical distinctions between the biological and the social) or any other systematic social sciences (which were all in their infancy); instead, they adapted ideas from the natural sciences about organisms, systems, harmony, growth, and decay and applied them to the workings of society. Given this impulse to "biologize the social," it is not surprising to see considerable overlap between social medicine and eugenics during this period.[124]

Up to this point, social medicine was mostly unconcerned with analyzing the structure of national political economies, or the causes of social injustice, or collaborating with social movements or civil society organizations, like the labor movement, which did take up such concerns. Instead, its agenda centered on reshaping environments, inculcating biomedical and hygienic knowledge, encouraging behavioral change, fortifying the state's public health role, and providing medical services to a population in need. Social medicine thus mixed a broad and ambitious sense of purpose with the realization of targeted interventions, some popular and successful (e.g., the *Gotas de Leche* promoted by puericulturists), others not politically viable at the time (e.g., the push to improve rural health conditions). The anarchist alternative, offering an ethos of self-care and empowerment, less paternalistic relationships between doctors and the working class, and the possibility of small-scale medical cooperatives, gradually died out, replaced by state institutions led by technocratic elites. Overall, political socialism was decidedly marginal in the early development of Latin American social medicine.

In this chapter, I have proposed a new narrative of social medicine's intellectual roots, one that does not depend on a diffusionist account of social medicine ideas traveling from Europe to South America via particular individuals. Instead, I propose that a flourishing Latin American intelligentsia was operating in the same transnational field as European and North American thinkers, scientific experts, and policymakers.[125] In the countries I have highlighted in this chapter—especially Argentina, Chile, Peru, and to a lesser degree, Uruguay—reform-minded elites concentrated on scientific solutions to *national* problems, and this is how social medicine emerged, and quite early in the twentieth century. But the protagonists of early Latin American social medicine were part of larger international networks, movements, and epistemic communities, not just in medicine itself, but also eugenics, feminism, labor organizing, anarchism, and conscious procreation, among others.

The next few chapters show how social medicine began to change, moving away from foundations in hygiene and eugenics toward something distinctly different. During the latter part of the interwar period, in the 1930s, the international crisis of capitalism had local economic effects that prompted reconsideration of liberal political-economic models and the rise of powerful leftist and populist political movements in some parts of Latin America. Social medicine was caught up in this ideological ferment and some began to more closely examine the political-economic roots of health crisis and engage a different kind of social politics. Through formal international networks, anchored by institutions like the LNHO, the ILO, and the Pan American Sanitary Bureau, experts in social medicine developed and circulated concrete policy tools to improve the distribution of health services. The ILO, especially, promoted the tool of social insurance, a forerunner of more comprehensive welfare states that would be realized, albeit imperfectly, in some Latin American countries. Chapters 3 and 4 then trace the fitful translation of social medicine ideas into health and social policy in Chile and Argentina, respectively.

CHAPTER TWO

Networks

How Social Medicine Traveled Internationally, 1920s–1940s

In chapter 1, I argued that social medicine emerged from the milieu of modern Western scientific and political thought—from eugenics and positivism, to anarchism and socialism—advanced by a medical elite in some parts of Latin America. In this chapter, I turn to examine the international institutional networks that influenced ideas and policy in social medicine in the interwar period.[1] In short, how did social medicine ideas "travel"?

Social medicine thought was certainly "in the air" internationally during the interwar period. As Randall Packard and other historians of global health have described it, the integrative frameworks and equity concerns of social medicine found advocates in nascent international organizations, such as the League of Nations (LN).[2] In Western democracies, this was also a period of policy experimentation to construct modern welfare states, motivated, at least in part, by pressure from leftist movements. After World War II, the momentum of welfare state politics continued in the West. However, the postwar geopolitical order, US dominance in science and technology, and antagonism toward socialist ideas in Western institutions sent international health on a different path—one dominated by disease-specific and technologically intensive strategies.[3] From this perspective, international social medicine appears as an aborted movement, emerging in a time of ideological ferment—especially during the Great Depression, which stimulated a search for alternatives to capitalist development models—but unable to adapt to the harsher conditions imposed by Cold War geopolitics.

The goal of this chapter is to explain how social medicine ideas traveled through networks shaped by the architecture of international institutions during the interwar period. I argue that international networks were not just "conveyor belts" for policy ideas in these domains from the industrialized countries of the North Atlantic into Latin America.[4] Rather, international meetings were sites of contestation over the causes of health inequalities, the universality of liberal welfare-state policy models, and the role of science in policy. Latin Americans' participation in these networks tended to reinforce perceptions of difference between Latin America and the global geopolitical core regions; prompted the search for "national solutions to national problems" in some Latin American countries; and fostered stronger intraregional ties among progressive doctors, scientists, and other intellectuals interested in social medicine. Social medicine ideas did not need to be transferred from abroad—there was already an established group of hygienists and other professionals receptive to what was being proffered through the expanding networks of international health.

To develop this argument, I focus on the workings of distinct but sometimes overlapping networks during the 1920s and 1930s, starting with European-based networks, centered on Geneva, the headquarters of the League of Nations and the International Labor Office (ILO). Proposals in occupational health, nutrition, and particularly social security (or social insurance) traveled through these networks and found a receptive audience among some Latin American professionals and technocrats. At the same time, networks dominated by the United States through the Pan American Sanitary Bureau and the Rockefeller Foundation focused on a different set of issues, especially infectious disease, while also sponsoring activities, such as international conferences, that facilitated conversations on broader social policy questions. Latin American experts were often caught in between conflicts or rivalries between the US- and Geneva-based institutions, although the philosophical divergences between them have perhaps been overstated. In the final section, I explain the role of a small group of Latin American socialists, who were mostly peripheral to the episteme of international health, but would influence social medicine in the 1930s and even more so in the long run. But first, it is important to offer some theoretical framing for how to analyze the circulation of ideas in international expert networks.

Situating Social Medicine Networks, in Time and Space

Historians of science and technology have long been concerned with how knowledge travels internationally. An early, dominant frame was a "center-periphery" model in which innovations "flowed" from wealthier, more technologically advanced countries of the Global North to the Global South, or from the metropole to the colonies. The deficiencies of this perspective led to theories based on circulation, contingency, mutual influence, and multidirectionality.[5] As John Krige puts it, "The scientific and technological knowledge that flows from one node to another in a network can take many forms, is mobilized in diverse social and institutional settings, and transforms social relationships on different scales. It can be tacit or propositional, cutting-edge or mundane. It is expressed in multiple practices—experimental, educational, managerial, policy oriented—as well as in modes of control and domination. It engages universities and corporations, missionaries and philanthropic foundations, national governments as well as regional and international organizations."[6]

At the same time, Krige (with Michael Barany) cautions that the use of terms like "circulation" or "flow" "risks minimizing the problems of crossing in transnational undertakings"—the frictions of travel, communication, language barriers, and so on in the real world.[7] In addition, while it may be true, at one level, that "transnational networks connect remote places where knowledge is produced, exchanged, and appropriated" and, therefore, "do not respect borders," power is uneven and concentrated in specific places. Networked ties may erode or break, due to internal issues, such as the breakdown in reciprocity or mutual benefit that maintains personal or professional relationships, as well as "unexpected and unplanned-for developments," such as loss of funding sources, geopolitical tensions, or pandemics that complicate or impede travel across borders.[8]

These general conceptualizations of international expert networks have been adapted in studies of health and social policy in Latin America. Given the shortcomings of core–periphery or imperial–colonial models, Anne-Emanuelle Birn also advocates a model of "circulation," meaning that "health and scientific ideologies, policies, and practices undergo an intricate process of give and take among multiple actors who are linked in particular professional, political, and practical circles."[9] Similarly, with reference to the Cold War era in international health, Birn argues that via "varied entanglements— which involved back-and-forth expert communication, conferences, and sponsored research—Latin American physicians, scientists, and social reformers did not simply digest European, North American, Soviet, and one another's ideas and approaches, but debated them furiously, forged their own variants suited to domestic problems, and projected them internationally."[10] Teresa Huhle, borrowing from scholars of transnational movement of social policy, such as Daniel Rodgers and Christoph Conrad, suggests a variety of "vectors of transnationality" to analyze, including the "circulation of [policy] models," "the 'transnationalizing' role of international institutions and organizations," the roles of "individual expert actors, their communities, and networks," and "the languages of cross-border communication, such as statistics and law," which provide a common framework for exchange of policy ideas.[11]

In analyzing how ideas travel, it is also important to consider the conditions and possibilities of specific historical periods. The events and connections described in this chapter span from World War I, through the Great Depression, and into the maelstrom of World War II. By the end of this period, the influence of Europe on Latin America—culturally, economically, and geopolitically—had diminished considerably. As Olivier Compagnon, among others, has suggested, the mass slaughter of World War I revealed the dark side of European modernism.[12] The imitative, Europhilic tendencies of Latin American elites did not disappear overnight, but reaction to the war provoked a distancing from, and diminishing of, the European modern project among the region's intellectuals. Latin American modernists' search for a "new civilizing order" that drew on autochthonous New World influences has been well studied in the realm of arts and literature, but this framing has been relatively less important in analyzing scientific research, or health and social policy.[13] Yet I will argue that Latin American experts who were engaged in transnational networks were gaining confidence in the possibilities of homegrown science and policy, while cultivating a sense of regional identity. Paz Soldán, for example, saw the European war as a marked contrast to an emerging spirit of peace and fraternity among Latin American countries, and even the development of something like an American race based on new ideals of science and progress.[14] The concomitant rise of US geopolitical hegemony in the Western Hemisphere and the consolidation of regional interests under the rubric of "Pan-Americanism" would also help to diminish the influence of Europe in the health and social policy arenas.

The Great Depression further opened up political possibilities for Latin American countries. As one historian of the ILO's role in Latin America suggests, "It would be hard to find another period that presents itself as completely as a field of political experimentation. To the extent that the world economic system seemed to reach a state of collapse, a series of political possibilities emerged to manage this situation. . . . From communism to fascism, the New Deal or corporatist tendencies, all these options would have some kind of impact on the region: some [proposals] to replace democracy or capitalism, others to breathe new life into them."[15] International multilateral institutions, based in Geneva, were key players in this effort to rejuvenate both liberal democracy and capitalism—with the United States serving as "a safeguard against ideological extremisms."[16] Even though, as Alan Knight warns, it is possible to fall into the trap of overgeneralizing about the regional experience of the Depression, it was a time of political awakening and possibility in many places.[17]

At first glance, it might seem as if focusing on two major science/policy networks, one based in the United States and the other in Europe, would tend to reinforce the center–periphery model (albeit with two centers) and its many defects. Clearly, these two overlapping networks do not represent the totality of networks that nurtured social medicine thought. Still, the US- and Geneva-based institutions offered structure, resources, opportunities for travel, and concerted attention to specific policy issues (like social security). These particular networks tended to be populated by scientists and technocrats. They were not established or sustained just for the spread or circulation of "scientific knowledge." Even though we can characterize them as "transnational (techno)scientific networks," these were also networks for the exchange of policy ideas, ideology, and professional culture.

Analysis of formally structured networks around social medicine is complicated by the fact that there were no prominent international organizations for the promotion and advancement of social medicine per se, despite the fact that the interwar period is understood as a period of florescence for the field. Generally rising usage of the term in noun (*medicina social*) or compound adjective (*médico-social*) forms during the 1930s—in journal, book, and article titles; academic departments; conferences and conference sections; and government programs in Latin American countries—is a cue that the concept was gaining relevance. While few international meetings on social medicine, as such, were organized in the region during this time, it was a cross-cutting approach employed to analyze an array of health and social problems.

One might wonder whether expanding networks of political leftists of different stripes (anarchists, socialists, communists) had an influence on social medicine. No doubt, there was a flourishing network of leftist intellectuals, artists, and activists in Latin America during this period, but, as I suggest below, they were mostly focused on things other than health and disease. Still, this generation of Latin American leftists had a short-term effect on social medicine, by creating political pressure for welfare state policies; as well as a delayed effect, laying the conceptual groundwork for a more rigorous regional Marxism that was integral to "second-wave" social medicine starting in the early 1970s.

European Influences: The Geneva Institutions

Major Geneva institutions of the interwar period, the LN and the ILO, were idealistic experiments to sustain an international liberal political order. Due mainly to its failure to prevent the catastrophe of World War II, the LN particularly has long been dismissed as a failure in international governance, but more sympathetic analyses emphasize the Geneva institutions' role as pioneer in humanitarian internationalism and as a laboratory for social policy.[18] The Geneva institutions developed a technocratic approach to governance, and an ostensibly nonideological style of policy innovation and transfer, which made them forerunners to postwar international institutions such as the WHO, the United Nations, and the World Bank.[19]

The League of Nations Health Organization became a significant player in international health during the interwar period. The economic dislocations of the Great Depression moved the LNHO toward a "social medicine" orientation in the research it sponsored and policies it supported.[20] Ludwik W. Rajchman, a Polish bacteriologist who served in the key role of medical director of the LNHO from 1921 to 1939, was known for promoting a "conception of a social medicine serving humanity" and the LNHO paid "growing attention to social medicine in the 1930s, when [member] governments turned toward social welfare policies."[21] The LNHO's activities shifted, from a focus on technical assistance in programs to combat specific diseases and epidemiological surveillance, to a "broader inquiry into disease etiology that encompassed the roles of nutrition, housing, working conditions, agricultural production, and the economy."[22] In Europe, this new orientation was especially evident in rural hygiene and malaria policies.[23] Andrija Stampar, of Yugoslavia, became a leading voice for land reform and improving the standard of living in rural areas to produce better health conditions, based on his experiences in Europe and East Asia.[24] But institutional weaknesses and concerns over political neutrality tempered the LNHO's leftward tilt.[25]

Similar to the LN, the ILO—known in Latin America as the OIT, Organización (or Oficina) Internacional del Trabajo— had a high-minded purpose: that "lasting peace can be established only if it is based on social justice," and social justice—often used interchangeably with the concept of "social peace"— could be achieved only through agreements between labor, capital, and the state, meeting together on equal footing.[26] Intrinsic to the ILO's governance practices was the "tripartite" format, whereby representatives of three parties (labor, employers, and the state) were supposed to negotiate and hammer out resolutions, which initially dealt with regulating industrial working conditions, at regular meetings in Geneva. With its program in industrial hygiene, the ILO interfaced with public health, for example, in studies of silicosis and drafting of conventions to ban the manufacture of poisonous chemicals, such as white lead (basic lead carbonate) and white phosphorous, responsible for the notorious "phossy jaw."[27] In the 1930s, the ILO increasingly looked beyond questions of occupational safety, workplace conditions, and fair labor contracts toward broader questions of worker health and security.

The Geneva institutions, especially the LNHO, were notoriously Eurocentric, and relations with Latin America were sporadic and slow to develop. Partly due to the costly and time-consuming travel to Geneva, Latin American presence in the LNHO was weak, although notables such as Carlos Chagas of Brazil and Gregorio Aráoz Alfaro of Argentina represented their countries at its meetings.[28] In dialogue with the French school of "puericulture" (whose prominence in the region is discussed in chapter 1), the Latin American contingent pushed for LN involvement in child and maternal health issues. An LN-sponsored conference in 1927 on this subject, held in Montevideo, led to the creation of the IIPI, also based in Uruguay. The IIPI served as a "bridge" between the LN and American states, including the United States though mainly Latin American countries, but at the same time it had considerable autonomy, both in financial terms and in setting an agenda on child health.[29] Meanwhile, ILO involvement in Latin America officially began in 1925 when Albert Thomas, the organization's director, visited Chile to recognize the progressive labor and social laws its government had enacted in 1924. These included the creation of the Caja del Seguro Obligatorio (CSO), a large social insurance fund that offered medical services, and Chile's prompt ratification of several ILO declarations (see chapter 3).[30]

Others in the Geneva crowd, such as René Sand, are often cited as evangelists for social medicine in Latin America.[31] Sand, a Belgian doctor, was a kind of liberal internationalist policy entrepreneur, defining new spaces of action and placing himself in them. On the international stage, he served as general secretary of the League of Red Cross Societies from 1921 to 1927 and as a member of the LN's Child Welfare and Health Committees in the 1930s. After World War II, he helped establish the World Health Organization.[32] Sand wanted doctors to be more like social workers, and he gravitated toward the field of social work later in his long career.[33] Always on the move, Sand traveled to Santiago in 1924 to give a series of lectures at the University of Chile, published the following year in Chile as *Medicina social y progreso nacional*.[34] Since Chile's government pushed through a spate of welfare-state legislation around the time, it is tempting to think that Sand introduced progressive social medicine ideas from Europe to Chile. But his view of social medicine—with assumptions from positivism and eugenics, a concern with promoting health to protect a nation's human capital, a focus on puericulture, a concern with the "social illnesses" of tuberculosis, alcoholism, and venereal disease—was already widespread in the region, as an offshoot of the hygiene movement, as discussed in chapter 1. Indeed, Sand cited Paz Soldán of Peru as an influence, and they clearly shared a vision of social medicine.[35] In other words, Sand carried a mildly reformist message to receptive Latin American audiences, like so many other European liberal internationalists.

During the tumultuous 1930s, in a push for legitimacy and to ensure their survival, the Geneva institutions increased their activities outside of Europe.[36] ILO leadership "was aware that the organization was in dire need of Latin American support if it wanted to survive the looming European crisis."[37] The ILO also recognized that, in comparison to Europe, many Latin American countries were relatively peaceful and politically stable, and already showing demonstrable advances in social policies.[38] With much of the world's territory still colonized by European powers, Geneva found it hard to ignore Latin America's independent states, which were already involved with closely allied US-led health institutions, the Pan American Sanitary Bureau and the International Health Board of the Rockefeller Foundation. Such engagements "would provide the principal blueprint for the fully 'international' health apparatus that emerged in the post–World War II era, when the nation-state became the global norm," as Cueto and Palmer suggest.[39]

Social Security and the Welfare State

Representing the lines of tropical medicine and public health, the US-led networks tended to focus on scientific and technical solutions to infectious diseases. The European networks, however, provided more space for discussion of complex social policy issues. Study tours organized by the LNHO in the 1920s brought together experts from various countries (including Uruguay), who traveled through Europe to learn about school hygiene, health-care administration, malaria control, industrial hygiene, puericulture, nutrition, nursing, and sexually transmitted diseases.[40] Both the LNHO and ILO developed an interest in the issue of nutrition, sponsoring conferences and supporting expert missions to Latin America on the subject.[41] All these social policy questions fell under the purview of a hygiene movement that defined its domain even more broadly under the name of social medicine, as explained in chapter 1.

Here, I want to focus on the Geneva institutions' role in laying the foundations for welfare state policies like social security and state-regulated health insurance in Latin America. The ILO, particularly, was pivotal in disseminating the policy model of social insurance, a product of liberal Western European statecraft, around the world. ILO leaders viewed social insurance as one means to adjust the social contract between labor, capital, and the state, and thus to promote social peace. For some Latin American governments, social insurance was attractive since it offered a practical way to fund the expansion of health-care services to reach a greater share of national populations. Indeed,

one reason for governments to be involved with the ILO was to avail themselves of the technical expertise necessary to launch, finance, and administer
these complex social insurance systems.[42] The ILO's social insurance model
found support among a new cadre of technical experts (in finance, actuarial
science, law, and administration), even more than the support of doctors and
hygienists. However, the push for social insurance also inspired skepticism
among some in the Latin American labor movement.

Not surprisingly, the Latin American governments most involved with the
ILO already had some semblance of a social insurance system, and Chile
stands out in this respect.[43] The official publications of Chile's CSO, *Acción
Social* and *Boletín Médico-Social*, closely followed news of ILO policy resolutions, meetings and conferences, and the travels of its functionaries during the
1930s. In Chile, sustained involvement with the ILO depended on the entre-
preneurial energy of people like Francisco Walker Linares, who served as a
"correspondent" to the LN, and Moisés Poblete Troncoso, a lawyer and one
of the few Latin Americans to actually hold a position in the central office of
the ILO in Geneva.[44] Poblete Troncoso was recommended as a candidate for
this position because of his immersion in social and labor policy in Chile,
along with his avoidance of partisan politics, and he would go on to serve as
adviser to other Latin American countries, such as Costa Rica, on social insurance issues.[45] Poblete Troncoso and Walker Linares also created a Chilean
association in support of the LN; it was a small group, but one composed of
influential members of a progressive Chilean political-intellectual elite.[46]

Given Chile's already high level of participation in the ILO, Santiago was a
natural choice for the first ILO Regional Labor Conference in Latin America,
in January 1936.[47] Unlike other networks around social medicine—such as eugenics, puericulture, hygiene, and nutrition, which were largely dominated by
members of the medical profession and allied sciences—the ILO meetings
brought together a wider range of professions, interests, and outlooks. Lawyers,
economists, accountants, actuaries, and an increasingly professionalized labor
union sector convened to discuss the intricacies of social insurance and industrial labor conditions, while medical professionals, who were protagonists in
other expert networks, were mostly at the margins. Labor leaders, for their part,
used the occasion of the 1936 Santiago conference to collaborate, strategize, and
organize their own networks while adopting a cautious stance toward the ILO
governance process.[48] Coincidentally, the first Chilean National Medical Convention, a landmark in the history of the development of social medicine in the
country, was held at the very same time, in Valparaíso, which could also explain
the low turnout of physicians at the ILO meeting.

Despite several months of planning for the conference, led by Poblete Troncoso, the deliberations of the meeting largely departed from the narrow agenda
set by the ILO. Adrien Tixier, the head of the ILO social security office, wanted
to focus on moving Latin American countries toward ratification of declarations on just two issues: "social insurance" and the "working conditions of
women and children," but delegates covered a wide range of subjects in their
speeches, including immigration, monopolies, international trade, minimum
salaries, the special problems of Indigenous groups, and housing conditions.[49]
Labor union representatives made use of conversations outside of sessions to
discuss the common interests of labor across the hemisphere and signed a pact
to form a Latin American labor confederation, eventually realized in the formation of the Confederación de Trabajadores de América Latina (CTAL).[50]

The discussion of social insurance policy was marked by a general affirma-
tion of the ILO's objectives, but there were also intriguing silences, divergences, and skepticism, particularly from organized labor. The ILO's social
insurance model centered on adjusting the labor contract to include "sickness
insurance" that encompassed, first, "compensation" for lost wages, and second, "restoration" of "health and working capacity."[51] The Latin American
delegates at the Santiago conference offered a more expansive concept of social insurance, in line with social medicine, "especially the need to link social
insurance to other policies such as medical services" and "to prevention, worker
education on hygiene, and nutrition."[52] Voicing the concerns of the conference's social insurance committee, Edgardo Rebagliati, the governmental
delegate from Peru, pointed to the special circumstances of Latin American
countries, "still in the critical stages of their organization," which called for integrating social insurance into "the fight against diseases, [which are] the eternal
source of poverty, desperation, and decrepitude of nations."[53] Some labor delegates viewed social insurance programs with suspicion. Luis Solís Solís, the
Chilean labor representative, rather than praising his country's social insurance
system, argued that the CSO was underfunded (due mainly to the meager contribution required from employers), ineffectual (the country continued to suffer from rampant infectious diseases and high infant mortality, giving Chile
"one of the lowest life expectancies in the world"), and did nothing to address
the underlying structural problem for Chilean labor, the gap between low
wages and the very high cost of living.[54] In the following decade, the ILO
continued to strengthen its ties to Latin American states, by holding two
more regional conferences in Havana in 1939 and Mexico in 1946, establishing
several branch offices in the region, and working to develop a cadre of technical experts in social security.[55]

Pan-Americanism in Public Health

During the interwar period, innovations in public health and medicine increasingly traveled through Pan-American networks anchored in universities, foundations, and government offices in places like New York, Baltimore, New Orleans, and Washington, DC. As Marcos Cueto has written, "The First World War debilitated Europe's preeminence in many areas; but above all, it undermined the cultural supremacy the continent had long enjoyed in universities and medical schools throughout the Americas. Through scholarships and grants, learning institutions in the United States began to attract promising young students of science and medicine from the Region."[56] Two organizations in particular, the Pan American Sanitary Bureau and the Rockefeller Foundation's International Health Board, played an essential role in the development of much of Latin America's public health infrastructure (we could also mention a third US institution, Johns Hopkins University, whose school of public health had a close relationship with the RF, and trained many Latin American sanitarians starting in the 1940s). While their influence has been much discussed and debated, here I want to focus on how these US-based institutions propagated a public health philosophy that countered social medicine. Shared roots in the turn-of-the-century ideals of public hygiene may have obscured, at the time, how social medicine differed from the increasingly hegemonic American influence in international health. Over time, leftist social medicine advocates were marginalized from major Pan-American health networks, as the US-based institutions promoted technical, apolitical interventions and bioscience research that were pillars of mid-twentieth-century international health work.

Founded in 1904, the PASB is cited as the first international health organization. From its inception, the bureau focused on controlling infectious diseases such as yellow fever and the plague to ensure they did not impede expanding commerce between Latin America and the United States. The old-fashioned methods of preventing the international diffusion of infectious disease, particularly quarantines in ports of arrival, were no longer economically viable. Instead, officials of the PASB advanced the idea that proactive surveillance and sanitation in the port cities of Latin America and the Caribbean, from Havana to Guayaquil to Rio de Janeiro, could guarantee safety and stabilize the international system of maritime trade. With the usually enthusiastic support of Latin American hygienists, the PASB soon carried its purview beyond ports and drafted model sanitary codes for member states. As an organization based in Washington, DC—indeed, as an arm of the US

Public Health Service, which itself was part of the Department of the Treasury until 1939—the bureau was uninterested in social insurance, occupational health conditions, and similar social policy issues.

Although Latin American officials were well represented in the PASB (for example, at biannual meetings of national ministers of health), Washington controlled the organization's purse strings, and its internal hierarchies followed a neocolonial logic. The longtime director of the PASB, Hugh S. Cumming, though lauded for his diplomatic and tactful consideration of Latin American public health officials, was also concurrently the US surgeon general (from 1920 to 1936). In effect, the bureau was an early (and successful) experiment in the geopolitical model of Pan-Americanism: promoting the peaceful relations between Latin American states, coordinating international exchanges, and limiting the influence of European powers, but under the wing of the US government. Throughout the twentieth century, the organizational apparatus for Pan-Americanism grew more elaborate: the Good Neighbor Policy, the Institute of Inter-American Affairs, the Organization of American States, and the Alliance for Progress, to name just a few well-known endeavors.

Compared to the PASB's official agenda, the occasional Pan American Sanitary Conferences it sponsored were relatively more open and receptive to progressive social policy ideas presented by Latin American representatives. The reports presented at the Pan American Sanitary Conferences usually stuck to a scientific-technical discourse, but ruptures, in the form of politically provocative pronouncements, occasionally showed through this veneer. For example, at the Ninth Pan American Sanitary Conference, held in Buenos Aires in 1934, the Chileans Eugenio Suarez and Victor Grossi explained that their national health ministry was bringing an epidemic of exanthematic typhus under control through expansive (and somewhat invasive) delousing and disinfection measures. Yet, back in Chile, this epidemic was causing widespread chaos, galvanizing the social medicine movement, which saw the root cause of the epidemic in deteriorating economic conditions. Grossi also alluded to the fact that, in the context of the worldwide economic depression, "few countries have suffered such an intense crisis in recent years as Chile" leaving "a huge part of the population deprived of shelter, clothing, and food."[57] And he fearfully alluded to how "political elements interested in disturbing social order" were taking advantage of the epidemic, with masses of unemployed people "roaming from one place to another in search of work."[58] Thus, while alluding to social crisis, the Chileans represented and reflected the values of officialdom, privileging stability for the sake of sustaining the dominant economic model.

Arguably, the Rockefeller Foundation was even more powerful than the PASB in promoting an American perspective on public health. The philanthropic work of the RF expanded quickly after the end of World War I, and the International Health Board (known after 1927 as the International Health Division) was its centerpiece. The IHB operated according to some clear and straightforward precepts. First and foremost, its directors viewed infectious disease as a major cause of economic underdevelopment around the world (and in "backward" regions of the United States). As a consequence, the IHB poured most of its resources into studying and controlling disease, as a tool for reducing poverty. Diseases like hookworm and malaria were framed as "diseases of laziness" and "debilitating illnesses" that sapped the energy and ambition of its sufferers and silently devastated the economic prospects of entire regions. The IHB framed its interventions as investments in national development and made arrangements with national states that were meant to be short-term, with government partners taking on a larger share of the burden over time. The scientists and public health experts sent from the United States to Latin America tried to stay out of domestic political issues and stick to the terms of the agreements with national governments. The constant cycling of IHB officers through tours of duty in various countries, similar to the practice of a diplomatic corps, was intended, in part, to prevent the formation of loyalties outside of the foundation. Nevertheless, Americans could hardly avoid entanglements with their counterparts in countries like Brazil, Argentina, and Peru; and, although the IHB exercised considerable power, with its vast financial resources, scientific expertise, and highly efficient organization, there was a process of give-and-take or negotiation between Americans and their Latin American counterparts.[59] In any event, the RF was one of the most widely respected international organizations of its time, and scarcely an ill word was ever said about it—publicly, at least—by Latin American public health leaders.

It is easy to see an antagonism between social medicine and the RF's public health philosophy, and this tension was perhaps most evident in the realm of malaria control. In the interwar period, the RF's strategy for malaria control, eventually glossed as "the American model," became dominant. RF malaria experts like Fred L. Soper or Lewis Hackett saw social problems as intractable, while biological pathogens and their environments were, in principle, susceptible to control. This outlook translated into a strong and almost exclusive emphasis on attacking the vector to control malaria, initially through multiple tactics, but eventually settling on the application of chemical insecticides like DDT. The proving grounds for eradication, arguably, were in Brazil, where Soper and his Brazilian colleagues carried out an effective campaign to annihilate the invasive *Anopheles gambiae* mosquito, and before DDT was available. Even in countries where relations with the RF were more contentious, like Argentina, the American model for malaria control dominated because of its technical and scientific credentials.[60]

By contrast, the "European model," associated with some schools of malariology in Southern Europe, was endorsed by the LNHO during the 1920s and 1930s. From this perspective, malaria was not so much a mosquito-borne illness as a social disease, primarily a product of poverty. Improvements in housing stock, better nutrition, access to preventive treatments for malaria, and regulation of certain kinds of agricultural labor were seen as ingredients for reducing vulnerability for people who lived in malarious areas. The LNHO made these sorts of recommendations as part of a broader effort to improve what we would today call the "social determinants of health." To simplify their differences somewhat, the American model was technology-oriented and narrowly focused on the biological aspects of the malaria transmission cycle, and the European one saw malaria primarily as a social disease.[61]

Historians' evaluation of the Rockefeller Foundation has been divided. Sympathetic analyses emphasize the productivity of the IHB's scientific work and its many successful public health interventions, while critics assert that such philanthropic efforts propped up an unjust and exploitative international economic system. Juan César García, a central figure in the 1970s revival of social medicine in Latin America, helped initiate the more critical line of analysis, by suggesting that the RF's work supported US commercial interests in places like Central America, where the production of export commodities such as coffee or bananas required a healthy workforce.[62] García, who was immersed in the language of dependency theory, further argued that the RF and PASB promoted the growth of Latin American states' power in public health, an effort driven by a local "bourgeoisie that emerged from the capitalist production of raw materials and export agricultural products."[63] From this perspective, the "American" school of public health fostered an ideological apparatus that was biologically reductionist, favoring disease-specific (vertical) interventions. And yet, the RF was responsive to rural medical and sanitation services in a way that national governments often were not, as explained in chapter 1, in the context of rural medicine. The RF overcame the urban biases and centralized power of many Latin American countries by being largely indifferent to those political dynamics, and its scientific interest in vector-borne disease and "tropical medicine" drove RF personnel to the hinterlands of the region. In some countries, such as Costa Rica, the RF developed infrastructure that served as the foundations of national health systems.

However, that strong insistence on a scientific paradigm in health, and a resistance to getting entangled in politics, meant that the RF was skeptical of social medicine in a general way. The RF also commanded sufficient financial resources and technical expertise to exert a powerful influence on national-level health policies and medical training in the region, by spreading the "Flexnerian" model of US university education in medicine, public health, and sanitary engineering.[64] Nevertheless, it is important to stress that during the interwar period, among Latin Americans in the health and medical fields, the RF was held in high regard and its frequent successes were celebrated.

Latin American Experts, between Geneva and Washington

Relations between the US- and Geneva-based institutions were complicated and inconsistent. While the United States remained outside of the League of Nations system, some Americans were well-placed within the LNHO's advisory body, and the RF enjoyed a "symbiotic relationship" with the LNHO, supplying about 30 percent of its budget and covering much of the cost of travel for delegates to international conferences or study tours.[65] And while the ILO's relocation to Montreal, Canada, during the war facilitated its work in the Americas, its leadership had to be mindful of Washington's desires and "the competitive force of Pan-Americanism."[66] Meanwhile the United States reasserted its hemispheric hegemony with the soft diplomacy of initiatives like the Good Neighbor Policy of 1933 and an attempt to create a Pan American Labor Organization to supplant the ILO in the Americas. As a result, the planning of meetings to discuss seemingly innocuous and technical policy matters often entailed fraught diplomatic negotiations behind the scenes.[67]

Ultimately, friction with the United States kept Geneva's health institutions from developing strong and sustainable ties with Latin America. For example, the PASB was initially indifferent to child health initiatives, so it did not block the LN's sponsorship of the IIPI. However, just a few years later, the PASB director Hugh Cumming (of the United States) influenced the composition of the expert team conducting the LNHO-sponsored nutritional survey of Chile in 1935 and intervened to block LNHO sponsorship of a rural hygiene conference in Mexico the same year.[68] The IHB's heavy involvement in the control of infectious and vector-borne diseases in Latin

America deterred all LNHO efforts in this domain, except for its support of a leprosy research center in Rio de Janeiro.[69]

Thus, during this period Latin American social policy experts, bureaucrats, and sympathetic politicians were often required to gauge and triangulate their interests against those of Europe and the United States. However, the root of these tensions did not necessarily lie in philosophical differences about health and social policy; the European agencies were not automatically more "progressive" or less "reductionist" in their outlook, compared to US institutions. During the 1930s and 1940s the United States supported the expansion of welfare states in Latin America, by promoting its own model of social security developed during Roosevelt's New Deal.[70] No doubt, the United States had outsized influence in the PASB, but at the regular Pan American Sanitary Conferences, US representatives exercised only loose control over the meeting agendas, and these meetings became a forum for discussion of a wide range of policy approaches, including some inspired in social medicine. As discussed above, at international conferences on social security, Latin American experts seldom took their cues from European social medicine, and offered their own integrative and politically sophisticated analyses of social and structural causes of local public health crises.

Meanwhile, social security was integrated into the hemispheric public health agenda, as a means to guarantee what was coming to be framed as a *right* to health. However, there were incipient tensions surrounding the proper roles of the state and the organized medical profession in the health sector. The declaration of the Tenth Pan American Sanitary Conference in Bogotá in 1938, sponsored by the PASB, offered express support for social security as a "means to defend collective health."[71] After World War II, the rights-based framing of a new liberal international order took hold. Notably, the preamble of the WHO charter was written, with its famous guarantee of a right to health (crafted mostly by Andrija Stampar) in early 1946.[72] In December of that same year, the First Pan American Social Medicine Conference, held in Havana, produced the "Carta Médica" of Havana, which included the statement, "Every individual in the Americas has a right to live in health" (*Todo individuo en América tiene derecho a vivir en salud*).[73] Although very little has been written about it, this Pan-American conference brought together the leaders of doctors' unions—*gremios médicos*—from Latin America, including representatives from the Asociación Médica de Chile (AMECH) in Chile and Confederación Médica de la República Argentina (COMRA) in Argentina.[74] In terms of network structure, this group seems totally outside the orbit of the

Pan-American health mainstream; however, some of its goals, including the continued strengthening of national social insurance systems, were becoming more mainstream. At the same time, the composition of the membership suggests that not all were on board with the program of socialized medicine. Notably, one of the eleven delegates from the United States, Dr. Harrison H. Shoulders, president of the American Medical Association, was then leading the fight against a national health insurance system in the United States.[75] Alongside the conference's strongly worded declaration of a right to health for all Latin American citizens, there was an equally strongly worded statement that "every doctor in the Americas has a right to the respect of the free exercise of the profession," implicitly a rebuke of government-directed health systems.[76]

In any case, the ideological and material commitments of the United States to promoting social security systems and labor rights more generally in the region, through its influence on the ILO, diminished rapidly after World War II, while the PASB (reborn as the PAHO) largely neglected social insurance as it concentrated efforts on the control of infectious and vector-borne diseases.[77]

The Networks of the Radical Left

In this discussion of international social medicine networks during the interwar period in Latin America, the near absence of the political left is perhaps surprising. The ILO, PASB, LNHO, and even the RF were all multilateral institutions, either formed by member states or working with governments, to shape public health and social policy. In this terrain of government officials, technical experts, and diplomats, the radical proposals of the Latin American left were excluded or at the margins. Yet, while these official institutions were doing their work, there was a growing network of leftist intellectuals and political activists that would eventually come to constitute a more cohesive Latin American socialist movement; their influence on social medicine in the region would be most strongly felt in its second wave, a few decades later.

During the interwar period this leftist network was in its infancy, and its members were themselves often quite young. Many of this generation of leftists emerged from student movements for university reform. Successful protests at the University of Córdoba in Argentina in 1918 were followed by radical student demonstrations in Santiago, Chile, and Lima, Peru, in 1919. Student activists aimed to transform the deep-seated traditionalism of the universities and make them more than places for the reproduction of the national ruling class. In the long term, "university reform inspired an intellectual movement announcing 'the dawn of a new civilization whose home would be based in America,'" according to Lance Selfa.[78] For example, in Peru the student movement was led initially by Victor Raúl Haya de la Torre, who with his comrades hoped to transform one of the most ossified and conservative institutions of Peruvian culture, the University of San Marcos. While Haya de la Torre would become a legendary figure of Latin American socialism, he had no evident connection to social medicine. Some student activists in Santiago (such as Juan Gandulfo, the anarchist doctor introduced in chapter 1) and in Córdoba (Juan Lazarte) identified with social medicine. Student organizations, such as the FECh in Chile or the Federación de Estudiantes del Perú, continued to agitate for open, socially active, and intellectually adventurous universities.

During this time, new publications launched by the same university student activists brought fresh ideas and polemics. The French literary and political journal *Clarté!* founded by Anatole France and Henri Barbusse in 1919, soon inspired imitators in Mexico, Guatemala, Peru, Chile, and Argentina, published under the title *Claridad,* often with an eponymous book publishing house attached to it.[79] Haya de la Torre founded the Peruvian *Claridad* as the "organ of the free youth of Peru" and with a call for a "spiritual revolution."[80] After a few years, Haya de la Torre passed the editorial reins to José Carlos Mariátegui, perhaps the most creative and original leftist intellectual of the era, who introduced a truly rigorous Marxist analysis of the social problems of his native Peru.[81] The different national versions of *Claridad* involved some of the best-known intellectuals and leftist political figures of that era: Mariátegui and Haya de la Torre, José Vasconcelos, José Ingenieros, Miguel Ángel Asturias, and, again, Juan Gandulfo.[82]

For their literary and political actions, many within this radical left group became dangerous enemies of the state. Several were forced into political exile, starting in the early 1920s. Arguably, the experience of exile only strengthened international leftist networks. The Alianza Popular Revolucionaria Americana (APRA), a political party founded by Haya de la Torre in 1924 during his exile in Mexico, had a major influence on Chilean socialism; something like three hundred Peruvians, most of them Apristas, were exiled to Chile between 1930 and 1945.[83] Haya de la Torre's political strategy influenced Allende, particularly the notion that "the ballot box was the best political strategy for remedying the widespread poverty and social injustice affecting their people"—in other words, the political and parliamentary path to socialism.[84] Exiled Apristas like Luis Alberto Sánchez, Manuel Seoane, and Magda Portal integrated themselves into the leftist intellectual and artistic circles of cosmopolitan Santiago during the 1930s.[85]

International socialist and communist networks had both short- and long-term impacts on social medicine. In the short run, the pressure from leftist groups prompted a political accommodation of working-class interests. As Paulo Drinot and Carlos Contreras explain, in Peru center-right governments borrowed liberally from the APRA platform to prevent the party's ascent to power during the tumult of the Great Depression; this included the creation of a "social insurance system for blue-collar workers."[86] Some governments of the region responded with authoritarian maneuvers to silence political dissent and quash labor unrest, but often they yielded to pressure from the left to construct or reinforce the trappings of a modern welfare state (almost always focused on urban sectors). But the labor movement also accommodated itself to changing circumstances; as Patricio Herrera González has argued, on the eve of a second world war, labor leaders of the region focused on maintaining hard-won social protections and "there was no space to call for revolution."[87] This helps to explain a center-left consensus around expanding the welfare state in many countries, which harmonized with the reformist attitude of social medicine at the time.

In the long term, the dynamic leftist movements of the interwar period laid the intellectual and ideological foundations for second-wave social medicine in Latin America. The student-led reform movement opened up the universities to young people of many class backgrounds and led to new experiments in popular education and the development of new fields of study (including sociology and other social sciences). Although Marxist teachings were often proscribed, a serious, theoretically rigorous kind of socialism began to circulate. In some well-known instances, these networks helped bring about revolutionary change; famously, Dr. Hugo Pesce, of Peru, passed along the ideas of Mariátegui, his close ally, to a young Ernesto "Che" Guevara in the early 1950s.[88]

But during the 1930s, at least, there was little direct and sustained interaction between social medicine proponents and those who were committed to socialism as a political project. Put a different way, the networks of social medicine and the political left were mostly not articulated, although there were some points of intersection, like Allende. Ideological alignments between social medicine and political socialism are hard to decipher; in journals like the *Boletín Médico de Chile*, specific political figures or parties were rarely mentioned, although as the 1930s wore on, due to the rise of fascism, the Spanish Civil War, and World War II, urgent political statements became more frequent. These included an eloquent declaration of support for the Frente Popular (FP) party in 1938, an election framed as a conflict between reactionary and progressive forces.[89] Mariátegui, who died in 1930, would not live to see the political action of Salvador Allende and the Vanguardia Médica of Chile, but there are clear echoes of his ideas in their work, as I explain in chapter 3. Nevertheless, very few medical doctors took part in the Communist International (Comintern), the institutional embodiment of the kind of revolutionary socialism that Mariátegui advocated, with the exception of a group of communist doctors in Havana.[90] Marxism's influence would be felt much more strongly in social medicine's second wave, many decades later.

Untangling International Networks in Social Medicine

How did ideas from abroad influence LASM? With a "circulation" model of international networks in mind, we can see that there was no programmatic diffusion of social medicine thought from Europe to Latin America. If the ILO and the League of Nations offered something like a "social medicine" perspective and advanced the development of strong welfare states, they did so in a Latin American context where such proposals were already gaining acceptance. If anything, the Latin Americans presented a more politically radical and epistemologically integrative view of social medicine and the welfare state that exceeded the modest and technocratic recommendations of the Geneva institutions. Still, the occasional presence of European notables like René Sand probably helped raise the prestige of social medicine in Latin America. And it is fair to say that the "circulation" of ideas was not reciprocal, as Latin America's influence on European social medicine appears to have been minimal.

Thus, if these networks were not so crucial, how did ideas in social medicine travel? Since the occasions for personal encounters between European and Latin American experts were sporadic, the latter's awareness of international health and social policy trends resulted more from a lettered culture of scientific publication and diffusion; interpersonal contacts in professional networks at specific events like conferences may have been secondary in importance. Journals such as *Acción Social* or *Boletín Médico-Social* in Chile reported constantly on health and social policy innovations elsewhere in the region, the United States, the Soviet Union, Western Europe, and even Asia. The ILO and LN worked most effectively in countries with existing pro-Geneva associations and energetic policy entrepreneurs, like Chile and Argentina. Unlike international development institutions of the Cold War era, the Geneva institutions had almost no financial or geopolitical leverage to promote their agenda in the region.

Instead of emulation, there was contestation and adaptation of European social policy ideas. By and large, Latin American experts favored *internationalism*, in the sense of exchanging ideas across borders, but they were skeptical of *universalism*, the notion that good policies would be effective anywhere.[91] The ILO, in particular, tried to spread social policy models, such as social insurance, that it saw as universally viable. Latin Americans at the regional labor conferences were not convinced, instead contending that many ILO resolutions were not relevant for Latin American countries, where industrial development was incipient. At these meetings, Latin American delegates had the eye-opening experience of finding some common interests and even a common frame around the experience of international economic depression from a dependent, semicolonial position. These core–periphery tensions were subtle at the ILO meetings, but they reflect a larger intellectual project of Latin American identity construction of the 1930s. Put differently, the "Latin Americanness" of these networks is not only evident, objectively, in their spatial contours; these networks also helped foster a subjective sense of Latin American identity, around shared problems and conditions of peripherality.

While the US stance toward Geneva institutions was often aloof, it is important not to exaggerate philosophical and policy differences between them. Packard, among others, has suggested that the Geneva institutions championed social medicine's program of broader, systemic social and economic reforms, in sharp contrast with the outlook of the PASB and the IHB, which tended to support laboratory research and narrow, technical public health interventions, especially against infectious and vector-borne disease.[92] But at least into the late 1940s, the United States lent support to welfare state initiatives in Latin America, through the example of its own progressive social security legislation and the wide-ranging agendas of the Pan American Sanitary Conferences. To the extent that the RF and PAHO's preference for vertical (disease-specific) interventions later became dominant in the region, it may have been due as much to the size of their budgets and ability to develop technical expertise, as to the quality of their policy ideas. These financial and technical advantages of the US-based institutions over their European counterparts would only become more pronounced after World War II.

Still, the Geneva-based networks may have had an important ancillary influence in shaping the discourse of social medicine in Latin America. As the Geneva institutions' social policy models made inroads in the region, the influence of Latin American eugenics—which blurred at times with social medicine, as explained in chapter 1—appears to have declined. Ideas about the racial degeneration of national populations were widespread during the interwar period, but not at the Latin American conferences sponsored by the ILO and the LN. There, calls for eugenicist measures to raise the quality of the population were infrequent. Experts in social security apparently saw little explanatory power in eugenics. Quite possibly, as the 1930s progressed, the Latin American eugenicists' network became tighter but also more isolated, cut off from more important currents in health and social policy, and out of step with the movement toward more expansive welfare states, a key legacy of social medicine.

Networks outside the boundaries of international scientific technocracy were also important for the development of social medicine, though with delayed effects. As Paul Weindling and Corinnne Pernet each point out, most of the Latin Americans involved in Geneva-sponsored policy networks were well-established public health officials; they valued stability and order, and thus looked for ways to manage and reform society scientifically.[93] Both the Geneva-based and Pan-American networks in health and social policy employed technocratic strategies to stay above the fray of ordinary politics, eschewing political radicalism and anchored in liberal political and economic precepts. Yet, outside of these official channels, other transnational networks were building and coalescing to advance more radical, leftist political proposals. While groups like the Apristas in exile probably influenced their left-wing counterparts in Chile, such as the Vanguardia Médica, which included a young Salvador Allende, it is difficult to substantiate these connections. However, there is little doubt that, after a longer period of gestation, development, and diffusion, structural Marxist frameworks would have a strong effect on the second wave of Latin American social medicine, as I discuss in chapter 6.

To fully understand the intricacies of social medicine ideas and their translation into policy, it is necessary to shift the scale of analysis, back to the nation-state as a social, economic, and political unit. Chapters 3 and 4, centered on Chile and Argentina, respectively, illustrate how health professionals under the banner of social medicine achieved dramatically different policy outcomes, as they worked through distinct conditions and circumstances.

CHAPTER THREE

Politics
Social Medicine and Health Reform in Chile

In 1939, Salvador Allende published *La realidad médico-social chilena*, a diligently researched exposé of the punishing toll of grinding poverty on the lives of the Chilean people. With simple and direct prose, Allende painted a grim portrait of this national "reality." Out of a cohort of four newborn babies, one would die in its first year, while the three survivors would likely be subject to a childhood of empty stomachs, recurrent illness, and deprivations of all sorts—no shoes, warm clothes, or a roof over their heads. Worse still, due to illness, accident, or abandonment, some would be left with just one parent, or none. This was a "socio-medical" crisis rooted in the inequitable and unjust structure of Chilean society, a problem that Allende traced to the dynamics of an international capitalist system that extracted not just the wealth but the lifeblood of poor countries like Chile. To begin to solve the crisis at a national level would require the concerted effort of government to stimulate broad-based economic development, provide for basic needs of Chilean citizens, and, not least, centralize health insurance and medical services, making them universally accessible to all Chileans.

Allende's book has been appraised as a "classic expression" of Latin American social medicine.[1] As it articulated the social program of the government of the Frente Popular—in which Allende served for two and a half years as minister of health—the book exemplifies the health policies of rising welfare states in Latin America. Some have praised Allende's Marxian analytics, which framed health crisis as a predictable, perhaps intrinsic, outcome of cycles of capitalist accumulation, dispossession, and labor exploitation.[2] And while *La realidad médico-social chilena* shares the urgent tone and graphic accounts of human misery that typified the social medicine genre at the time, Allende's fame would transcend this field. The book marked an early episode in Allende's political trajectory, which culminated in the democratically elected socialist government he led from 1970 to 1973, followed by his overthrow in a bloody coup and sixteen years of a repressive and pro-capitalist authoritarian regime. Thus, Allende and his program of universal health care symbolize, to many, *the Chile that could have been*—one guided by principles of social justice.[3]

However, without the benefit of foreknowledge of the rest of Chile's twentieth-century history, would we see Allende as such a central figure in national social medicine? In reality, Allende was just one player in health policy debates in Chile over a period of several decades. As noted in chapter 1, social medicine in Chile developed along with the notion of the "social question," starting with the essay of the same name by Augusto Orrego Luco in 1884. By the 1920s, within a highly combative and sometimes violent political scene, anarchist doctors like Juan Gandulfo proposed radical alternatives to address the health problems of the working class. And, as explained in chapter 2, increased interactions between Chilean technocrats and figures of European liberal internationalism helped shape an expansion of the Chilean welfare state.

Socialist partisans like Allende were but one element among advocates of social medicine. His group, which called itself the Vanguardia Médica in the mid-1930s, published incisive polemics in journals like *Medicina Social* and *Boletín Médico de Chile*, organized important conferences, and took over the leadership of the AMECH, the Chilean medical association. Still, there were many centers of political action in health reform. Some politically conservative doctors called for increased state involvement in the health sector, not simply as a reformist strategy to short-circuit more radical interventions from the political left, but as the praxis of a coherent vision of social transformation inspired by Catholic social doctrine. A centrist and corporatist agenda, embodied for a time in the Chilean Radical Party, saw the state's role as balancing competing interests, to be accomplished, in part, by allocating parts of the state apparatus to a professional class of technical experts. Meanwhile, Allende's program was pragmatic compared to that of anarchists (or libertarian socialists), whose visions of gender equality, sexual liberation, emancipation through consciousness-raising, and radical democracy were mostly nonstarters in Chile. Across the political spectrum, in Chilean social medicine few disputed the necessity of a modern welfare state, and Chile became one of a group of so-called pioneers, along with countries like Uruguay and Argentina, in developing modern social security systems in the region.[4] Rather than the social medicine movement driving the creation of the Chilean welfare state, existing government structures for the health-care system created the political conditions for social medicine to grow and make an impact.

This chapter analyzes the politics of social medicine and its role in the expansion of the welfare state in Chile during this period of change. I argue that socialists, though influential, were not the key protagonists in Chilean social medicine. Rather, social medicine was a relatively open domain that encompassed varied analytics of the political, economic, and social causes of health crisis, while entertaining a world of alternative models for constructing a strong welfare state to protect public health under the guidance of technical and scientific experts. Amid ideological conflicts, comity was maintained through practices of professional deference, attitudes of mutual respect, well-developed social networks, and recognition of shared class interests. This harmony broke down only when controversial issues arose, such as abortion. Generally, members of the social medicine episteme understood themselves as leaders somehow above the fray of politics, as scientific managers of society. This elitist attitude reinforced class cohesion and did not keep doctors from offering cogent, empathetic, and impassioned portrayals of the deep misery of ordinary Chileans, but it may have stood in the way of undoing imperfect institutions and moving Chile toward a universal regime of socialized medicine. Simultaneously, gremialismo—labor union politics—developed as a political strategy. Doctors, through collective effort, could better control their workplace conditions and gain substantial power in steering the national health system.

To develop this argument, I draw on a rich primary source base, from popular, political, and scientific journals and newspapers, and build upon a growing historiography on the roots of the social medicine movement in Chile. Soon after Chile's return to democracy in 1990, María Angélica Illanes initiated the contemporary national historiography on public health, treating Allende and his fellow socialists as the prime movers of health progress, and adopting Allende's analytical approach, a sort of historical materialism, in which conservative, traditional factions aligned with international capitalist interests thwarted broad-based development and real democratization, thus defining the tragedy of modern Chile.[5] This perspective has been amplified by Howard Waitzkin, a sociologist and physician who has situated Chilean social medicine in a long chronology dating back to Rudolph Virchow in mid-nineteenth-century Germany.[6] Drawing on feminist and post-structural approaches, the historian Karin Rosemblatt has positioned Chilean social medicine as part of a broad project to develop a state-employed cadre of experts, "welfare professionals," to manage the population in the 1930s. The Frente Popular's governing program embodied this objective, which was part of a "gendered project" to create a society of "honorable [male] workers and wives" to "ensure the demographic health of the nation, enhance industrial productivity, and secure national progress."[7] When the medical profession began to organize itself, not as a scientific association but as a labor union, it mostly aligned itself in support of the state project of socialized medicine.

Drawing on the work of Illanes and Maria Eliana Labra, Carlos Molina Bustos (who served in the Ministry of Health in the early 1970s under Allende) interprets social medicine as a broad field with various political strains (conservative, socialist, radical, Falangist) in the 1930s and 1940s.[8]

This chapter also confronts the thorny question of whether, and how, to differentiate "social medicine" from "socialized medicine." As Jadwiga Pieper-Mooney explains in a discussion of Chile's public health politics of the mid-twentieth century, these two ideas were often "contested and conflated"; there was a "politically and ideologically fraught relationship between social medicine and socialized medicine" at the time.[9] Why was it so fraught? On the one hand, social medicine, especially in the eyes of groups like the Vanguardia Médica, was a movement that called for transformation of Chilean society. The government of the Frente Popular attempted a coordinated effort to achieve broader transformation on many fronts, but this moment was short-lived. Stymied in that process, the social medicine movement became more focused on fixing the workings of the health system: uniting disparate health insurance, medical care, and public health functions into one government body; ensuring adequate funding for the system; and moving toward universal health coverage for all Chileans. These efforts eventually culminated in the creation of Chile's National Health Service in the early 1950s. It would be a mistake to say that there was a sharp distinction between social medicine and socialized medicine during this period, and such conceptual differences need to be assessed as historically contingent, not permanent and universal.

Foundations of the Chilean Welfare State

The construction of the Chilean welfare state was forged not in democracy but in a short-lived dictatorship. Arturo Alessandri had been elected president democratically in 1920 (although only a small minority of Chileans were able to cast a ballot) on a platform of progressive social change, promising reforms to calm the chaotic political atmosphere shaped in part by Gandulfo and his fellow anarcho-syndicalists. However, Alessandri found his agenda frustrated by a powerful Congress dominated by conservative interests.[10] As a result, the national government was effectively paralyzed in the face of growing public discontent and social disorder. In September 1924, a military junta led by General Luis Altamirano established control over the parliament and sent Alessandri into temporary exile, while pushing through the social and labor reform laws he had sought. These included a new labor code, a sanitary code, a Ministry of Hygiene, and the creation of the Caja del Seguro

Obrero Obligatorio (usually abbreviated as CSO), a national social insurance system covering health care, workers' compensation, and retirement pensions. Despite the dubious constitutionality of its origins, the enabling legislation, Law 4054, became the basis for new layers of expansion of social security and socialized medicine in Chile, into the 1970s.[11]

The CSO was the brainchild of Dr. Exequiel González Cortés, a physician who, as a representative of the Conservative Party, introduced the idea to Congress in the early 1920s. The structure of the Caja was adapted from what would come to be called a Bismarckian social security model, due to its origins in nineteenth-century Germany, based upon a tripartite financing mechanism, with workers, employers, and the state making roughly equal, salary-based contributions to the CSO's central fund. CSO beneficiaries were entitled to medical services in the Caja's own facilities (or from doctors contracted by the Caja), prenatal services and limited maternity leave for female workers, insurance for worker disability, funeral services, and an old-age pension.[12] However, most of these benefits (including, notably, medical services) covered workers only, and not their families. The CSO was also just one institution—albeit the one with the largest number of beneficiaries—in a fragmented system of social insurance programs. By 1939, as Allende would observe, there were forty-four different *cajas* that covered special categories of workers (e.g., members of the military, state employees, journalists, railroad workers, the merchant marines, and so forth), although over 80 percent of wage earners were enrolled in the CSO.[13]

Early on, the CSO faced opposition from many sides. Some "conservative liberals"—that is, defenders of the program of economic liberalism—hoped to transform the cajas from social insurance programs into personalized insurance plans, where individual workers would keep the benefits that accrued from their mandatory contributions to their own accounts, while the state would continue to provide medical assistance to the indigent under the older model of *beneficencia*, or charity care.[14] Organized labor—ostensibly the principal beneficiary of social insurance benefits—was initially opposed to the CSO. Some labor unions called Law 4054 the Ley del Garrote (roughly, the Law of the Cudgel) and opposed the CSO on multiple grounds: their anger at "confiscation" of their hard-earned wages, skepticism that employers and the state would comply with their required contributions to the fund, and concern about *empleomanía* or bloating of state employee rolls.[15] In March 1926, the Federación Obrera de Chile (Federation of Chilean Workers) organized a general strike calling for the repeal of Law 4054 and elimination of the new Ministry of Hygiene, arguing that the budget for the health ministry could be better used for other social purposes, including housing and education.[16] According to Illanes, "in an environment of overwhelming poverty and revolutionary social agitation, it was logical to think that the laws in general, and the law of social security in particular, were perceived as legalized theft of workers' salaries or as a scam."[17] Law 4054 was, in a sense, a flash point in a larger crisis of state legitimacy.

Under these circumstances, what saved the CSO from early demise? For one thing, the CSO had a natural constituency in a medical profession with an orientation toward social reform that was motivated, not least, by class interests. With some urgency, they desired a state that could mediate class conflict and calm revolutionary threats, not by force but by providing essential services to a large segment of the population. This was essentially the "social democratic" project, supported by the efforts of the ILO and League of Nations in the interwar period, which aimed to enhance public welfare and build the resources necessary for broad-based economic growth, while providing workers a modicum of security from the vicissitudes of capitalist development.[18] In Chile, according to Labra, "this project was incorporated into the nationalist and eugenicist vision of the era, within which the object of health is human capital, which should be valued, protected, and multiplied by the state for the glory of the nation."[19] "Political doctors," such as Julio Bustos, Arturo Lois Fraga, and Isauro Torres, aligned with the centrist Radical Party, worked toward perfecting the technical and administrative aspects of Chile's social insurance system.[20]

After withstanding early political opposition, the CSO achieved a firmer financial footing and a clearer sense of purpose by the early 1930s. Its journals, the *Boletín Médico-Social* and *Acción Social*, became important forums for promoting the gradually expanding work of the CSO and diffusing international social policy ideas.[21] For example, from 1934 to 1935, *Acción Social* reported on social security, labor, and public health policy in the United States (under Roosevelt's New Deal), the Soviet Union, Germany, Italy, Denmark, and Great Britain, as well as Latin American states such as Peru, Mexico, and Argentina. The CSO began to provide not just insurance but also its own medical services, essentially creating a more vertical structure to internalize health-care costs. The capital reserves of the Caja grew steadily, multiplying roughly tenfold from 1926 to 1934, although the Great Depression had a severe impact on the salary pool and thus reduced the Caja's rate of growth in the early 1930s.[22]

The CSO was controversial throughout its existence. Its supporters, which included a large part of the medical establishment, considered themselves "authoritatively responsible for taking on the direction of social movement and political change" and believed that the CSO would maintain social peace, safeguarding the liberal model of economic production by offering "the physical-biological protection of the national labor force."[23] The CSO's long-time chief administrator, Santiago Labarca, saw the CSO as an exemplar of a "new politics," in which a technical agency, shielded from everyday politics by its autonomous fiscal status, would not simply "build a bridge" between capital and labor, but harmonize their interests through rational and efficient organization.[24] (Years before assuming the directorship of the CSO, Santiago Labarca had been one of the key student leaders of the FECh, along with Juan Gandulfo, in the revolutionary years of the early 1920s. His brother, Miguel Labarca, was one of Salvador Allende's closest political confidants. These connections exemplify the "small world" of Chilean politics of that era.) The CSO's leaders, by the mid-1930s, could confidently assert that they were part of an expansionary international trend in state social insurance systems to safeguard liberal democracy by saving capitalism from its worst imbalances.

Promoters of the CSO viewed it as more than a social insurance program that needed to be merely solvent; it was also a model and resource for the exercise of Chilean economic sovereignty. In a 1934 retrospective on the first ten years of the CSO, its financial directors argued that the reserves of the Caja were "a powerful nucleus of national capital formation. For the first time, the country was forming its own capital."[25] In other words, the Caja created a new, large, reliable, domestic source of investment capital for national projects.[26] The CSO directors believed they had found at least a partial remedy to a classic problem of Chilean development, the lack of domestic capital for investment, due to extraction by foreign interests and the passive, risk-averse practices of local elites. During the leanest years of the Depression, the Caja stood out for its large cash reserves accumulated during better times that Labarca hoped to use for diversified investments in Chilean enterprises.[27] The development of the Caja foreshadowed the shift toward explicitly Keynesian economic policy under the Frente Popular government at the end of the 1930s, particularly the creation of CORFO (Corporación de Fomento a la Producción), a state corporation that became the basis of three decades of state-directed economic development policy in Chile.[28] Labarca envisioned the CSO's becoming a state conglomerate doing business in other sectors, making it, "in a sense, a large workers' cooperative" that could expand beyond health insurance and pensions into affordable home loans and clothing stores.[29]

At the same time, criticism abounded, particularly from leftist sectors of social medicine, such as the Vanguardia Médica. As we will see further on, what Labarca saw as the Caja's great virtue, its moderating effect on class relations under capitalism, the Vanguardia Médica saw as a defect, insofar as it avoided a deeper questioning of the failing capitalist development model. Others assailed the CSO's inadequacies as a health system. In 1931, José García Tello, an avowed communist, wrote an exposé of life and work inside one of the CSO polyclinics in Viña del Mar, which he directed. While he offered a litany of complaints, the gist of the critique was that the CSO offered a sham of social medicine. The CSO had made medical services more accessible to a sizable segment of the population, but medical care could only address the symptoms of the problem, not its root: the inhumane living conditions of working-class districts.[30]

The caja system had many other problems: a multiplicity of cajas with widely differing financing structures and benefit plans, a complex nonsystem that seemed designed mainly to satisfy the demands of politically organized groups; the general lack of health insurance coverage, in any of the cajas, for workers' families; a demonstrable lack of results in addressing Chile's severe health crisis; the financial squeezing of the doctors who worked for the cajas; and a failure to fully incorporate public charity hospitals, insurance funds, and public health agencies into a single, unified system. As Salvador Allende would articulate better than anyone, the cajas were an obstacle to the necessary complete socialization of medicine under a unitary national system that would provide equal benefits for all Chileans.[31]

Nonetheless, the CSO remained active until the early 1950s. Chile could rightly claim to have created the first national system of social insurance in the Americas, and despite its defects in practice, the CSO served as a blueprint for other national social insurance and socialized health-care systems, most notably Costa Rica's.[32] Meanwhile, a steadily increasing share of the medical profession, just part of an "expanding corps of state-employed experts," whom Karin Rosemblatt has called "welfare professionals," would be drawn into the cajas, further entrenching the system while generating growing discontent within it.[33]

The Vanguardia Médica and the Organization of the Medical Profession

While the directors of the CSO were cautiously optimistic about the progress of their agency, many doctors in Chile were growing increasingly restive and agitated in the 1930s. In their journals, books, and speeches, they painted a portrait of a society near its breaking point, with public health conditions deteriorating under the strain of world economic crisis and government inaction. Sparked by the crisis, a growing faction of doctors began to reassess their role in society, picking up where the anarchist doctors of the 1920s had left off. They were aware that the CSO and the other cajas were already undermining the free-market model of "liberal medicine" and transforming labor relations in the medical field. As the Argentine *gremialista* Juan Lazarte observed firsthand in a 1936 visit to Chile, many doctors united to resist their own "proletarianization" or reduction to mere functionaries in larger bureaucratic systems.[34] Efforts to organize the medical profession reflected the chaotic atmosphere of Chilean politics in the 1930s, conditioned by the devastating impact of the Great Depression. During this tumultuous decade, the Chilean Medical Association, AMECH, became the hub of labor organizing in the health sector, a forum for social medicine thought, and the vehicle for the Vanguardia Médica to channel its political efforts.

The unionizing of medical workers had begun with founding of the Sindicato de Médicos de Chile in October 1924, in Valparaíso, a hotbed of anarcho-syndicalist activity. Until then, Chilean doctors had been organized in what was a "scientific" organization, the Sociedad Médica, ostensibly removed from ordinary politics, which was sometimes called *politiquería*. The Sindicato had been formed in response to the creation of the CSO, which rapidly incorporated the services of physicians in major cities. For reasons that remain unclear, the Sindicato failed to unite Chile's medical profession, but the AMECH would be more successful. Medical students in the FECh (which Juan Gandulfo and Santiago Labarca had led, around 1919 to 1921), their professors, and medical staff of public hospitals joined together to form the AMECH in 1931.[35] In the winter of that year, students of the FECh, which now included Salvador Allende, took over the administration building of the Universidad de Chile, organized a nationwide general strike, and fought in the streets against the dwindling ranks of supporters of the unpopular president Carlos Ibáñez del Campo. The opposition to Ibáñez in the worst year of the Great Depression was multifaceted, but the AMECH was incited specifically by a presidential decree in June 1931 that transferred funds from the CSO and other cajas to cover other government expenditures.[36] For some in its ranks, the AMECH carried the banner of "civilismo," a short-lived coalition of the parties of the political establishment (Conservative, Liberal, and Radical), desperate to restore a limited democracy after several years of dictatorship and to maintain order in the face of left-wing (socialist, communist, and anarcho-syndicalist) threats.[37]

The Vanguardia Médica, which brought together many of the FECh insurgency leaders, such as Allende, splintered the AMECH into factions for several years. Leaders of the Vanguardia Médica were intimately linked to the Socialist Republic.[38] This memorable "government of ninety days" was formed through a curious alliance of socialists, military men, and supporters of the recently deposed Ibáñez, who came together to overthrow the ineffective "civilista" president Juan Esteban Montero on June 4, 1932. Roughly two weeks later, two of the coup plotters, the military leader Marmaduke Grove and the Freemason attorney Eugenio Matte, were exiled to Easter Island as the Ibáñez ally Carlos Dávila seized power. Meanwhile, the Sindicato de Médicos relaunched its journal, the *Boletín Médico de Chile* (*BMC*), as a weekly for the "workers of medicine," and before long, the main forum for the Vanguardia Médica. Several weeks later, in August 1932, naval officers in Valparaíso arrested as a group Marmaduke Grove's brothers Eduardo and Hugo (the editor in chief of the *BMC*), Carlos Gómez Baltra (a leader of the Sindicato Médico), and Salvador Allende, and placed them on trial by a military tribunal, for seditious acts.[39]

From their jail cells, the group christened itself the Vanguardia Médica and issued their defiant declaration of principles, announced dramatically in the pages of the *BMC*.[40] This statement offered a radical vision of the nation's future. They declared that "the destruction of the actual social system is inevitable" with the "revolutionary action of the oppressed minority giving rise to a scientific organization of society." The near-term goal of the Vanguardia Médica was to transform the AMECH into a union that would govern the health sector, its legitimacy deriving not from political alliances but from technical competence, not just in the clinical practice of medicine, but in the organization and coordination of medical services.[41] When all the dust had settled, after the end of the Socialist Republic and the restoration of democracy in early 1933, the Grove brothers, Matte, and Allende, along with Oscar Schnake (also a physician, and former anarchist student leader) came together to form the new Socialist Party of Chile, which was no longer proscribed by law.

It was only in 1936, after a pivotal National Medical Convention, that the AMECH overcame internal divisions to take on the form a federation of collective bargaining units of medical workers employed by government agencies, hospitals, and the social security system (principally, the CSO). The convention was held in Valparaíso in January 1936, and its main objective was to develop a solid organizational structure that would place the medical profession in a position to steer the dynamic process of the socialization of medicine. While the AMECH would emerge revitalized from the convention with a clear commitment to socialized medicine, it was abortion, an issue not originally on the meeting's agenda, that would attract the most attention and divide the medical establishment for years to come. Plans to openly discuss decriminalizing abortion alienated conservative Catholic physicians, many affiliated with the Universidad Católica and the Asociación Nacional de Estudiantes Católicos (ANEC), who boycotted the conference, leaving the left wing of the AMECH firmly in charge of the proceedings.[42] Its mission became more defined, as an organization that sought to advance the interests of the medical profession as a *labor union* under the wing of the state with a centralized national system of health care. Nevertheless, we should be cautious not to view the AMECH as the conduit for all social medicine thought or policy proposals, nor did its role in representing the interests of the medical profession go unchallenged.

AMECH and the Embrace of Socialized Medicine

The AMECH was the most durable institutional expression of a leftist social medicine movement that had been channeled ephemerally through the Sindicato de Médicos and the Vanguardia Médica. Throughout, despite internecine conflicts, their analysis of Chile's public health crisis and the solutions to it remained largely the same: the miserable health conditions of Chileans required an overhaul of the economic and health systems, to overcome the deficiencies of capitalist development and imperfect state management of the health sector. More unification and centralization of health services under the umbrella of the state were necessary, but only with the leadership of a unified medical profession.

The worldwide economic depression, which hit Chile especially hard between 1931 and 1933, had multiple effects. Poverty became deeper and more widespread, and its impact on health more pronounced.[43] Skyrocketing unemployment—from just under 7,000 unemployed workers in January 1931 to around 125,000 by the end of 1932—deepened the crisis of poverty, sparking mass internal migration from the northern mining district to the slums and conventillos (tenements) of Santiago.[44] The budgets for charity hospitals and the CSO were stretched more than ever. Doctors despaired over the ineffectiveness of their arts in the face of such misery. And many began to question the foundations of an entire economic system and the state that sustained it.[45]

A nationwide typhus epidemic from 1933 to 1935 accentuated Chile's deficiencies in public health and provided a focal point for calls for reform.[46] The spread of this flea-borne disease, on top of Chile's other troubles, represented a national humiliation: as Senator Guillermo Eliseo Azócar put it in 1935, this "epidemic is a stigma for our country, since it [typhus] only develops in those nations where the proletarian classes live in misery, dress in rags, have homes that belong in the Stone Age, and lack sufficient food."[47] In the same parliamentary session, Hugo Grove, the Socialist Party leader and member of the Vanguardia Médica, lamented "two years of the absence of planning and the abandonment of a poor people decimated by hunger, filth, poverty, and diseases!" He implored his fellow senators to support government action in the face of the typhus epidemic, which he calculated had killed some 7,500 people, and sickened 30,000 more, over the previous two years.[48] Health workers were severely affected by the typhus epidemic: in early 1935 the *BMC* published a long list of dozens of health workers killed by typhus, mainly orderlies and other lower-level hospital staff, rather than doctors, demonstrating again the social hierarchy in the death toll from the epidemic.[49]

Viewed from one angle, the typhus epidemic was merely a symptom or superficial expression of deeper economic crisis that reverberated across the world, deepening poverty, putting costly medications out of reach, and limiting the fiscal basis for a government response.[50] As discussed briefly in chapter 2, Chilean representatives to the 1934 Pan-American Sanitary Conference framed the typhus epidemic as a natural outcome of massive poverty, malnutrition, homelessness, and internal migration of families in search of work.[51] Aquiles Machiavello, the head of the Dirección de Sanidad, pleaded that his agency was helpless to act when the economic crisis, the "primary factor" behind the typhus epidemic, was beyond his control.[52] For others, ascribing the typhus epidemic to underlying economic conditions was a defeatist stance that excused the Chilean government's lack of coordination and downright incompetence in the face of the epidemic. In particular, in the middle of 1935 the government had allowed the distribution of a useless vaccine in a hasty response to public panic. What was now turning into a crisis of authority and expertise led the *BMC* to demand "ALL POWER TO THE AMECH" (the original headline was indeed in all capital letters, boldface type, about ten times the height of the ordinary print).[53] A few years later, now as minister of health, Allende would single out the typhus epidemic as a deadly consequence of the lack of coordination of government health services.[54]

Such calls for the reorganization of medical services were just part of a broader agenda: AMECH wanted to hasten the demise of "liberal medicine" and steer the process of moving toward a socialized health system, which had begun with the creation of the CSO. Liberal medicine, according to the AMECH, operated on the presumption of the individual autonomy of the doctor, "trying to better his own interests in the solitary retreat of his private clinic."

But, "the new medicine" was "diametrically opposed" to this so-called priestly model of medicine, because collective efforts of a variety of medical personnel and support staff were necessary not only to cure a patient during sporadic episodes of sickness but also to practice preventive medicine. In addition, continuous progress in medical science led to the development of new specialties, so that best practices lay beyond the capability of any one doctor. Only higher-level organization could effectively coordinate the efforts of specialists.[55] José García Tello, cited earlier for his exposé of the CSO polyclinic in Viña del Mar, proposed granting vast coercive powers to the state's medical apparatus, to the point of suspending an individual's right to *refuse* medical care. This particular proposal went nowhere, but it speaks to the medical profession's rising self-regard and belief in the possibility of the scientific management of society at large, as well as the institutional imprint of the CSO.[56] Already in 1935, an editorial in the *BMC* proclaimed, "The liberal profession is over. The independent doctor is already an exception, respectable, evidently, but a rare bird. And this change has come about in the short span of ten years!"—that is, from the beginnings of the CSO.[57]

In its effort to control the supply and distribution of medical personnel in the country, AMECH disputed the common assertion that there was a "plethora"—that is, an oversupply—of doctors in Chile. Such claims arose frequently starting in the 1930s, both in Chile and neighboring Argentina. Political conservatives, including some doctors, used the specter of a "plethora" to prevent an increase in the number of doctors in the country, arguing against a proposal to open a new medical school in Concepción, Chile's second largest city at the time.[58] Doctors affiliated with AMECH contended that what appeared to be a plethora was actually a sort of market failure (though that precise term was not used): Santiago, it was true, was full of doctors, thanks to the draw of higher salaries, a steady customer base, and adequately equipped hospitals and clinics. In large expanses of poorer parts of Chile, however, there were no doctors or medical services to speak of. An editorial in the *BMC* in 1935 calculated that the country would need about one thousand additional doctors just to reach a national ratio of one doctor per two thousand inhabitants.[59] At the same time, Chile was generally so poor that many doctors struggled to get by financially. Garcia Tello saw through the rhetoric of plethora, characterizing it as a problem that only made sense within the framework of capitalism's law of supply and demand.[60] Garcia Tello lamented "the superabundance of workers of medicine that have nothing to eat and no work to do, while men die in the thousands due to poverty and disease, which has led individualist medicine to its complete bankruptcy."[61] The editors of

BMC hoped that "all of the sick would have a doctor, and every doctor would have work." But this would require a change in "regime," from a liberal to collectivist economic system.[62]

To realize such radical change would require doctors and other health workers to become more intensely involved in politics. Evaluating the appropriate role for doctors in politics was another contentious issue in social medicine circles. The AMECH and especially the Vanguardia Médica promoted an activist political praxis and, as we have seen, some were persecuted for their beliefs and actions. Despite the growing influence of AMECH, many conservative Chilean doctors hesitated to join it because of its political radicalism. But even some among the vocal left called for doctors to stay out of the political arena. Angel Vidal Oltra of Viña del Mar, who labeled himself a committed socialist, pleaded with his fellow doctors to draw a clear line between politics and medical practice: "Medicine in itself," he wrote, "has nothing to do with social doctrines, given that it is a science, and as a science it is independent from our moral or social conceptions. When a doctor enters the hospital or the home of a sick patient he ought to leave his sociological doctrines hanging by the door and concentrate all of the forces of his spirit in his role as a health technician."[63] A critique of the Vanguardia Médica, written by an anonymous group of "young doctors from Santiago" in 1935, suggested that the power of the medical profession resided in its scientific and technical expertise and warned that this valuable political capital could easily be squandered in partisan battles.[64]

Yet Allende, among others, argued that political engagements were unavoidable. How else could government health services become unified, or more physicians be placed in the higher echelons of public administration?[65] To overcome this dilemma, one typical stance was to capitalize on the profession's high social status and its monopoly over medical education and practice, to push for progressive reforms and consolidate union power over the state's health apparatus, while maintaining a separation between the medical sphere and the world of low partisan politics—the "politiquería" that privileged political connections over technical competency and scientific knowledge.[66] In any case, between the end of the Socialist Republic in 1932 and the election of the Frente Popular in 1938, several progressive doctors were elected to the Chilean Congress, moving health policy issues up the legislative agenda. Even though few concrete policy changes were made during this period, leftist political doctors, such as Hugo Grove, Allende, and Schnake, made the country's ugly sanitary conditions a focus of national debate, as chronicled in 1934 and 1935 in the *BMC*, which regularly reported on congressional debates.

How do we read the achievements and rising influence of the AMECH in the 1930s? On the one hand, we can see it as a real force for change, infuriated by the limits of politics-as-usual, responsive to Chile's grave health crisis, and capable, suddenly, of building effective institutions to promote the principles of social medicine. On the other hand, AMECH leaders seemed unconscious of their arrogance, manifest in the conflation of their own interests as a professional organization with the interests of society at large. In pressing for a socialized health system independent of political oversight and minimizing the values and concerns of those outside the expert professions, the AMECH sometimes aligned with a benevolent rationalist authoritarianism, even leading to strident pronouncements on abortion and sterilization to regulate society by correcting its demographic imbalances, according to transparently eugenicist principles.[67] With the AMECH and Vanguardia Médica staking out such extreme positions, yet with social medicine thinking in wide efflorescence, it is not surprising that there was an alternative, influential position in health politics, conservative reformism, typified by the renowned Chilean doctor, Eduardo Cruz-Coke.[68]

Conservative Reformism in Social Medicine

Eduardo Cruz-Coke was an eminent and widely respected figure in mid-century Chile. Although his name barely registers outside of the country, he was the epitome of the political doctor, one who wore many hats in an era of only nascent professional specialization. Cruz-Coke was a prolific scientist, a respected university professor, practicing physician, government minister, senator, and diplomat. He even ran for president in 1946, but lost in a close election (Cruz-Coke's presidential campaign of 1946 was a key moment in the rising influence of the National Falange, a conservative Catholic youth movement, which would eventually metamorphose into the major Christian Democratic Party led by Eduardo Frei Montalva).[69] Politically, Cruz-Coke was a center-right reformist and longtime member of the Conservative Party, but with an underlying philosophy that defied easy categorization.[70] While his time as minister of health was short-lived, he would have lasting influence on Chile's health system, through his own continued political action and the work of his disciples, including Jorge Mardones Restat and Benjamin Viel, who helped establish and build the SNS.[71]

Cruz-Coke was born into a wealthy family, descended from British aristocracy, in Valparaíso in 1899. As noted by all his biographers, Eduardo was an excellent student and matriculated to the Facultad de Medicina in Santiago at the age of sixteen, graduating in 1921 and accepting a position as a professor of biochemistry and pathology in 1925. He spent most of the rest of his life based in Santiago, practicing at the Hospital San Juan de Dios, one of the principal teaching hospitals of the city, teaching at the university, and maintaining a private practice as personal physician to Chile's elites. His early political action began in the university, with his leadership of the ANEC, which gained public attention for its boycott of the 1936 Chilean medical conference, over the inclusion of the abortion question on the agenda.[72] The ANEC provided a forum for the discussion of philosophical bases of medical practice and national health policy informed by Catholic social doctrine, originating in the 1891 papal encyclical known as the *Rerum Novarum*. It was also often opposed to the FECh, an incubator of secular-leftist Chilean social medicine.

Cruz-Coke was immersed in Catholic social doctrine and he also followed young, progressive Catholic philosophers such as Pierre Teilhard de Chardin, who presented a distinctive vision of humanity's place in the evolution of the entire cosmos, and Jacques Maritain, who developed a "new humanism" based on a revival of the teachings of Saint Thomas Aquinas.[73] Cruz-Coke believed that the doctrine of the Catholic Church could be constantly renewed and could serve as an instrument of social progress. At the same time, Cruz-Coke saw no conflict at all between his religious devotion and his intense dedication to natural science. Still, in his politics, Cruz-Coke was committed to the Conservative party, and worked from "the heart of his [political party] ... to reform society from within."[74] Notwithstanding his party loyalty, he felt limited by the conventional ideological divisions of Chilean political life; to him, "what differentiated political and social forces had its roots not in the labels of left/right, but rather their position in relation to change."[75] As María Soledad Zárate puts it, Cruz-Coke appeared to many as a centrist in the world of social medicine, someone who was widely respected and not strongly attached to party doctrines.[76]

According to Carlos Huneeus and Maria Paz Lanas, Cruz-Coke was the first "genuine" minister of health, meaning the first to be appointed for reasons other than political patronage (as they describe it, the minister of health position was used frequently as a "wild card" to balance partisan and factional interests within presidential cabinets).[77] Though this assessment may not be fair to all his predecessors (twenty-five ministers over the course of fifteen years), Cruz-Coke made innovative use of his office, from January 1937 to September 1938, bringing forward significant policy initiatives, particularly the establishment of a national commission on nutrition and the passage of the Law of Preventive Medicine (Ley de Medicina Preventiva). Cruz-Coke's interest in nutrition as a cornerstone of public health grew out of his scientific research specialty, endocrinology. Policy reports crafted by his students, such as Mardones Restat, Aurora Rodriguez, and Ricardo Cox, were informed by the rising science of nutrition. Their research offered precise accounting of macro- and micronutrients and the extreme deficiencies of the everyday Chilean diet, with most calories derived from limited sources of carbohydrates, such as processed grains and alcohol, and scant proteins from meat, fish, and dairy. The immediate stimulus for the national commission on nutrition was a sensational report on the desperately poor state of nutrition in Chile issued by two European scientists representing the League of Nations, Etienne Burnet and Carlo Dragoni, in 1935.[78] Cruz-Coke's commission was similarly clinical in its dissection of the wide-ranging effects of nutritional deficiencies, but it also recognized the need for cross-sector collaboration—especially in reforms of agriculture and the marketing and distribution of food—to make successful reforms.[79]

The Ley de Medicina Preventiva was intended to improve the medical services of the CSO. The core rationale behind the legislation, as Zárate explains it, was to use the government's medical services as an investment in labor productivity. The Caja's doctors would "seek out disease" in those who appeared to be well rather than waiting for the ill to appear at the clinic—a true exercise in "preventive medicine."[80] Cruz-Coke saw this as a rational and far-sighted use of scarce medical resources that would prevent more costly treatments and reduce the expense of disability, unemployment, and old-age pensions later in life. The law established an annual medical exam for those covered by the CSO. The exam would focus on three conditions, syphilis, tuberculosis, and cardiovascular problems, which, as Cruz-Coke and his fellow researchers had determined, produced a severe yet "hidden" burden of morbidity and mortality. To varying degrees, these medical problems could be addressed through medication, other therapies, and rest, if detected early enough. The law also allowed paid time off for rest and rehabilitation for people diagnosed with one or more of these problems. (Since these conditions did not usually impede work, they were not covered previously under CSO disability insurance.) The law also established sanctions against workers who refused the exam or treatments, and against those who did not respect medical confidentiality, to prevent companies from choosing only the healthiest workers.[81] Another aspect of the law was the concept of "medicina dirigida," or directed medicine, by which Cruz-Coke intended to coordinate and standardize the work of doctors who were contracted by the CSO. Cruz-Coke, too, objected to liberal medicine and the esoteric mystique of the

doctor-patient relationship. Continuing medical education and collaboration, along with a sort of evidence-based medicine, would ensure consistency
and accountability in medical practice.[82]

Criticism of the law focused mostly on technical aspects, but it also exposed
some key philosophical differences between Cruz-Coke, on one side, and the
Vanguardia Médica and the AMECH, on the other. Cruz-Coke believed that
the new law suited the conditions set by Chile's political economy: Chile was,
after all, a poor country with low wages and severe fiscal limitations. Where socialists saw the exploitation of labor by industrial capitalists, Cruz-Coke perceived an unproductive working class unlikely to be motivated by salary
increases. In a critique of the new law, AMECH leaders questioned narrow biological interventions and reiterated the AMECH's foundational declaration
that Chile's economic structure required "fundamental modifications" to ensure the public's health and welfare, starting with an equitable distribution of
the fruits of their labor.[83]

But what rankled the AMECH most was that it had been left outside of the
process of devising and drafting the law (although Allende represented
AMECH's point of view in parliamentary debates). In AMECH's view, Cruz-
Coke lacked allegiance to the mission of gremialismo (medical union organizing); moreover, the exigencies of the law, especially the obligatory annual
exams, would only create more work for Caja's medical staff without a corre-
sponding increase in compensation. In other words, the labor of *physicians*
was now being exploited to square the accounting of the CSO. And although
AMECH leaders respected Cruz-Coke's credentials as a scientist and teacher,
they saw the law as a kind of eccentric and impractical concoction that only
someone removed from daily clinical practice could devise.[84]

Cruz-Coke withstood such criticism, but his term as minister of health was
upended by one of the most peculiar events of Chile's tumultuous 1930s,
known as the Matanza del Seguro Obrero—the massacre at the CSO building.
In September 1938, a homegrown Chilean faction of the National Socialist
(i.e., Nazi) party marched into central Santiago and occupied the new art
deco headquarters of the CSO, as part of an attempted coup d'état. Possibly,
President Arturo Alessandri, directing government troops from the nearby
presidential palace, La Moneda, gave the orders himself to kill all the demon-
strators, even after they had been disarmed; in any case, sixty men were killed
by rifle and bayonet. Cruz-Coke resigned from the government in protest, with
three months remaining in Alessandri's term. The massacre also shifted public
sentiment decisively to the antifascist Frente Popular candidate, Pedro Aguirre
Cerda, who as president would continue many of Cruz-Coke's initiatives,

further expand the capacity of Chile's welfare state, and, in short order, appoint Allende as minister of health.

Allende's *La realidad medico-social chilena*: A Critical Reading

Throughout his career, Allende combined medicine and politics. Following the example of Juan Gandulfo, Allende immersed himself in university politics at the medical school of the University of Chile, with leading roles in the medical students' association, Avance (a student group linked to the Communist Party), and the FECh, which was revived in defiance of the Ibáñez dictatorship.[85] In 1931, Allende led a group of students that seized the administrative building of the university, declared a national strike, and took up arms against the dictatorship that was then in power. Soon after, he cofounded the Chilean Socialist Party, while continuing his medical studies, and wrote his thesis on the social causes of mental illness in Santiago, which was based on his experience as an intern in the city's psychiatric hospital. After medical school, he worked in the morgue of a large hospital in the port city of Valparaíso, performing, by his account, hundreds of autopsies—an experience with the actual viscera of the Chilean people that he would allude to repeatedly during his long political career. While also shaping the Vanguardia Médica and the AMECH, Allende continued as a Socialist Party leader and was elected to Congress representing Valparaíso in 1937. In 1938, Allende, just thirty years old, played a crucial role in bringing the Socialist Party into the Frente Popular coalition, and he gave up his congressional seat to join the FP government as minister of health in its second year.

Thus, Allende was well-suited to write a book like *La realidad médico-social chilena* (*LRMSC*). Social criticism was common in the world of Chilean social medicine as far back as Augusto Orrego Luco's essay on "the social question" in 1884.[86] But *LRMSC* also presented the health plan of the new FP government. The report crystallized social medicine thought of that era, comprehensively captured the health and socioeconomic conditions of Chile in 1939 and offered a path toward policy frameworks to address these problems. Most of what Allende reported was not new; he primarily reiterated the damning studies and incisive critiques that circulated at national medical conferences, in the AMECH newsletter, and in other Chilean social-medical journals. However, he may have been the first in Chile to develop a unified analytical framework based on historical materialism to explain the root causes of the health crisis.[87]

The bulk of the report's 200-plus pages consisted of a statistical compendium to demonstrate the depths of Chile's awful public health crisis, something that was already widely recognized in national politics. Chile, at the time, had the highest infant mortality rate in the world—at least in the part of the world that kept statistics about it—around 200 per 1,000 live births throughout the 1930s.[88] Much of the infant mortality problem could be traced to chronic malnutrition; here Allende drew on the well-known Dragoni–Burnet survey, which found that about 70 percent of the Chilean public did not receive an adequate caloric ration, and that many subsisted on 900 to 1,000 calories a day, even as the typical Chilean worker spent something like 90 percent of his or her wages on food.[89] Among the dozens of countries where the League of Nations had done surveys, only China, Morocco, and Poland had comparable levels of malnutrition.[90]

As Allende put it, the Chilean masses faced outright food scarcity and constant nutritional deficits, which held true for urban and rural workers alike. National milk production was only about 50 liters per capita, compared to 363 liters per person in the United States and 569 liters per person in the Netherlands at the time. Taking what were then accepted nutritional requirements of 1 liter of milk daily for every child, and a half liter per adult, Allende calculated that Chile produced only about one-fifth of the milk required to reach basic nutritional standards.[91] Allende also reeled off a number of other problems: Chile had an alarmingly high maternal mortality rate and a very high incidence of illegitimate births, which he framed not as a moral condemnation of single mothers, but rather as a predictable result of Chile's fraying social fabric, marked also by alcoholism, prostitution, rampant venereal disease, and the world's highest tuberculosis mortality rates.

The thrust of Allende's political-economic analysis hinged on two concepts: human capital and imperialism. Allende wrote, "Human capital, which is the fundamental base of a nation's economic prosperity, has been underappreciated and the people have been left to fend for themselves. . . . Any government plan requires a numerous, healthy population, capable of production and of making industrial and economic development flourish. This is the mission of human capital."[92] While there are examples in Allende's early writing of ethical and human rights-based justifications for state action to address Chile's health problems, his main argument was economic: disease and poverty and lack of education worked together to weaken Chile's productive capacities. Put another way, Chile was not fully utilizing its economic potential because of a failure to "invest" in human capital. Such a notion of human capital was already well established in social medicine, as shown in the economistic analyses of Carlos Paz Soldán, René Sand, or Andrija Stampar, long before it became a keyword of late twentieth-century neoliberal doctrine.[93]

According to Peter Winn, Allende was not an "original Marxist thinker, nor did he claim to be."[94] But his understanding of human capital, and a Marxist turn in his thinking about social medicine, might possibly have emerged from, or been reinforced by, conversations with Peruvian socialist intellectuals—Apristas including Manuel Seoane and Luis Alberto Sánchez—in exile in Chile in the 1930s.[95] There are also interesting parallels between Allende and José Carlos Mariátegui, who died in 1930, in their approach to health, human capital, and national development. In 1923, Mariátegui had analyzed the role of "human capital" in Peru's development, and how poor health undermined the growth of this human capital. Reviewing a recently published treatise on the medical geography of Peru by two hygienists (Sebastián Lorente and Raúl Flores Córdova), Mariátegui remarked on the shocking "realidad médico-social del Perú"—a phrase echoed almost perfectly in the title of Allende's famous book. In the same essay, Mariátegui despaired over the problems highlighted by Lorente and Córdova—high infant mortality, infectious diseases, stagnant population growth—but criticized the hygienists' narrow vision: "The sanitary problem [of Peru] cannot be considered in isolation. It is connected to and mixed up with other deep Peruvian problems in the domain of the sociologist and the politician. The diseases, the morbidities of the Sierra and the Coast, are fed primarily by poverty and ignorance."[96] For Chile, Allende saw things much the same way and he adopted Mariátegui's Marxist vocabulary and analytical scheme, while never citing him explicitly.

To Allende, the degradation of Chile's human capital through poverty, overwork, malnutrition, and disease had its roots in the unequal exchange of goods of services in the international economy.[97] Chile's economy was highly dependent on a few natural resources, which encouraged the transfer of wealth abroad and its concentration in the hands of a few in Chile. In essence, Allende's analysis linked the workings of global capitalism directly to the bodies of the Chilean working class. Allende anticipated the Uruguayan Eduardo Galeano's famous work, *Open Veins of Latin America*, itself a classic in Latin American dependency theory. For both Allende and Galeano, the body is not just a metaphor; the bodies of workers are a physical, integral component of an economic system, their corporeal sacrifice a source of capital accumulation.[98] Here Allende borrowed from Lenin's interpretation of imperialism, as an advanced stage of capitalist development, although he does not specifically mention Lenin or any other Marxist thinkers by name in the text.

In comparison with his radical analysis of the political-economic origins of Chile's health crisis, Allende's view of gender roles was more conventional. Early in the book, Allende identifies the essential object of Chilean social reform, the *binomio madre y niño* or "mother-child unit" (or "dyad").[99] One of Allende's first acts as minister of health was to create the Departamento Central de la Madre y el Niño to coordinate maternal and child health efforts within the ministry and outside of it, including with the ministries of education and justice. Illanes, a historian generally sympathetic to Allende, judges this concern to be proportional to the scope of Chile's alarming maternal and child mortality problem at that moment, exacerbated by the fact that around 30 percent of children were illegitimate; not only were such children not covered legally by the benefits of the CSO, but also a sizable fraction of young mothers were left to fend for themselves, taking on the dual role of mother and worker.[100] The historian Karin Rosemblatt, however, has situated such efforts within a larger project of the FP to develop a populist politics of welfare state expansion predicated on the subjugation and disciplining of women, or at least the narrowing of their social roles. In its rhetoric and policy proposals, the Frente Popular confined women to the domestic sphere and aspired to build their capacities as mothers, ostensibly the defenders of the national race. Meanwhile, men were supposed to be given preferential treatment in the job market, a tactic supported by labor union activists; a man's role as a disciplined head of a nuclear family was incentivized by social security policies (through the Caja) while women were domesticated and educated through the visitadoras sociales (female social workers).[101] Such attitudes or ideologies preceded the Frente Popular, but the government of the Frente Popular transformed the way the state was expected to support these gender norms.

To conclude the book, Allende presented the government plan, titled the *Programa Médico-Social* or Socio-Medical Program. Much of this program was outside of the domain of public health. The FP government stressed policies to guarantee salaries sufficient to cover the rising cost of living; increase agricultural production and subsidize the production of milk in particular, to guarantee that the population meet minimum nutritional requirements; invest heavily in new government housing, to build thousands of hygienic homes for the working class; and institute rent control. These economic and social policy strategies were coupled with a call for centralizing the different elements of Chile's health system under one ministry to improve the efficiency and distribution of services. The FP government's rapid response to the January 1939 Chillán earthquake, with emergency powers to provide food, shelter, medicine, and other supplies consolidated under a single authority—*mando único*, as in a military campaign—only deepened Allende's commitment to the centralization and unification of services.[102]

Allende's health sector reform proposals largely went nowhere in the decade that followed, only to be revived in the face of mounting social crisis. During his tenure as minister of health, Allende's view of the social determinants of health harmonized with a government focused on elevating the health, safety, and dignity of ordinary Chileans, so he was able, for a time, to lead cross-sectoral efforts, for example, to improve the state of public housing or facilitate farmers' markets to lower the cost of fresh, nutritious food for urban consumers.[103] Yet the Frente Popular coalition was fragile and fell apart quickly after the untimely death of Aguirre Cerda from tuberculosis. Allende moved on to the Chilean senate in 1945, where he would occasionally spar with Cruz-Coke in debates over health and social policy. However, Allende's health policy reform proposal found little support; indeed, it has been described as merely gathering dust, tabled indefinitely.[104] The passage of two laws in 1948 and 1951 governing the medical profession paved the way for the unification of government health services. Fulfilling a long-standing desire of the AMECH, the association was dissolved into the Colegio Médico, the exclusive organization for licensing medical professionals and negotiating terms of employment with the state.[105] The Beveridge Report and the subsequent creation of the British National Health Service provided a new inspiration for reform. Benjamín Viel, one of Cruz-Coke's disciples and professor in the School of Public Health at the University of Chile, and Francisco Pinto, a legal expert and political scientist, offered up a plan for a Servicio Nacional de Salud (SNS) based on their fact-finding trip to Great Britain.[106]

And yet the law creating the SNS, which was enacted with a broad political consensus, satisfied only some of Allende's goals of centralization and rationalization of a convoluted and underfunded system. In the end, the new SNS did not offer universal coverage, nor did it preclude the growth of a parallel private system in the decades that followed. Meanwhile, the pension system, administered in the new Servicio de Seguro Social, maintained class-based inequalities, with salaried professionals and government employees gaining much more favorable retirement benefits than ordinary laborers.[107] Still, the new SNS internalized many of the contradictions of the old system, by creating the conditions for the design of unified health policy that encompassed sanitation and hygiene, infectious disease control, nutrition, improvements in maternal and child health, preventive care, and emergency services, under a single authority. Over the next few decades, Viel and his colleagues from the School of Public Health, such as Hernán Romero and Abraham Horwitz, would shape the SNS according to centrist values and technocratic logic: careful planning, budgeting, and emphasis on preventive services would gradually enhance the health and welfare of all Chileans.

Health Politics: Pluralism and Paradoxes

During this period of Chilean history, from the early 1920s to the early 1950s, *social medicine*, as an analytical lens or discursive formation, promoted a politics that led toward an increasingly robust (but far from perfect) system of *socialized medicine*—that is, a regime in which the state plays the central role in designing, managing, and financing the health sector.[108] However, while this movement was accelerated by leftist political figures, most notably Salvador Allende, it was not an exclusively socialist project. Early on, in a time of considerable political chaos and weak state health institutions, anarchists or libertarian socialists, such as Juan Gandulfo, questioned the necessity of the state and pushed to help the working class emancipate itself through grassroots consciousness-raising and health promotion. Progressive physicians, often channeling Gandulfo's rebellious energy, if not always his ideology, attempted to organize via the Sindicato de Médicos, the Vanguardia Médica, and the AMECH. Although characterized by internal ideological divisions, these groups ultimately prevailed in defending the economic interests of the medical profession and its privileged role in managing the transition away from a "liberal" model of medical practice toward a system of socialized medicine. But socialized medicine first found institutional form in the Caja del Seguro Obrero (and the other cajas) in the mid-1920s, well before Allende and the Vanguardia Médica. The CSO was perhaps a reaction to volatile labor agitation, but it was not really desired by organized labor, nor was it created through democratic mechanisms. Parallel to the well-known leftist current in social medicine, a group of relatively conservative doctors influenced by Catholic social doctrine, led by Eduardo Cruz-Coke, worked steadily to improve health conditions through such measures as the Law of Preventive Medicine and the establishment of the National Council on Nutrition.

The ideological diversity in Chilean social medicine helps explain why, when the legislation that would eventually create the SNS was introduced to the national Congress in 1950, deputies from almost every political party, whether Socialist, Radical, Traditional Conservative, or Falangist Conservative, stood up to

cite their own group's historic role in constructing the national health system.[109] All could claim, more or less legitimately, some role in developing and
improving the system. Despite often contentious disagreements, the parties
converged in granting priority to the development of human capital, social
justice, and the socialization of the health sector.

The Chilean case illustrates the old dictum, attributed to the political scientist Theodore Lowi, that "politics follows policy." One might imagine that
different groups offered health policy proposals that derived, logically and
consistently, from coherent political principles—in other words, a "socialist"
policy, a "conservative" policy, and so on. Instead, it makes more sense to
view social medicine as a fluid field of policy experiment, where participants
drew inspiration from a hodgepodge of internationally available health policy
options, and worked to adapt them to their subjective impressions of Chilean
realities. At the same time, existing policy structures, especially the CSO, imposed considerable inertia and shaped the scope of reform proposals. As Labra
has argued, "just as in other nations, the transformations of the Chilean health
system . . . were the combined product of the functioning of political democracy, of the institutional rules that framed the decision-making processes, of
external influences, of previous decisions, of internal contingencies, and a
complex pattern of negotiations and agreements. As a result, the agreements
achieved were always imperfect, due to the multiplicity of interests in play at
every juncture."[110]

All the while, the arena of health policy was dominated by a profession,
medicine, which built its own identity on the premise that their work existed
outside of—or above—conventional politics. This pretension that society
could be scientifically managed by a cadre of experts was not only tenable
within Chile's increasingly technocratic systems, but it also created a class of
professionals interested in sustaining imperfect institutional structures like
the CSO, and who were, with some noted exceptions, ill-equipped and disin-
clined to engage the political system to undertake substantive reforms.

Lastly, we can observe in Chile one of the great paradoxes of the politics of
social medicine, namely, that successful strengthening of the state's health institutions tends to narrow the expansive and integrative domain of social
medicine. Allende and his cohort saw disease and illness as the end result of a
web of causal factors, a fraying of the social fabric that lay mostly outside the
domain of medicine. This exercise in causal analysis took political doctors
beyond the space of the clinic—either in their mind's eye or in their daily
practices—into the slums, the conventillos, the rural shanties, and the northern mining towns. The creation of the SNS, while viewed as a successful

(though delayed) accomplishment of first-wave social medicine, also signified a retreat from this larger political scene. In the SNS, medical services would be apportioned in a more egalitarian fashion, to be sure, but the old spark of subversive and revolutionary possibilities in social medicine largely disappeared, supplanted by the apolitical analysis and technocratic routines of the postwar period.

CHAPTER FOUR

Fragmentation

The Politics of Health and the Welfare State in Argentina

In Chile, the Vanguardia Médica and the AMECH channeled the energy of progressive and left-wing doctors to enact, with time, a program of health reform based on social medicine. During this same period, there was no coherent epistemic community organized around the idea of social medicine in Argentina. Instead, there were, in a sense, micro-epistemes, where different visions of social medicine were laid out: the still-active realm of the higienistas continued to seek the extension of medical science into the regulation and control of social life; an overlapping community of eugenicists argued that biological control of the population was crucial to the building of a strong and vigorous nation; socialists used health inequalities to illustrate the injustices of an exploitative capitalist economy and make a push toward socialized systems of health care; and doctors' associations or unions sought to control the conditions of their incorporation into such socialized systems. These disparate, parallel conversations rarely coalesced into coherent reform proposals, in part due to prevailing political conditions in the 1930s, the so-called *década infame*, or infamous decade, marked by undemocratic and ineffective governments. For social medicine, an absence of democratic governing institutions, the lack of effective forums in the public arena, and the repression of anticapitalist political activity made it a challenge to channel dissent into policy.

This all changed with the rise to power of Juan Domingo Perón, starting in 1943. As many scholars have suggested, he not only placed public health at the center of a populist governing agenda but also created the political conditions that brought the relevant parties to the negotiating table. This relatively open political strategy made Argentina's modern welfare state possible and legitimate. Under the capable direction of Ramón Carrillo, the Ministry of Health was able to materialize many of the demands of social medicine, including a more powerful centralized agency for health, a hospital-building campaign to ameliorate interregional disparities in health conditions, investment in effective disease control campaigns, and more attention to "preventive medicine" to support healthy living for middle-class families. Beyond the health sector, Peronist politics tended to improve economic circumstances and address social medicine's concerns with hazardous workplace conditions, availability of affordable, high-quality housing, and improvements in nutritious diets. However, Perón was never able to resolve a central contradiction of welfare-state populism: how to extend health insurance and medical services to fully cover the whole population, while satisfying the demands of his key political base, public- and private-sector unions, demands that included the maintenance and multiplication of what came to be called *obras sociales*, independent health insurance funds. Thus, the classic Perón era set the structural conditions for what continue to be fragmented and "stratified" health and social security systems of highly uneven quality in Argentina.

This chapter traces the development of the social medicine milieu and its political consequences, from the 1920s through the "classic" Perón era from 1945 to 1955. This period of profound transformation of Argentine society has generated an immense historiography, which is impossible to summarize in its entirety and has provoked scholarly debates that are complicated by the lasting influence of polarized pro- and anti-Peronista camps.[1] Nevertheless, to simplify drastically, there are two schools of thought on the development of social policy in Argentina in the period leading to the Perón era, as recently summarized by the historians Carolina Biernat, Juan Manuel Cerdá, and Karina Ramacciotti. First, in the view of historians such as Juan Suriano, "social conflict drove the conformation of state and political institutions." Conflict was generative of change, and Perón did not eliminate competing interests, but sometimes inflamed them and then managed to bring them into balance within a corporatist governing strategy.[2] As Perón put it, "In politics first one needs domination, and then conciliation comes as a result of it."[3] Under Perón, labor interests, in particular, were channeled through the state, to the advantage of unions but generating conflict with other sectors. The other school of thought, embodied in the work of the historian Eduardo Zimmermann, maintains that Peronist social policy built on a line of reformist liberalism, wherein intellectuals advocated a scientific approach to managing national society, with increasingly technocratic modes of action—in other words, an extension of the hygiene movement and eugenics in their many guises (puericulture, social hygiene, occupational medicine, and so on).[4] This historiographic dichotomy implies distinctive modes of state action: a state whose main role is to negotiate conflict between groups, in contrast to a state that builds capacity for top-down expert management of social problems.

I would argue that both interpretations have some truth, and together they help explain the incomplete development of the Argentine welfare state and the lasting fragmentation of the health system. A move toward a universal health-care system was stymied, in large part, by other priorities within the Peronist governing regime. Specifically, trade unionists were temporarily empowered to secure amenities, such as health insurance for themselves and their comrades, which prevented a full socialization of medicine. Meanwhile, the unions and other sectors, such as women's organizations, chafed at the top-down agenda of national health ministers who wanted to extend the domain of scientific knowledge (especially biomedicine) into the realms of family, procreation, sexual conduct, nutrition, and food. Public health technocrats, steeped in ideas of social medicine, thought such interventions were necessary and right. However, they underestimated the resistance of newly empowered groups to such efforts, and more broadly, these vociferous sectors believed strongly in prioritizing other policy changes to deliver their vision of an economically just, productive, and dignified modern life. As militants in a struggle, a role that Peronism facilitated and depended on, they took ownership of the projects they cared about, building the welfare state, in a sense, from the ground up.[5] The medical profession, meanwhile, either offered active or passive resistance to many of the gestures toward centralization of health services of the Perón government.

This chapter begins with an analysis of the historical roots of Argentinean social medicine, which must begin with the hygiene movement. As discussed in chapter 1, hygienists believed that the social question could be solved with the tools of modern medicine and other rational sciences. They set a pattern for the top-down management of social problems by cadres of technical experts, which would be intrinsic to Peronist health policy as well. Next, I examine the variety of schools of thought in social medicine of the 1930s, including the influence of eugenics, leftist social reform, and preventive medicine. Special attention is given to Juan Lazarte, an anarchist doctor from the province of Santa Fe, who articulated a radical program of social medicine that would contrast sharply with what Perón and Carrillo envisioned. I then turn to an assessment of Peronist health and social policy changes, which delivered on many of the hopes of social medicine as it developed over the previous three decades. These successes, however, were undermined by internal contradictions in the politics of the Peronist welfare state.

Health, between the Public and the Private

A profound sense of health crisis in Chile motivated a large segment of the medical profession to engage in political action under the rubric of social medicine, with this movement intensifying in the 1930s. In Argentina, the situation was somewhat different, since the mobilization around a perceived health crisis came much earlier, with intensive (but inconsistent) state efforts to manage and improve public health. Some of Argentina's gains in public health during the early twentieth century were probably a by-product of economic development, but there was also a more purposeful effort to improve public health, embodied in a vigorous "hygiene movement," initially a response to disease epidemics starting around the 1870s. It is worth examining the hygiene movement and its history in some detail, because of its ambiguous relationship to social medicine. Hygienists often spoke of their work in terms of "social medicine," yet they usually defended the political-economic status quo, promoting moderate reforms to prevent upheavals that would undo the liberal (free-market) model that shaped Argentina's development. Many proponents of social medicine from diverse ideological backgrounds also embraced eugenics, which, in its conception of society as a biological superorganism, favored the use of scientific knowledge to solve social problems. As we will see, though, the many social medicine proposals of this era found little traction, due to prevailing political conditions, which would change somewhat abruptly with the rise of Perón in the early 1940s.

From around the 1870s until the 1920s, these hygienists and other "liberal reformers" not only offered their response to the "social question" but also helped shape the question itself. They perceived that a modernizing and rapidly urbanizing society was marked by dislocation, insecurity, and anomie, problems that could be recast as "social ills" that flourished in the dark and overcrowded ethnic enclaves of large cities and the remote hamlets of Argentina's vast countryside. Hygienists took it upon themselves to bring enlightenment and the conditions for healthy living to the benighted classes, in a paternalistic and technocratic fashion, sealed off as much as possible from the combative arena of Argentine politics.[6] No Latin American country invested more than Argentina in public health and sanitation, and at such an early stage.

Still, historical interpretations of the hygiene movement are divided; from one perspective, this was a golden age in which wise leaders managed scientific and technological progress for the benefit of society, investing in public goods, such as potable water, sewage treatment, parks, and hospitals, that were integral to a modern, clean, safe urbanism. On the other hand, hygiene has been portrayed as an elite project to exercise social control, maintaining social hierarchies based on race, class, gender, and region, that went hand in hand with other new positivist social sciences, from criminology to social psychology. Hygiene procedures at ports of entry were used as a tool of ethnic selection in a country being rapidly populated by immigrants.[7] Tuberculosis was one of the leading causes of death in Argentina during the early 1900s and a focal point of hygienists' efforts. Yet, as Diego Armus has shown, bacteriology, which promised a more "scientific" approach to controlling tuberculosis, did little to eradicate the moralizing discourses around the disease.[8] Meanwhile, in Northwest Argentina, the national government invested in malaria control to open new land to agricultural production through drainage and reclamation for mosquito control, and with the hope (mostly unrealized) that malaria-free zones would attract European immigrants to displace deficient local laborers.[9]

Overall, whatever their accomplishments, the hygienists supported the broader national development strategies and cultural perspective of the elite class to which most of them belonged. They were a well-connected group, developing a nexus of power between the Medical School at the University of Buenos Aires, the National Department of Hygiene (Departamento Nacional de Higiene, or DNH), other government agencies, the national Congress, and scientific and philanthropic organizations—which Julia Rodriguez calls "an alliance of state and science for the advancement of hygiene."[10] Men (and this milieu was predominantly male at the time) such as Gregorio Aráoz Alfaro, an ardent promoter of puericulture, hygiene, and eugenics were often prolific essayists, leaving a mark on Argentine intellectual life, and leaders in international hygiene networks. Before the era of mass electoral politics, they were often tapped for elected office at the provincial and national level. This network of hygienists was tight-knit, had a relatively narrow ideological range, and also controlled what counted as legitimate thinking in the realms of medicine, public health, and related areas of social policy.

The period of Radical Party dominance and expanded political rights from 1916 to 1930 did not bring significant changes in patterns of health or social spending. Under the leadership of Hipólito Yrigoyen, the Radicals brought about universal male suffrage and then capitalized on it electorally. However, Yrigoyen and his successor Marcelo T. de Alvear, also from the Radical Party, generally continued the export-oriented political-economic direction of previous administrations, partly due to the intransigence of conservatives in the national senate. Health policy experienced a similar sort of inertia. The well-connected network of hygienists continued to oversee matters at the DNH, and some Radical Party politicians promoted hygiene and social medicine. Among them, the most prolific was Leopoldo Bard, a physician who turned to politics and became a Radical Party loyalist, serving in the lower house of the national Congress from 1922 to 1930, representing the Buenos Aires district of Flores. He authored dozens of bills—few of which became law, due to conservative opposition—to regulate labor conditions and improve public health, including legislation on malaria, tuberculosis, and sexually transmitted disease, legalization of divorce, and women's suffrage.[11] (Bard made another consequential contribution to Argentine culture when, in 1901, at the age of seventeen, he cofounded River Plate, one of the country's most important soccer clubs.)

In the period of Radical Party dominance, social demands were typically satisfied not so much by scientific social policies like those that Bard presented, but rather by "a clientelistic logic" of what the historian Ricardo D. Salvatore calls the "creole politics" of the era—a combination of "partisan clientelism, nepotism, and republican rhetoric" that led to swelling national government payrolls.[12] In the eyes of Jeremy Adelman, Yrigoyen "treated legislation as a lower form of politics," compared to the efficiency and simplicity of clientelism.[13] The fracturing of the Radical Party in the mid-1920s into pro- and anti-Yrigoyen factions also shaped the administration of public health: Alvear took a stronger interest than Yrigoyen in health policy, and appointed Aráoz Alfaro to lead the DNH. The renewed energy of this period, which included budget increases and a cooperative agreement with the Rockefeller Foundation, was dashed with the return of Yrigoyen in 1929, who "purged the public administration of all Alvear sympathizers," compelled Aráoz Alfaro's resignation, stocked the DNH with political loyalists, and forced the withdrawal of the RF just when its work on malaria control in the Northwest was finally bearing fruit.[14]

During this time, how did Argentineans access and pay for medical care? Generally, those with sufficient means paid "out of pocket" for appointments with doctors in their offices, but the average person would receive care at public hospitals. This care was initially administered and funded by the Sociedades de Beneficencia, philanthropic organizations usually run by women from elite families, which received gradually greater subsidies from municipal, provincial, and national governments.[15] Thus, under the prevailing model of "liberal" medicine, patients and doctors were linked together either by cash exchange or bonds of charity. Under these circumstances, coordinated efforts in preventive medicine or health promotion were minimal, except for the efforts of the DNH or philanthropic initiatives such as the Gotas de Leche.

In the space between the private and public spheres in health care, the so-called mutualista movement galvanized collective action to provide greater livelihood security and protection from risk of illness—for some. Mutual-aid societies (mutualidades) were initially organized around ethnic immigrant communities, starting in the early nineteenth century. With the purchase of a membership and a small regular premium, members could insure themselves against unemployment or disability, and defray the costs of doctor visits, medications, hospital stays, and funerals. These societies were concentrated especially in major cities of the littoral region, inhabited by the Spanish, Italian, and French immigrant communities; the 1914 national census showed 1,202 different mutual-aid societies, with over 507,000 members, representing approximately 16 percent of the economically active population, with an even higher proportion among immigrants.[16] Into the 1920s and 1930s, the ranks of the mutualidades continued to swell, with membership increasingly linked to belonging in the same professional guild or labor union, although those based around ethnic/national groups persisted. The more successful societies developed their own networks of clinics, hospitals, and drugstores. Some of the most renowned private hospitals of Buenos Aires—the Hospital Suizo and Hospital Alemán, for example, in the city's affluent northern zone—are a legacy of these groups.[17]

The mutual-aid societies embodied the potential of an international "labor solidarity" movement that differentiated itself from socialism by resisting state intervention and control.[18] Nevertheless, these societies were beset by financial problems from the late 1910s onward. The proportion of spending on doctors' fees remained stable, but the cost of medicines, lab tests, X-rays, and other technologically intensive procedures rose precipitously. Some funds, like the railroad worker's retirement fund, were badly mismanaged to the point of insolvency.[19] The typical member of a mutual-aid society was also using more services, partly due to the rising capabilities of medicine, but also because of a change in culture. Earlier in the century, many had paid into their mutual-aid society in solidarity with the neediest members of their ethnic or national group, but members began to view medical care as an entitlement and sought care more frequently.[20] Some observers criticized the inefficiency of the mutualista system; for example, in the city of Buenos Aires, there might be a dozen mutualidades with clients and clinics in the same district, with totally uncoordinated services; likewise, other clients might have to travel miles across town to obtain service at their members-only clinic. Of course, for all their influence, the mutualidades only served a portion of the population, and most of the working poor did not benefit at all from them. Regardless, each of the mutualidades was protective of its own interests, and various attempts at forming a federation to coordinate these societies or placing them under state control were failures.[21]

Thus, by the 1930s, Argentina had a fragmented health system—really, no system to speak of—that excluded most of the population from reliable, quality care. Then again, in the international context of that era, the country had the healthiest population in Latin America (by measures such as life expectancy, and general and infant mortality). As was widely noted at the time, Buenos Aires, in particular, enjoyed better health conditions than many European capitals. In addition, the medical profession commanded considerable prestige, autonomy, and political power. The hygiene movement led by "liberal reformers" from Emilio Coni to Aráoz Alfaro demonstrated the possibilities and pitfalls of the scientific management of society. Perhaps, as Julia Rodriguez has argued, the hygienists led an elite project that tended to reinforce existing hierarchies in the nation's social structure. But many of their achievements were actually *infrastructural*, compelling a refashioning of urban environments— water, sewage, parks, hospitals, emergency services—that decisively diminished the threat of many infectious diseases and built health promotion into the urban fabric. To a large degree, the hygiene movement was also successful in stimulating a popular culture of healthy living, which only raised expectations for better medical practice and medical technology, for broader segments of the public.

The 1930s: Crisis and Critique

To understand the development of social medicine in Argentina, it makes sense to treat the 1930s as a period of multiple crises and rising discontent that led to the social and health policy transformations of the first Perón era. There was a notable rise in usage of the term "social medicine" in countless proposals and schemes. As Susana Belmartino explains, the medical profession of the 1930s perceived a severe crisis, even an existential crisis—*malestar*, a pervasive discontent or malaise. Doctors felt a declining sense of shared interests, as they were divided into different workplace sectors (public, private, mutualista) and challenged financially by the rising complexity of medicine.[22] At the same time, hygienists and other social reformers had not really resolved the so-called social question. Rather, signs of social decay, poverty, and inequality were everywhere. For medicine and public health, this was a period "with an abundance of inconclusive projects and unsatisfied social demands."[23]

In response to this sense of crisis, a new legitimizing discourse developed. Inspired in part by ideas from a reinvigorated eugenics movement, the medical community held itself up as the guardian of national fitness and strength, expressed in terms of racial improvement or growth of human capital, and as proponents of social justice.[24] Along a somewhat different track, the idea of preventive medicine gained influence, as more attention was paid to the chronic conditions of an aging population. The repression of democratic process during this so-called infamous decade did not seem to impinge on the production of social critique, although under these circumstances making progress on health policy was a challenge.[25]

Argentina's eugenics movement experienced a resurgence in the 1930s as it meshed with hygiene and social medicine. The "late eugenics" of this period in Argentina was intellectually eclectic but propelled mainly by activity in the Italian school of biotypology, which used biometric techniques to identify defective or dangerous social types. In 1933, a group of leading hygienists and other scientists, mostly affiliated with the DNH or the Facultad de Medicina in Buenos Aires, formed the Asociación Argentina de Biotipología, Eugenesia y Medicina Social (AABEMS). The fact that that eugenics and biotypology were grouped together with social medicine suggests that these fields had some common ground.

How much was Argentine social medicine influenced by this movement, whose mainstream reputation probably peaked in the 1930s? The Argentine eugenics episteme, which coalesced around the AABEMS, could be viewed as an offshoot of hygiene, since influential hygienists, such as Aráoz Alfaro or Nicolás Lozano, were avid participants in the association. One of the leaders of AABEMS, Gonzalo Bosch, made it clear that the group's work in social medicine, specifically, was a continuation of the "science of biotypology" crafted by the Italians Giovanni, Viola, and Pende.[26] From this perspective, the role of social medicine was to identify the defects and deficiencies of individuals as early as possible, then to correct or modify these tendencies to prevent further contamination of society or degeneration of the race. In their tendency to "biologize the social," the AABEMS group seldom examined the political-economic roots of poverty, because such an analysis did not fit with their model of how society was organized and functioned.[27] Quite different from the social medicine discourses of, say, the Vanguardia Médica group in Chile, undergirded implicitly by the dialectics of historical materialism, the AABEMS group viewed society as a superorganism where all conflict and criminality was aberrational and in need of control by rational scientific processes.

Thus, eugenics was an extreme manifestation of a common belief in the hygiene movement and social medicine that society could and should be managed by a cadre of scientific elites. The AABEMS group, by and large, was drawn from the existing elite sector of Argentine medical education and public health administration. They moved comfortably in international networks of like-minded professionals, exchanging ideas in conferences often attached to other health-related meetings—for example, the Pan American Sanitary Con-

ferences, the Pan American Red Cross, the IIPI, and Argentina's First Conference on Population, held in 1940.[28] They also formed numerous new spaces
in civil society to advance eugenics, not only the AABEMS but also the Liga
Argentina de Higiene Mental (headed by Bosch), the International Federation of Latin Eugenics Societies, and a polytechnic institute for Biotypology,
Eugenics, and Social Medicine in Buenos Aires.[29]

Yet, for all their recorded activity in these quasi-official spaces, very few of
their concrete initiatives to impose state controls on reproduction actually
became policy.[30] Within the eugenics community, there was strong concern
about the racist and militarist agenda of fascism, especially after the start of
World War II in September 1939. At the First Argentine Conference on Population, held in October 1940, attendees discussed various eugenic measures,
but the group ultimately made a declaration "to express its conviction in the
essential unity of the human species" and "to reject the racist doctrines of
blood and race . . . for being scientifically false."[31] Nevertheless, eugenics
would serve as the "ideological matrix" for Peronist health planning, rooted
in a new kind of biopolitics where an interventionist state could manage reproduction, child-rearing, nutrition, hygiene, and sanitation, to strengthen
the vitality and potential of an Argentinean national race.[32]

A small group of social reformers in the national parliament maintained
the agenda of the scientific-hygiene movement and intensified efforts to expose and regulate the social causes of Argentina's continuing health inequalities. One of the most widely recognized, vocal figures of this group was
Alfredo Palacios, arguably the most enthusiastic supporter of social medicine
of anyone outside of the medical profession. Remembered best as the first
Socialist Party member of the national Congress, Palacios served in this capacity in a long career, off and on, from 1904 to 1965.[33] One of his early legislative accomplishments was to draft the regulations for the new Department of
Labor, and he campaigned tirelessly for the rights and protection of the working class.

Though he served a constituency in the Boca district of Buenos Aires, Palacios made occasional, extensive tours of the Argentine interior, on fact-finding
missions that revealed the poverty and disease afflicting rural laborers. Building on the turn-of-the-century exposés of Juan Bialet Massé, Palacios took a
special interest in the Northwest and its public health problems, which he
detailed in books such as *El dolor argentino* (Argentina's Sorrow, 1938) and
Pueblos Desamparados (Forgotten Peoples, 1944).[34] Palacios's conception of
social medicine, articulated in such works, construed the nation as an organic
entity, debilitated by unjust working and living conditions that made it

vulnerable to the ravages of infectious disease and nutritional deficiencies.[35] As time went on, inspired by Latin American literary nationalists such as José Vasconcelos (Mexico) and Gabriela Mistral (Chile), Palacios used a rhetoric of the "degeneration of the race" to convey his almost mystical notions of the formation of the national race as an organic whole. Preventing such degeneration began with the protection of mothers and infants, similar to Allende's arguments in Chile around the same time, and a point of continuity that linked hygienists, social medicine, and Peronist health doctrine.[36]

By all accounts, Palacios did not form political alliances easily and his fierce defense of his political and intellectual independence might have worked against productive legislative action. Palacios was a leftist social reformer and ran on the Socialist Party ticket, yet he disavowed Marxism, mainly because of what he perceived as the limits it placed on individual conscience, consciousness, and action as motors of history.[37] He maintained loose ties to the Socialist Party hierarchy, and his charisma, more than his doctrine, carried him to electoral victories. He was a prolific writer with a great love of learning who also served in university administration; especially in the 1930s, with real limits on the capacity of the national Congress to act, Palacios made little headway in legislative terms but left a record of his policy positions: "During long sessions, Palacios would recite from his studies in the senate, which was transformed into his lecture hall."[38] The military junta sent Palacios into exile and he remained a political outcast during the Perón era, even as that administration took up and put into effect many of the public health projects Palacios had initiated.[39]

A rising group of scientific experts worked within the new paradigm of preventive medicine, which, as in Chile, tried to address the chronic health problems of a modern population. For example, Pedro Escudero emphasized maintaining health over the life course through the application of nutritional science. He founded the Municipal Institute of Nutrition in Buenos Aires, which became the National Institute of Nutrition in 1938 and a model for the study of biological and social aspects of nutrition in Latin America.[40] The institute served multiple, integrated roles as clinic, laboratory, social research center, school, and public-outreach center.[41] Under his supervision, the institute carried out well-organized, richly detailed surveys of the food spending and consumption habits of working and middle-class families in Buenos Aires and Mendoza.[42] Escudero repeatedly emphasized that the institute was concerned mainly with the "monitoring and protection of the healthy man," in other words, "researching the means to maintain health in the absence of all disease."[43] The work of the National Institute of Nutrition fit within the internationally rising emphasis on preventive medicine, the goal of which, according to Escudero himself, was "to maintain a vigorous and useful [state of] health, avoiding not only the diseases that originate with living agents or specific causes, but also those illnesses that appear due to the simple act of living."[44] The prolific Germinal Rodriguez, the chair of Hygiene and Social Medicine at the Medical School of the University of Buenos Aires, promoted the philosophy of preventive medicine in his academic and political endeavors.[45] (He was also a congressional representative from the Independent Socialist Party in the late 1920s and early 1930s, with an anticommunist and pro-union "guild socialism" stance that anticipated some aspects of Peronism.[46]) The work of Escudero, Rodriguez, and others marked a transition toward concern for maintaining the relatively good or standard health of increasingly affluent and stable middle-class populations.

By the early 1940s, then, pressure was building for a new national health policy and the ideological terms of Peronist health policy were largely in place. From all quarters of the medical profession and public health came clear frustration with the organization of health services and calls for their unification and coordination. The hygiene movement and then eugenics helped supply a biopolitical discourse of national economic power dependent on the health of its citizens. Social reformers like Bard and Palacios exposed the dire health conditions that existed outside of Buenos Aires and made the case for intensified state action to promote public health and provide needed medical care. Advocates of preventive medicine (like Germinal Rodriguez) and nutritional science (Enrique Pierangeli, a disciple of Pedro Escudero), were well-positioned to soon become key policy advisers in the Perón administration.[47] In retrospect, all the ingredients were in place for social medicine to transform health policy—expertise, ideologies, and policy proposals. But only Perón, it seems, was able to exercise the political will to realize these transformations.

Juan Lazarte: A Forgotten Voice in Social Medicine

Not everyone fit the trajectory of social medicine's development and culmination into Peronist health policy in the 1930s and 1940s. In this sense, Juan Lazarte, a doctor from Santa Fe province, stood out, both for his ideas and his vehicle of political action, gremialismo médico, the organizing of doctors into unions. While often categorized as an "anarchist doctor," Juan Lazarte's philosophy defied easy description. He was a prolific writer and polymath, immersed deeply in political theory and active in socialist and libertarian politics, forming various political groups, starting up periodicals and independent publishing houses, and creating an international network among anarchists, feminists, antifascists, and progressive physicians that stretched from Chile, Uruguay, and Brazil to Spain. As a union organizer, he helped form gremios at the local, provincial, and national levels, including leadership of the COMRA, the Confederación Médica de la República Argentina. From this position, for a time in the 1940s he became a protagonist at conferences and in other discussions of redesigning the Argentine health and social security systems. Lazarte stood opposed to increasing state control of the medical profession, and instead desired a health system managed by doctors collectively in a unified system without interference from the government. His views were too radical for Peronism, which was culturally conservative and dedicated to the expansion of state power for the benefit of the masses in a populist mode. Thus, he was increasingly a voice of opposition to Peronism and became thoroughly marginalized politically by the end of his career.

Lazarte studied medicine at the University of Córdoba, where, like many contemporary figures of social medicine, he became a student activist, leading the protests that ultimately resulted in the University Reforms of 1918.[48] The strikes that added pressure for the milestone reforms were a rare example of an alliance between students and industrial workers.[49] After finishing medical school, he settled in San Genaro, in the province of Santa Fe, not far from Rosario, the city where he had been raised in a middle-class family.

While known as an anarchist, perhaps the label of *librepensador*—a freethinker—is a better fit for Lazarte. His intellectual influences were varied, and included Georg F. Nicolai (a German physician and pacifist, who spent the second half of his life in Chile and Argentina, where he and Lazarte developed a close friendship during the 1930s), Lisandro de la Torre (a fellow *rosarino* and defender of Argentine federalism), and Carlo Rosselli (the Italian antifascist and theorist of "liberal socialism").[50] His idiosyncratic ideas, especially his penetrating analysis of unequal gender relations as the basis of social injustice, put him outside of the mainstream of social medicine thought in Argentina.[51] In his book *La revolución sexual de nuestro tiempo* (The Sexual Revolution of Our Time, 1932) and other writings, he proposed emancipating women from their traditional roles as wives, mothers, and caregivers, by disconnecting the reproductive function of sex from its pleasurable and sensual aspects. Accordingly, he fought against the "double standard" of sexual morality between men and women. This message apparently resonated with working-class men and women, who made the "scientific" sexual guide, *El matrimonio perfecto* (published by Claridad, a press with anarchist and libertarian leanings), a best seller.[52]

Compared to the hygienists, eugenicists, and social reformers who dominated Argentine social medicine, Lazarte presented a vision of a society that required a radical restructuring of interrelated institutional foundations of repression: not just the economy and the state but also sexual and gender relations, domestic life, and religion.[53] Sexual liberation and gender equality, Lazarte argued, would lead to the "liberation of great human forces, [now] hidden and imprisoned by centuries of Catholic capitalist slavery."[54] This perspective came from Lazarte's experience as a medical inspector in the regulated brothels of Rosario, and his engagement with an international network of libertarian socialists and anarcho-feminists advocating "conscious procreation."[55] In *Chile en la Vanguardia* (1936), he lauded the Chilean Vanguardia Médica, discussed in chapter 3, for its scientific and broadminded views on the abortion question.[56] Lazarte sometimes advocated eugenic controls on reproduction, but he could not reconcile a program of state eugenics with his "libertarian socialist" disposition.[57]

Perceiving a crisis in the "liberal" economic model of medicine, Lazarte gave voice to the "malestar" afflicting the Argentine medical profession in the 1930s. His incisive analysis of the structural problems of Argentina's health sector helped lay the groundwork for Peronist health reform proposals.[58] In medicine, Lazarte argued, the market was incapable of allocating resources in a way that would maximize collective welfare, a problem that derived from unique characteristics of economic relations in medicine. For starters, episodes of illness set the conditions for exchange: "The sick person is the individual who pays; the doctor is the individual who charges. This union is established by illness."[59] From this condition flowed two problems: uneven capability to pay and the neglect of prevention. As Lazarte figured it, about 40 percent of the Argentine population had no capacity to pay for medical care, so they depended on public hospitals or the goodwill of private doctors; some 30 percent had "limited" capacity to purchase doctors' services; and around 30 percent, known as "enfermos pudientes," were capable of paying for care. Doctors competed, in essence, for this small sliver of the public, which drove down their own salaries and left them barely able to maintain middle-class status.

The free-market model of medicine also created a geographical imbalance, with shortages of care in some places and an abundance of doctors in others. According to Lazarte's analysis, the city and province of Buenos Aires, with about 46 percent of the national population, had around 62 percent of the nation's doctors; in the national capital, there were 625 inhabitants per doctor, while in the province of Santiago del Estero, one of the nation's poorest, the ratio was 5,569 people per physician.[60] In rural areas, and especially in the northern provinces, "sick people die without medical assistance. Doctors can't live there, not for a lack of sick people, but because the capacity to pay when one needs a doctor does not exist."[61] He continued: "In capitalist terms, these towns cannot maintain a doctor. . . . Unemployment of doctors is due to a poor organization of the profession, better said, a disorganization."[62]

Lazarte drew on the example of Chile's caja system to demonstrate what a rational distribution of medical personnel would look like. When he was writing in the early 1940s, the city of Rosario had approximately 420 physicians, out of a population of 550,000. If, he argued, Rosario had a system similar to the Chilean cajas, only about 100 doctors would be necessary.[63] To his mind, comprehensive social insurance schemes could foster an equilibrium between supply and demand, mainly by removing competition between medical providers. Rosario (for example) had so many doctors because they were essentially chasing the small fraction of clients who could pay and were likely to be concentrated in a densely populated (and, in those days, relatively affluent) city.

These evaluations of the failure of liberal medicine and the recognition of rising needs for more collaborative or collective efforts were part of Lazarte's labor activism, or gremialismo. With his founding of the Federación Médica de Santa Fe in 1933 and his long-term involvement with COMRA (from its founding in 1941 to his death in 1963), Lazarte sought to organize doctors into unions for their own betterment and the good of society.[64] He worried about the exploitation of doctors' labor and their reduction to cogs in a bureaucratic machine. Lazarte saw a stark choice: doctors faced either their "proletarianization" in a free-market model or their relegation to "functionaries" without control of their own practice in a government-managed system.[65] Unionization, then, was the only way for doctors to maintain individual conscience of practice, professional autonomy, control over working conditions collectively, and bargaining power over mutual-aid societies, government agencies, and hospitals. Moreover, since doctors were guided by science and professional ethics, they were the only legitimate agents to direct the socialized systems of care that were on the horizon. Lazarte's visit to Chile in 1936, where he engaged with activist doctors in the Vanguardia Médica and the AMECH, reinforced his convictions that gremialismo was the only true path to a health system that was fair to patients and doctors alike, and with the modern organization that could comprehensively address population health problems.[66]

Lazarte was always skeptical about the state's role in a system of socialized medicine. In keeping with his advocacy of a strong federalism—a concern that would increasingly occupy his thoughts and writing—he advocated for decentralized medical associations directed by doctors to design health systems appropriate for local circumstances, while the national state would be charged with financing the whole system.[67] Lazarte's resistance to state management of the health sector, however, would prove to be out of step with the times globally, where various manifestations of statism were on the rise. As I discuss further on, Lazarte's view of social medicine would prove too radical for the Perón era, not only for its resistance to state control but also in its revolutionary gender politics. Toward the end of his career, after the overthrow of Perón, in 1956 he was appointed to teach political-economic and sociological theory at the Universidad del Litoral in Rosario; he died in San Genaro in 1963.[68]

Peronism: Health and Populist Politics

Led by the minister of health, Ramón Carrillo, Peronist health reforms were a sort of culmination of discussions within the social medicine milieu. The social medicine proposals of the 1920s through the early 1940s had few channels available to convert ideas into policy, given the indifference of national leaders to public health problems and, particularly in the later part of this period, hostility to addressing working-class demands through open democratic channels. During the "classic" Perón era (1945–55), the government's health institutions were strengthened considerably, with an elevation in administrative status as the old DNH was transformed, after a series of changes, into a full-fledged Ministry of Health. With large budgets and an impressive expansion in personnel, it managed to make noteworthy strides in projects like hospital building and disease control. More broadly, Perón's populism broke through political logjams by constructing an "illiberal" democracy—a fusion of conservative, authoritarian, and nationalist tendencies, pulled back from the brink of fascism through the sanctioning power of electoral democracy and a quasi-religious relationship between the leader and his subjects.[69] The governing philosophy of "social justice" meant that the state should be the guarantor of economic and social equality; certain "social rights" could be enumerated and made effective through state action, including the rights to education, health, employment, and even to certain goods (housing, clothing, domestic items) that were seen as indispensable to dignified modern living. Ultimately, the sweeping social changes wrought by Peronism, by reducing poverty and deprivation, may have done as much to improve health as any specific interventions in the health sector.

The architect of a new Peronist health policy was Ramón Carrillo, a neurosurgeon with little experience in public health before 1946. It is important to note that Carrillo hailed from the interior province of Santiago del Estero. From an early age, mixing ideas from eugenics and an organicist conservative nationalism, Carrillo proposed that the criollo stock of his native Northwest embodied the essential national racial type, whose full potential could only be realized by resolving issues of poverty and disease in Argentina's interior.[70] Carrillo participated in the 1940 National Conference on Population, which confronted the problem of Argentina's ostensibly diminishing birth rate as a sign of declining national vigor.[71] Carrillo first met Perón in 1943, when he was working in the central military hospital of Buenos Aires; that same year, Carrillo began rising through the administrative ranks of the Facultad de Medicina at the University of Buenos Aires. According to Ramacciotti, Carrillo took advantage of the deep ideological polarization that affected the university, remaining loyal to Perón as scores of faculty resigned (or were forced out) due to their opposition to the government's heavy-handed interventions in academic institutions.[72] In this conflict-ridden atmosphere, many prominent hygienists and medical scientists viewed Carrillo as an interloper. One of Carrillo's main detractors, the Nobel Prize–winning physiologist Bernardo Houssay, viewed the kind of social medicine promoted by Carrillo (and Perón) as a vulgarization of the "pure" biomedical science he was advancing in Argentina.[73]

Recognizing his loyalty and intrigued by his comprehensive plans for a new health policy, as president, Perón put Carrillo in charge of the Secretariat of Public Health in 1946 (which became a full-fledged ministry by 1949). Upon assuming this role, Carrillo offered a bold vision for improving population health, based on his own coherent philosophy of social medicine, a doctrine that he articulated in speeches, radio lectures, articles, and books. In a May 1948 speech to a national conference on Hygiene and Social Medicine, Carrillo "posed the principal problem in social medicine of our time": how to take the advances in medical science and technology, which had enabled the incremental extension of the human life span, to make it possible for everyone to enjoy a life of "physical, mental, and social well-being—that is, health."[74] Here, Carrillo obviously echoed the definition of health articulated in the constitution of the new World Health Organization, which had been enacted only the month before. Carrillo explained that a "positive concept of developing health" was supplanting "the negative conception of hygiene of yesteryear, with a view towards avoiding illness" and that "today all of the sanitary expertise of the State—now that the basic stage of attending to the sick had been mastered—should be concentrated on . . . the healthy man."[75] The chronic health problems of modern life—stress, heart problems, diabetes, and mental anguish—called for a strategy based in preventive medicine, which in turn required a strong state active in the promotion of healthy conditions throughout the life course, action that extended beyond the limited realm of conventional medicine.

Concretely, as secretary and then minister of health, Carrillo pursued a few major objectives, mostly in harmony with the broader Peronist agenda of social and economic justice: the centralization of government health administration, a major expansion of public hospitals and clinics, the implementation of a social security program that covered medical services, and massive campaigns to control or eliminate infectious diseases. Centralizing authority over health policy had long been an ambition of hygienists. Carrillo sought central control (*comando único*) over the whole national system for reasons of status (public health was important enough to merit its own ministry, rather than being managed from a department within the large Ministry of Interior), professional authority (ministry-level status would presumably lead to management by trained scientists, rather than political appointees), efficiency (consolidating institutions that duplicated effort or required better coordination), and equity (coordinated national policy would create more consistent norms, practices, and resources for health across the country).[76] Under Carrillo, the staff of the national health agency went from approximately 8,500 to 22,400 employees between 1946 and 1947, and stayed around that level into the early 1950s.[77] Almost all the divisional directors within the ministry had medical degrees from the University of Buenos Aires or University of La Plata. And with very few exceptions, they were men. As discussed further below, women were important participants in Peronist politics, and they resisted some of the more paternalistic efforts of the new health ministry, from which they were largely excluded.[78]

Carrillo also launched an ambitious hospital-building campaign. In 1948, he calculated that Argentina as a whole had fewer than half the hospital beds it required to effectively serve the public (based on the benchmark goal of having at least one hospital bed per hundred inhabitants). There was also wide variation between provinces: the aforementioned Santiago del Estero had only about one bed per thousand residents.[79] To remedy this gap in hospital services, Carrillo successfully lobbied to have the government agency in charge of hospital architecture moved from the Ministry of Public Works, where it had long resided, to the Ministry of Health.[80] Carrillo aspired to do more than just build capacity, as he also envisioned hospitals as the key nodes of a coordinated network of health care. Unlike the model of "primary health care" that would appear a few decades later, Carrillo's plan defined the hospital as the point of first encounter with a health system that offered comprehensive and diverse services (polyclinics) to promote preventive health practices.[81]

The Ministry of Health also intensified efforts to control infectious diseases. Perón enthusiastically made large sums of money available for these campaigns, but their success also depended on the infusion of new technology and the imposition of technocratic administrative practices, somewhat dissociated from a more integrative "social medicine" approach. The rapid decline of tuberculosis in Argentina during the early 1950s, for instance, depended on a more thorough medicalization of the problem. In the past, tuberculosis had been a social disease understood in a moralistic framework, but the postwar approach to tuberculosis reduced both cause and cure to biomedical terms. The availability of cheap and effective antibiotics in this period served as the technological catalyst for the dramatic reduction in tuberculosis, and the Ministry of Health committed to making the new medicine available to the whole public.[82]

The campaign against malaria in northern Argentina also distanced public health work from the framework of social medicine. Initially, the massive *Analytical Plan*—prepared in 1946 and released to the public in 1947 as the Health Secretariat's blueprint for public health policy— offered an integrative strategy for malaria control that involved cross-sectoral work. By the middle of 1947, though, Carlos Alberto Alvarado, the director of the government malaria service, was convinced that the plan should be radically overhauled, in favor of a rapid, massive campaign that hinged on house spraying with DDT. Carrillo and Perón enthusiastically supported this shift in strategy and offered unprecedented financial resources to support it. The near eradication of malaria in Argentina proved to be one of the most enduring symbols of the success of Peronist health planning, serving as fodder for government propaganda and becoming an achievement that even Perón's political opponents could approve of.[83] But it required no broader changes in political-economic structures or a concerted attack on poverty, quite unlike an integrative "social medicine" approach.

Still, the malaria campaign, like the hospital construction program, demonstrated the commitment of the Ministry of Health to deliver the highest quality care and the most current medical technology to the whole country.

With these programs, Carrillo looked to overcome what he termed a long-standing "health and demographic disequilibrium in the Republic," which had been a constant refrain of hygiene and social medicine.[84] Although much of the work of the Ministry of Health was still concentrated in and around Buenos Aires, under Carrillo's leadership there was a concerted effort to level health conditions across the country.

Even as Carrillo presided over the impressive growth of the Ministry of Health (in budget, personnel, technical capacity, and prestige), he sent mixed signals about how much the government needed to control and centralize all health services. Inspired by the Beveridge Report (and the subsequent creation of the National Health Service in Great Britain in 1948), at times Carrillo aspired to "turn doctors into functionaries" of a comprehensive national health system, which would also absorb the functions of hospitals that had been run by the Sociedades de Beneficencia with state subsidies, or by private, provincial, municipal, and mutualista entities.[85] Carrillo also recognized, through engagement with the medical community in venues such as the 1948 conference on Hygiene and Social Medicine (where an outspoken Lazarte made the most of what would be his last formal opportunity to influence Peron's health policy) that it would be difficult, if not impossible, to compel the nation's doctors to support their reduction to mere "functionaries" in a vast government system.[86] Thus, early on, the Perón administration staked out a compromise position: "It would advisable to *semi-socialize* medicine, respecting the free exercise of the profession and the free selection of a doctor by patients," with those capable of paying (*las clases pudientes*) continuing to engage in a system of private health care, and the government taking on a greater role in provisioning services for the poor.[87] Carrillo also insisted that social security and government health services should be managed by distinct agencies, even though they needed to work in harmony to provide full and efficient medical insurance coverage to the whole population. Confronting the limits of Peronist state power, Carrillo settled on a principle of "regulatory centralization and administrative decentralization," in other words, a national ministry with the expertise and capacity to plan initiatives that would be executed by provinces and municipalities, which was not so distant from Lazarte's "federalist" stance.[88]

Carrillo's invocation of the WHO charter demonstrates another important shift that occurred under Peronism: the use of a language of rights, especially "social rights," to redefine and expand the state's obligation to its citizens. The assertion of "social rights" could be seen as a late stage in the evolution of citizenship in Argentina, from guarantees of civil rights in the 1853 constitution, to the expansion of political rights with the Ley de Saenz Peña in 1912, culminating in the development of social (or "positive") rights under Peronism.[89] The 1949 constitution articulated an explicit right to health, along with other kinds of social rights that served the cause of public health.[90] Perón's opponents argued that he believed that social rights trumped political rights; populist autocracy could guarantee social rights while eschewing the political rights endowed by a liberal democratic model.[91] In other words, repressive means (such as silencing political dissent by purging universities of voices against Peronism) could justify the end of increasing social justice, and it was this kind of repression that frustrated leftist-libertarian voices like Palacios and Lazarte, or advocates of academic freedom like Houssay.

Overall, there is little doubt that the Perón government, at least in its early years, "was characterized by a notable economic redistribution in favor of the popular classes, measured as much in salary levels as in social services that offered a wide range of benefits. It was not only about material benefits; that phenomenon was accompanied by a decline in the deference that the underclass showed the higher echelons of society."[92] Carrillo believed that Perón's broader commitment to ensuring social welfare was "the cornerstone of an Argentine socio-medical policy."[93] Even as Perón significantly expanded the scope of state action to promote a new suite of social rights, according to Jonathan Hagood, "the Peronist state was willing to cede social rights and responsibilities to autonomous social groups.... While the rhetoric and policies of Peronism reframed citizenship and membership in Argentine society as a bundle of political, social, and economic rights, Peronism nevertheless frequently withheld or toned down state involvement in addressing some of the features of this newly-conceived vision of citizenship."[94] This is important, since Carrillo's plans for consolidation of state control over hospitals or health insurance would face opposition from labor unions, women's groups, and other autonomous groups newly empowered under Perón to articulate and defend a broad suite of social rights.

Contradictions of the Peronist Welfare State

The year 1949 was perhaps a high point in the expanding effort of the Argentine state to put the ideas of social medicine into practice. Perón's own power was peaking, new constitutional reforms established a right to health, and Carrillo assumed leadership of the new Ministry of Health, undertaking energetic interventions into public health, including the hospital-building program and the campaigns against infectious diseases such as malaria. In the years that followed, however, Carrillo's position would deteriorate and the most ambitious plans for a unified national health system would be abandoned, undone by internal rivalries within the government and the social policy contradictions of Peronism, even before the decisive disintegration of Perón's government in 1955. Managing the economy to satisfy the interest groups that composed the corporatist structure of Peronism took increasing precedence over social policy, particularly as the government faced real fiscal limits as a consequence of inflationary pressures.[95] However, in its basic contours, Argentina's modern welfare state would last for decades, producing the kind of broad-based improvement in well-being that social medicine advocates had long pursued.

Internal rivalries within the Perón administration and competing factions in the Peronist political base undermined the full development of a powerful, centralized public health agency. The strongest competing institution was the Eva Perón Foundation, created in 1948 as a means of channeling the largesse of the state more directly to those in need. Famously, Eva Perón herself would respond to letters, especially from children, with toys and other gifts, often in ceremonies broadcast on radio or filmed for newsreels. Such acts of charity were a visible expression of Perón's populist governing strategy, and before long the foundation grew quite large and began to take on some of the same functions as the Ministry of Health. The Tren Sanitario (Health Train) traveled across the country in 1951 to serve many of the same "abandoned" communities that Alfredo Palacios or Bialet Massé had surveyed before, delivering much-needed vaccines, life-saving medications, and dental care.[96] The foundation also began funding the construction of new clinics and hospitals, originally focused on pediatric care but soon encompassing large, comprehensive facilities in Buenos Aires and the interior.

Initially, the foundation and the Ministry of Health worked collaboratively and their efforts were complementary, but before long the two institutions were in direct competition for fiscal resources. In the foundation's first year, 1948, its budget was about one-tenth that of the Ministry of Health and all its resources came from private donations; by its fourth year, 1951, the foundation's budget was more than double that of the ministry.[97] Moreover, much of the expansion of the foundation came at the direct expense of the ministry: in particular, income from lotteries, casinos, and racetracks, originally earmarked for the ministry, was gradually transferred to the foundation, and labor unions—which Perón had empowered and taken under the wing of the state—also contributed a large share of the foundation's budget through an assigned portion of their membership dues. With the foundation sapping its resources in the midst of a more generalized fiscal crisis after 1951, the ministry lowered its horizons, significantly curtailing the hospital-building campaign and delaying the expropriation of hospitals managed by the Sociedades de Beneficencia and private entities.

Conflicting priorities in social policy from within the Peronist coalition were also apparent in the realm of food and nutrition policy, which had long been a contentious space in social medicine. During the interwar period, Latin American governments and the Geneva institutions began taking an interest in the problem of malnutrition.[98] Views on the causes of malnutrition were divided: many health experts focused on the nutrient content of food and how to guide the public toward more scientific diets, while organized labor emphasized the political-economic causes of malnutrition, essentially framing it as a problem of low salaries and inadequate protections for workers' rights. In the early 1950s, Carrillo directed the ministry to focus more on food and nutrition issues. Inspired by the work of Escudero's National Nutrition Institute and the findings of international conferences on nutrition, the ministry tried to promote "scientific" dietary habits and increase the direct intervention of the state in this area, notably in school meal programs. Such proposals prompted a negative reaction from the Unión de Mujeres Argentinas, a Peronist women's group, which felt that such policies undermined their social role as the head of the family and the value of their knowledge about food and diet. Organized labor argued that economic policies for higher salaries, price controls on food, and accessible domestic durable goods (e.g., refrigerators and stoves) were the key to improving diets. In this light, a right to health was all well and good, but it also competed with other equally important social and economic rights that Peronist politics sought to safeguard.[99] In reality, the Argentine public was eating better—for example, with a significant rise in meat consumption due to a growing internal market of middle-class consumers, whom Peronism had empowered to vociferously defend such gains in the political arena.[100]

The defense of expanding middle-class privileges also helps explain the noted long-term persistence of a fractured and stratified health-care system in Argentina, despite the Peronist regime's capacity to construct a more centralized system.[101] While there were many obstacles to a unified national health system, a principal impediment came from a countervailing force within Perón's corporatist political regime, powerful labor unions, which had been organized under the wing of the state in the Confederación General del Trabajo. As unions gained strength, and to reward their political loyalty, Perón took his cue from the existing institution of mutualidades to develop what would come to be known as the obras sociales, health insurance plans for union members and their families. These organizations not only provided health insurance but also might offer members access to home loans, cooperative retail outlets, and sporting clubs. The largest unions with the best-paid workers were even able to invest in hotels and resorts in vacation destinations like Mar del Plata, the Sierras de Córdoba, and Termas del Río Hondo. In 1954, the railroad workers' union built the Hospital Ferroviario, then one of the nation's largest, most modern facilities, and an enduring symbol of the golden era of labor power in the Peronist welfare state (it has been closed since 1999).[102]

Not surprisingly, workers who belonged to the obras sociales preferred their own members-only hospitals and clinics over the public hospitals. According to the historian Hugo Arce, who has studied the development of the obras sociales, unionized workers "felt like—in reality, they were—owners of those services, and this established a social phenomenon that went beyond the rationality of health planning."[103] In other words, a shift toward the use of obras sociales for health insurance and medical services occurred completely outside the purview of the Ministry of Health. Arce contends that Perón encouraged these efforts, not only due to the logic of political patronage, but also because a sense of exclusivity and belonging helped promote worker solidarity. This feeling of belonging—to a discrete community with common interests and a shared social position, but not to society at large—helps explain why the obras sociales became consolidated, permanent features of Argentine life.[104] The Peronist state (and its successors) "offered very heterogeneous social benefits to different occupational groups, depending on their powers of negotiation or proximity to the government," and left out domestic workers, rural laborers, and others in the informal economy (which was small during the 1940s and 1950s, in comparison to today).[105] Still, by 1980 approximately 45 percent of people in Argentina were insured through obras sociales, and another 8 percent through what remained of the older mutualidades.[106] The tendency of populist politics to create strong social ties within groups (of co-ethnics, or members of the same guild or labor union) led to the "fragmented" welfare state created under Perón that persisted, in its essential details, for decades.[107]

The forces of fragmentation under Perón were diverse. A variety of "pressure groups—unions, medical associations, private enterprises, etc.—reinforced their spaces of power and managed to keep the health system segmented, against the health reform project launched by Carrillo in 1947, which sought, in some way, to move towards a model of integrated medical services."[108] The physicians' unions resisted such reforms; Lazarte, who was originally included in negotiations on social security legislation, became vocal in opposition to state control of the health sector.[109] For the most part, though, the medical profession passively resisted its integration into the Peronist state. Lazarte's COMRA purposely distanced itself from Perón's government, and a series of medical unions sponsored by the Peronist government, intended to pull health workers into the regime's corporatist structure, failed to gain support from the medical community.[110] And, as much as Carrillo and other *sanitaristas* longed for the end of "liberal medicine" and its framing of health care as a commodity to be obtained in a market, such a move ran against the grain of another tendency of Peronism, most fully fleshed out by Eduardo Elena in his book *Dignifying Argentina*, which was to encourage a new kind of consumerist democracy, enabling the working class to acquire middle-class goods and living standards.[111] From this perspective, services provided by the obras sociales were akin to positional goods—markers of social differentiation or social status—that inhibited a sense of broad social solidarity that could provide the ideological base for universal health systems. The unions and their obras sociales typify what Carmelo Mesa-Lago called the "labor aristocracy," one segment with special privileges in a stratified Latin American welfare state model.[112]

In this manner, Carrillo's most ambitious plans were dashed and he lost legitimacy within the administration, being forced out by rivals in 1954 (and by 1956, he would be dead). Ramacciotti suggests that Carrillo's downfall resulted not just from such internal political conflicts, but also because of important philosophical differences, an issue that offers additional insight into the contradictions of social medicine. Carrillo advanced a vision of a society managed by technical experts, who were mainly, if not exclusively, male medical doctors. Public health was the paramount priority because disease and sickness undermined the formation of national human capital, but other centers of power in the Peronist regime, from the Eva Perón Foundation to the confederation of labor unions to women's groups, made different kinds of demands upon the state, in a quest for social and economic justice. Floreal Ferrara, an avid Peronist who started a long career in public health in the 1950s, later commented that Carrillo paid little attention to the need for public participation in the health sector; in contrast, labor unions channeled their advocacy with passion into their own health projects, and Ferrara cited the Hospital Ferroviario, again, as a prime example of this insularity.[113]

Perón was ousted from power in September 1955, in the so-called Revolución Libertadora. As a result, Perón's party was outlawed for the next eighteen years, and many members of his government were sent into exile or marginalized from public life. The new military government dismantled or abandoned many of the Ministry of Health's initiatives, and control of the national public hospitals was devolved to the provinces. At the same time, there was considerable inertia in the system that Perón and Carrillo had helped to establish. As Susana Belmartino puts it, from 1943 to 1955, the Perón government had taken existing fragmented and heterogeneous conditions of health-care provision and effectively institutionalized such conditions within the "interior of agencies of the state."[114] Organized labor, for example, managed to maintain its political power within the corporatist structure of the state, and the obras sociales continued to rise in prominence in the 1950s and 1960s (in fact, the official designation of "obras sociales" as a legal category came about in 1956, under the military government that had supplanted Perón).[115] The COMRA, now decidedly anti-Peronist, regained prominence in the late 1950s, defending the autonomy of the medical profession from the state and continuing to resist the occasional gestures to construct a unified, centralized health system.[116]

The Limits of Social Medicine

"Perón and Carrillo made social medicine into a policy of the state," according to Jorge Rachid, a public health doctor (and devoted Peronist).[117] Clearly, Perón and, especially, Carrillo managed to take ideas from social medicine and transform the conduct of health policy in Argentina, but as just one important element in the construction of a modern welfare state. Many of the health sector reforms enacted during the Perón administration, such as the transformation of the DNH into a Ministry of Health, had a long legislative pedigree. Previous efforts had failed because of the inability of people like Alfredo Palacios or Leopoldo Bard to make law in a vexing and conservative political structure. Peronism opened up and accelerated the political process considerably, even as anti-Peronist voices were sidelined. The Perón administration prioritized health policy, presented a coherent health doctrine, centralized (to some extent) the management of the national health system, and undertook successful campaigns to control infectious disease and build public hospitals, thus ameliorating some of the extreme geographical inequalities in health conditions between the city and the country and between the littoral region and the interior. Under Carrillo, social medicine became preventive medicine, intended to serve the needs of a usually health population over the life course, mirroring the analyses of Germinal Rodriguez and Pedro Escudero in Argentina, Eduardo Cruz-Coke in Chile, and René Sand in Belgium.

With a concept of a right to health within a suite of social rights, Peronism also fostered the expectation that the state would guarantee and strive to improve access to health care for the whole population.

Inevitably, the health policy reforms developed under the Perón government must be judged as a mixed success. Carrillo and his capable public health administrators were able to institute their own concept of social medicine, bringing some equity to the provisioning of health care across the country. Framed within a doctrine of "social justice" and reflecting international postwar trends, Peronism also made it possible to think about the protection and maintenance of health as one of many social rights that the state would guarantee. In Argentina today, it is well established that all citizens have a right to health care and that the state must play a role in provisioning medical services for those unable to pay. Then again, there is also little doubt that the public subsystem has been chronically mismanaged and underfunded, leading to second-class standards of care. The persistence of a fragmented and stratified system that does not serve the whole public well is also a legacy of the Perón era. As discussed, internal rivalries and conflicting priorities— including "the fragility of the alliance between doctors and politicians"— limited a comprehensive redesign of Argentina's health system.[118]

But this mixed outcome also demonstrates three political limitations of social medicine itself, at least as it was constituted in the mid-twentieth century. First, social medicine, for all its concern for the well-being of the poor and marginalized, continued the paternalistic, top-down management approach of an earlier generation of state scientist-bureaucrats, hygienists, and eugenicists. Carrillo's vision of society managed by a corps of technical experts clashed with the participatory modes of political action that Peronism also helped foster. Second, and relatedly, these sorts of democratic openings under Peronism helped build solidarity within interest groups that did not translate into a spirit of national solidarity that would enable a broad consensus for constructing state institutions that offer universal benefits in health care, social security, and other welfare-state goods. It is little wonder that labor unions' sacrifices—the hard work of organizing, protesting, filing grievances, going out on strike—would produce a sense of ownership of institutions like the obras sociales or the Hospital Ferroviario, and a defense of these hard-won privileges. As Hagood argues, "The true legacy of Perón's vision of Argentine citizenship was its articulation as membership in an autonomous social group—either ethnically-, labor-, or municipally-based—rather than citizenship in a social welfare state where such services are delivered by an autonomous nation-state itself."[119]

Lastly, this same tension between centrifugal and centripetal forces in social organization applies to the medical profession, which emerged from the first Peronist experience with renewed skepticism of centralization and a stronger sense of its power as an autonomous political force. While the first gestures in Argentina toward unionizing physicians—the Federación Médica de Santa Fe, which set the stage for the COMRA—came from an anarchist doctor, Juan Lazarte, by the end of the 1950s, gremialismo became a conservative force. But there is more continuity in the ideological orientation of gremialismo than might appear at first glance. As Lazarte conceived it, an organization like COMRA had to defend the rights of its members to fair salaries and working conditions, but also its autonomy from the state. Peronism challenged that autonomy, with the creation of what doctors perceived as sham medical unions inside of the corporatist structure of the state; and although there were many doctors who aligned with Peronism, the politicization of medical school faculties under Perón also soured a lot of doctors on the regime. Post-Perón, the defense of professional autonomy became the sine qua non of COMRA while its sociomedical agenda faded—one dimension of the decades-long hiatus in Latin American social medicine explored in the next chapter.

CHAPTER FIVE

Hiatus

Modernization and the Fading of Social Medicine in the Early Cold War

In 1952, the Rockefeller Foundation sent Johannes M. Bauer to conduct a survey of medical education in South America. In Peru, Bauer found the work of the Institute of Social Medicine, led by Carlos Paz Soldán, to be far from satisfactory. As the historian Marcos Cueto has recounted, Bauer saw little value in Paz Soldán's eclectic and holistic approach to medicine. He wrote caustically that "Dr. Paz Soldán has been a professor of something which he calls public health and social medicine for more than 30 years, and during this period he has not contributed anything to the development of this subject except being instrumental in having a building constructed."[1] Throughout the postwar period, the institute's staffing and budget declined substantially, while Paz Soldán was increasingly out of step with broader changes in the health field. In a speech to the national Academy of Medicine in Buenos Aires late in his career, in August 1945, he inveighed against "socialized medicine" (that is, state-run health systems), as a kind of "state demagoguery" that threatened "the moral grandeur and inalienable liberty of our Art"—that is, medicine.[2] The kind of social medicine he had strived to develop and institutionalize was under attack on many fronts—relegated to a project of socialized medicine by welfare-state and populist politics, questioned by seemingly more sophisticated and rigorous health social sciences, and bereft of support from international health institutions.

The fate of Paz Soldán and his Institute of Social Medicine was, in many ways, a microcosm of forces at work internationally. The first wave of social medicine crested in the late 1940s, and over subsequent decades the field and its integrative, holistic, and socially conscious philosophy were marginalized in favor of other, seemingly more "modern" models for improving population health. Examining this time of relative dormancy in social medicine during the 1950s and 1960s, rather than diverting us from the main story, is crucial for making sense of Latin American social medicine. Understanding the other health fields and policy models that covered similar terrain—like health planning, preventive medicine, and public health—sharpens our understanding of social medicine, what it meant, and how it was changing. It is important to understand trends that worked against social medicine—in particular, the new architecture of the international health and development technocracy, along with the rise of systematic social sciences in Latin America. Both international development and the health social sciences were strongly conditioned by modernizationist ideologies in the Cold War geopolitical context. Eventually, a growing dissatisfaction with the ideological, intellectual, and ethical confines of modern health and development discourses planted the seeds for social medicine's second wave, starting in the 1970s. We cannot really understand the past or present of Latin American social medicine without examining the reasons for its temporary decline.

In this chapter, I ascribe the ebbing of social medicine in Latin America to shifts in two mostly separate domains, international development and medical profession. During the postwar period, an expanding and powerful international development apparatus incorporated new social science theories and techniques that left little space for social medicine ideas and praxis in the health field. The apparatus of modern health planning drew the energy of public health personnel inward, into specialized professional fields, and away from engagements with the larger political realm to advocate progressive social policies. The idealism, passionate rhetoric, and politically conscious analysis of social medicine were at odds with the increasingly technocratic procedures of national health planning in the postwar era.

The medical profession also changed. In Argentina and Chile, doctors as a group became more conservative, partly in reaction to the expansion of welfare states, the perceived threat of socialism, and the rise of professional-class consciousness. In Chile, the Colegio Médico, descended from the once-radical AMECH, increasingly acted as a bulwark against further centralization of health services under the SNS.[3] In Argentina, the 1950s and 60s witnessed doctors' strikes, the strengthening of obras sociales as principal insurers and providers of care, resistance to the politicization of medical education, and a search for international prestige in medical specialties, all of which prevented movement toward more equitable, evenly distributed health services. Overall, the medical profession of the 1960s was quite different from that of the 1930s; in the earlier period, widespread economic depression and deteriorating social conditions put doctors in a position where they could barely make a living, thus causing many to place their chips on government-run, socialized medicine. But in the 1960s, with economic growth prospects improving, concerns over the threat of communism (which, after Cuba's revolution, no longer seemed abstract), and an expanding middle class (of which doctors were an important part), doctors pushed for greater autonomy from the state.

In addition to these specific factors, pervasive anticommunist rhetoric and persecution certainly diminished enthusiasm for social medicine across the international health field. As Nicole Pacino explains, Rockefeller's Bauer also visited Bolivia in 1952, just months after that country's significant political revolution, and his critiques of its medical education programs were colored by fears of the spread of communism.[4] Just a few years later, the United States would infamously intervene in Guatemala to help overthrow the left-wing government of Jacobo Arbenz. And throughout the decade, an atmosphere of "medical McCarthyism" aided by agencies of the US government served to silence leftist doctors, health social scientists, and health workers, especially those with international entanglements, like Henry Sigerist (who was forced to leave the United States for Switzerland in 1947 under a cloud of suspicion for pro-communist sentiments), Edward Barsky, Milton Roemer, and Lini de Vries.[5] Certainly this pervasive anticommunism undermined social medicine in the United States. It also seems to have destabilized international networks in the field, and probably discouraged leftists in the health field across Latin America.

In this chapter, I first explain how a Pan-American development apparatus that evolved in the early Cold War era was connected to larger geopolitical processes and how it conditioned the discourse and practices around international health. In the following section, I discuss a major health planning program sponsored by the Pan American Health Organization, the Organización Panamericana Sanitaria/Centro de Estudios del Desarrollo (OPS/CENDES) project. This program embodied the logic of mid-century developmentalism applied to problems of the health field, but it also inspired an internal critique that instigated the second wave of Latin American social medicine. I then turn to discuss the distinctive trajectories of two contemporaries in international health and development of the era. Abraham Horwitz of Chile, the director of the Pan American Health Organization for many years, was a consummate technocrat, invested in a modernizationist ideology and gradualist measures to improve population health conditions. In contrast, the Brazilian polymath and leftist political figure, Josué de Castro, with his integrative, structural analyses of social inequality and health, was increasingly marginalized from the development mainstream. The last part of the chapter explains why the medical establishment in two countries, Argentina and Chile, turned conservative, halting momentum toward universal health systems and setting up new political conflicts in the decades to come.

Health in the Pan-American Development Apparatus

This ellipsis in Latin American social medicine intersects with changes in the discourse and practice of international health in the postwar period. Inside the infant World Health Organization, the social medicine philosophy was influential at first, but increasingly supplanted by technology-intensive public health programs. The initial leadership of the Canadian Brock Chisholm, a left-leaning advocate of state-led universal health care and a rights-based approach to health, gave way to the US-approved technocrat Marcolino Candau of Brazil.[6] With Fred L. Soper leading the PAHO (known as the OPS in Spanish), the most powerful regional branch of the WHO, international health leaders focused efforts on technology-driven disease-control campaigns, most notably the global malaria eradication program launched in 1955. As Nancy Leys Stepan points out, this program, if not universally popular, was pragmatic in the postwar geopolitical context.[7] Malaria eradication was promoted as a technical package that could be launched anywhere that malaria was endemic. It seemed—in a word—"apolitical." This program epitomized the postwar approach to international health, with a proliferation of single-issue "vertical" interventions of a technical nature, some of which achieved success on their own terms, but which tended to ignore broader social (and environmental) conditions.[8] Increasingly, medical education internationally became more standardized (with a narrow and "rigorous" biomedical curriculum), thanks to the "Flexnerian" turn—prescriptions for medical education reform, based on the US Flexner Report, advocated by influential organizations like the Rockefeller Foundation.[9] Relatedly, the model of preventive medicine, with its emphasis on the monitoring and control of individual risk factors and behaviors, supplanted social medicine and its more political analysis of public health problems.

What was happening in international health was just one manifestation of a growing international development apparatus during the postwar period. A "development apparatus" has been defined as "a set of institutions, knowledge, methods, techniques, and technologies." During the Cold War, so-called functional international organizations—including "UNESCO, the UN's Food and Agriculture Organization (FAO), the World Health Organization (WHO), and PAHO, along with economic and financial aid bodies like the World Bank and the International Monetary Fund (IMF)," composed the development apparatus "but were also in good part responsible for producing the very conditions necessary for it."[10] With their "generalized confidence in science and technology and in planning methods," the "functional" organizations that were part of this apparatus promoted international norms, including measurable standards of living and quantifiable development targets that every nation ought to achieve, and had the financial leverage to do so, thanks to grants, loan packages, international exchange programs, and job security for globe-trotting technocrats.[11] Under these conditions, as Arturo Escobar explains, "Latin American social scientists and government officials faced [pressures] to transform radically the style and scope of their activities to fit the needs of the development apparatus."[12] Learning how to speak the World Bank's language of projects and planning and to use its favored analytical techniques and styles of presentation constituted more than just an academic exercise, since millions of dollars in development loans were at stake.[13]

The development apparatus was part of the Cold War economic order in the West shaped by US foreign policy. The US interest in funding development in Latin America intensified after the Cuban Revolution in 1959. The plan for a new Pan-American strategy against communism was forged at a meeting of members of the Organization of American States at Punta del Este, Uruguay, in August of 1961. One key point of contention was whether the United States should offer direct economic support for industrialization in Latin America or, rather, focus more on humanitarian projects.[14] Representing Cuba's new socialist government, Che Guevara resisted US plans for investment in public health (and education) as an imperialist subterfuge, a strategy to defuse revolutionary change and keep Latin American states in a subordinate economic position. Ultimately, the Alliance for Progress (AFP) that emerged from the Punta del Este meeting did, quite obviously, reflect a US strategy for limiting the communist threat via timely and adequate financial support for health, sanitation, education, agricultural production, and other development efforts. Latin American technocrats saw the Punta del Este charter as the blueprint for modernization and lauded "soft diplomacy" efforts via existing institutions (like the PAHO) or new US agencies (the United States Agency for International Development [USAID], the Peace Corps). The AFP also created new lines of funding for health and education projects, and in all, reinforced tendencies of the development apparatus to depoliticize social change and to reify sectors—agriculture, health, education, and so forth—as the natural units for development work. Some, like Eduardo Frei, the Chilean president from 1964 to 1970, believed strongly in the AFP as a homegrown regional project that would accelerate Latin America's modernization, but despaired as the program fell prey to opposition from the left and the right as well as shifting US foreign policy priorities.[15]

The social sciences in Latin America developed and gained prestige as part of the expanding Pan-American development apparatus. Broadly speaking, this new generation of social science research served the interests of a modernizationist national development agenda. In the first part of twentieth century, with social sciences in relative infancy, the intellectual foundations of social medicine were eclectic and unsystematic, a hodgepodge of political philosophy, medical humanism, biology, eugenics, and economics. The social sciences, with the familiar disciplinary boundaries we know today, became more established in Latin American universities during the 1950s. These universities, along with specialized research centers, like CEPAL and Facultad Latinoamericana de Ciencias Sociales (FLACSO), trained a generation of sociologists, anthropologists, and political scientists to observe the workings of national societies according to paradigms (positivism, functionalism, and modernization theory) that were broadly acceptable internationally and shaped the mindset of mainstream international development institutions. For progress in health policy, the new social sciences were a double-edged sword: robust research paradigms and investment in social science research programs helped refine and improve health policy, but at the same time, the emphasis on rational planning of interventions according to the economic possibilities of each nation tended to sideline concerns over equity and marginalize ideas of the political left. A new generation of pragmatic international technocrats came to power, tailoring their words and deeds to the dominant development discourse of the era.

Modernization theory was based in part on functionalist frameworks in sociology, political science, and economics that rose to prominence in the international and Latin American academies in the postwar period. Functionalism, or structural functionalism, as promoted by Talcott Parsons and David Easton, hinged on key assumptions about mechanisms of equilibrium and adaptation in a society. As Samuel P. Huntington wrote, from the functionalist perspective, "change is viewed as an extraneous abnormality. It is held to be the result of strain or tension, which gives rise to compensating movements that tend to reduce the strain or tension and thus restore the original state. Change is 'unnatural'; stability or rest is 'natural.'"[16] According to the sociologist David Harrison, structural functionalism held that "societies are more or less self-sufficient, adaptive social systems" and "the entire system, or any part of it, is kept together through the operation of a central value system broadly embodying social consensus."[17] Functionalism promoted the idea of individuals adapting to social conditions and offered a normative theory of social stability and gradual change shaped by consensus in democratic institutions. Its origins in models from biological sciences—physiology, in particular, with its concept of homeostasis—might help explain why it found an enthusiastic audience among public health professionals. In a way, functionalism seemed to formalize the organicist systems thinking of the hygiene movement and early social medicine.[18] Functionalist social science provided normative models of how societies should work, with variables to be manipulated through policy levers to enhance social and economic stability.

If the social sciences serving the development apparatus during the 1960s had a geographical nucleus, it was Chile. In Santiago, particularly, there was an impressive concentration of institutions dedicated to cutting-edge research in the social sciences and economic planning. Paulo Freire, who wrote the *Pedagogy of the Oppressed* while in exile in Santiago in the late 1960s, later recalled that Santiago was the undisputed center of advanced social and economic theory in Latin America, a place for invigorating debate and discussion, under a relatively stable and open government. The CEPAL, directed for many years by the Argentinean Raul Prebisch, was clearly the leader in economic research in the region. Although its researchers were recognized for their unorthodox economic theories suited to the problems of the Third World, they also laid down the norms of national economic planning that were vital to developmentalism, or *desarrollismo*. "Through their global vision," as the historian Margarita Fajardo has put it, "*cepalinos* created a Latin American-centered conversation about development."[19] Together, CEPAL, FLACSO (the Latin American center for graduate social science research), and Centro Latinoamericano y Caribeño de Demografía (CELADE, a demographic research center) agglomerated Latin America's social scientists in Santiago, initially to serve modernization, but later to question it, with the rise of the *dependentista* school of thought within the CEPAL.[20]

As a practical matter, the architecture of international postwar development created a financial resource base that had scarcely existed before. To draw upon these resources for health work required discipline, yielding or adjusting to the prerogatives of funding agencies to get work done. For health technocrats across Latin America, the new international health apparatus was appealing, as it offered an opportunity to circumvent the contentious and irrational arena of national politics to develop innovative health policies. For example, in Chile the ambitious legislative proposal to create the SNS—a concrete policy objective of the social medicine movement of the 1930s—languished in parliament for about a dozen years, an object lesson not lost on the younger generation of health planners like Horwitz, Benjamin Viel, and

Hernán Romero. They made the pragmatic choice to follow international trends in health planning, preventive medicine, and community health initiatives, with an "intentional detachment from the politics of 'left' and 'right'" in Chile.[21] Still, some projects, such as Viel's community health program in the Quinta Normal district of Santiago, viewed as a predecessor of the international primary health care (PHC) model, embodied a social medicine perspective and received support from a major US-based foundation (the RF).[22]

Adherents of functionalism believed it to be apolitical, but some applications of this modern social science approach were controversial, inspiring suspicion about the true motives of American or US-trained social scientists in Latin America. In this regard, the Project Camelot debacle, which took place in Chile in the mid-1960s, stands out. Although much has been written about this episode, I first came across reference to Project Camelot in a dissertation by Gary Filerman, an American who went to Chile to study its health system in the mid-1960s.[23] The US Army's Special Operations Research Office devised Project Camelot in 1964 to "determine the feasibility of developing a general social systems model which would make it possible to predict and influence politically significant aspects of social change in the developing nations of the world."[24] The whole project unraveled quickly when a Chilean American anthropologist, on a mission to recruit Chilean researchers for the project, unwittingly disclosed its US military backing, which caused a minor diplomatic row.[25] Although the CIA's involvement in Project Camelot was rumored but never confirmed, Chileans were right to be concerned; within a decade, Allende would be overthrown in a coup that the CIA helped sponsor. Furthermore, using insights from behavioral sciences, the CIA helped foment "social disorder" in acts of psychological warfare, in order to overthrow a democratically elected government.

The controversy over Project Camelot may seem to be a bizarre, one-off episode, but it signaled an emerging rift in the social sciences over the uses and misuses of the functionalist approach. Clearly, the architects of Project Camelot were highly invested in a normative theory that well-functioning societies are, above all, stable, and in the conviction that knowledgeable social scientists could intervene to prevent moments of discord from turning into political revolution. In 1965, the renowned American anthropologist Marshall Sahlins, reflecting the feelings of some on the New Left in the United States, explained at the annual meeting of the American Anthropological Association: "Most clearly in its characterizations of revolutionary unrest does Camelot reveal its basic valuations . . . what had been for some time a cultural common-law marriage between scientific functionalism and the natural interest of a leading world power in the status quo became under the aegis of Project Camelot an explicit and legitimate union." Shrewdly dissecting functionalism's hygienic metaphors, Sahlins continued: "Movements for radical change are in Camelot's view a disease, and a society so infected is sick. Here was a program for diagnosing social illness, a study in 'epidemiology,' called just that by a senior researcher. Another consistently refers to revolutionary movements as 'social pathology,' though disclaiming in a footnote that they are necessarily to be avoided. A third conceives of the growth of demands for change as 'contagion.'"[26] This reaction to Project Camelot was a harbinger of things to come. For left-wing academics, it exposed the work of social scientists in development work as anything but apolitical; even intellectually well-grounded research with advanced analytical techniques—"cutting edge" social science work—served to entrench the international development apparatus and US foreign policy priorities. This critique was slow to take hold, however, and for years to come, this development apparatus grew and increasingly colonized the discourse of public health, particularly through the new field of health systems planning.

Health Planning in Action: The OPS/CENDES Method

The OPS/CENDES method, developed in the 1960s, was intended to standardize a rigorous, evidence-based approach to health planning across Latin America and the Caribbean. Health planning arose directly from the emphasis on economic planning at the CEPAL and with the sponsorship of the Alliance for Progress. The cepalinos, as they were known, introduced not just certain kinds of economic doctrines and growth strategies but also a *culture of planning* that became widespread in the 1960s, affecting many other groups of technocrats, including those in public health. This planning gospel was diffused, in part, through the sanitarians who took the CEPAL course in *planificación en salud*, which was cosponsored by the Escuela de Salubridad at the Universidad de Chile. Invoking Arturo Escobar's *Encountering Development*, Fernando Pires-Alves and Marcos Chor Maio write: "The trend at that time was to make planning the panacea for all evils. As one of the most widespread 'development apparatuses,' planning was conceived to be as integral and comprehensive as possible and capable of functioning in accord with the various domains of social life in all their complexity; as such, it was designed to be the manifestation par excellence of the introduction of science and technology into government processes, guaranteeing the efficiency and efficacy of government action."[27] By 1970, the Chilean health expert Hernán Durán would write, "Planning, as a mechanism for development, is beyond question; the problem that is raised is how to do it."[28]

CENDES was a research institute at the University of Venezuela, focused on economic planning, the brainchild of the Chilean Jorge Ahumada, a founding member of CEPAL and one of the leading figures of Latin American developmentalism in the 1950s and 1960s.[29] Mario Testa, an Argentine doctor with a budding interest in public health, traveled to Caracas in 1960 to take the CENDES course, though at the time it was not focused specifically on the health sector. Soon after the famous Punta del Este meeting, in 1961 Horwitz met with Ahumada and Testa in Caracas to see if they could help him solve a problem: the AFP would make it possible for the World Bank and the Inter-American Development Bank (IADB) to offer national development loans to improve public health programs, but they required *plans* in exchange. Ahumada and Testa proposed adapting the CENDES planning method to the health sector, and this became known as the OPS/CENDES method.[30] Within a few years, Testa and his colleagues traveled across Latin America to host training sessions while others came to Caracas on scholarships offered by the PAHO. In this manner, a whole generation of health planning specialists was formed. During the 1960s, approximately five thousand officials from national governments in Latin America received training in the OPS/CENDES method.[31] By 1965, most Latin American states had health planning units in operation.[32]

OPS/CENDES focused on identifying priorities, creating targets, budgeting, and setting deadlines for planning milestones. A precept of the method, flowing from the functionalist paradigm, was that society was divided into different functional sectors, health being one of them. Available financial and human resources should be applied rationally to the problems where intervention would have the greatest effect. Thus, a starting point was the thorough diagnosis of national health problems and an auditing of available resources. Rational planning by experts was supposed to circumvent politically driven decisions. One of the practical reasons that planning had to be so detailed and rigorous was that, within the international development apparatus, not all decisions were being made autonomously by national governments. If the USAID, IADB, or World Bank provided funding for health projects, the destination of these funds had to be accounted for, carefully. Countries were subject to annual reviews by the Inter-American Committee for the Alliance for Progress, to verify advances in health planning.[33]

Before long, however, skepticism about the OPS/CENDES method grew. For the most part, these critiques circulated internally, since few outside the world of health systems planners knew or cared much about the method. One genre of critique was practical: the OPS/CENDES method seemed not to produce the predicted improvement in health services or population health conditions. As Testa told me: "After a decade, I realized that every three years a [health system] plan was made, and in each plan the country's diagnosis was exactly the same, nothing had changed. So if nothing changes in ten years after three plans, it means that the thing does not work. . . . This phenomenon happened in almost every country, in Colombia, Venezuela, Chile, or Argentina, repeatedly we made the same diagnosis."[34] Though health planners tried to remain "apolitical," decisions about the national health sector often remained in the hands of politicians, who had reasons to ignore the advice of planners.[35]

Another sort of critique, more in the realm of phenomenology, anticipated post-structuralist and Marxist critiques of development planning more generally. The normative practices of rational planning disguised the power of the "subject" behind the plans, usually technocrats in the Ministry of Health, trained in the CENDES method.[36] As Adolfo Chorny would later write, "This priority-setting function gave the method a scientific appearance which allowed [planners] to postulate, at least theoretically, that it was possible to assign priorities 'rationally,' without interference of the subject doing the planning."[37] Others, using a structuralist lens, focused on the role of health planners within the broader international political economy. The Chilean Clara Fassler, for example, writing in exile in the 1970s, echoed the dependentista critiques of the Alliance for Progress, as a sort of window dressing for US capitalist hegemony. The so-called crisis of health sector planning, she wrote, would be better termed a "demystification of health planning" that revealed a deeper "crisis of capitalist development in its dependent modality," the "incapacity of the system to satisfy the basic needs of the population," and the "failure of the technocratic and reformist project to reach the economic and social development it intended."[38]

Some in the public health field began to feel alienated from the technocratic institutions they had helped build, with the best of intentions. As political turmoil increased across the region, some questioned the need to sublimate all social conflict beneath the veneer of rational management. Floreal Ferrara, a professor at the Facultad de Medicina at the Universidad de La Plata (Buenos Aires), and a fervent Peronista, rejected the idea that health should be framed as a "complete adaptation" to social and environmental conditions. Such orthodox modernizationist thinking was well represented in PAHO reports, schools of public health, and popular public health textbooks such as *Salud, medicina y desarrollo económico-social*, by the Argentinean Abraam

Sonis.[39] Instead Ferrara proposed that health was a state of "vital optimum" (*óptimo vital*), that is, a healthy person would be ready to "fight [*luchar*] permanently" and engage in a divided and conflict-ridden society.[40] Ferrara developed this idea in dialogue with Milcíades Peña, a Trotskyite intellectual, who, incongruously, was also an expert in marketing research. (According to Ferrara, "no one fought harder against *desarrollismo* than Milcíades.")[41] As Ferrara later explained in a published interview, this conceptualization of health was intended, at its root, to demonstrate that "there was no aspect of daily life that was not a class struggle, a class conflict or a social conflict."[42] Testa also came to see things the same way: "So, trying to solve social problems with systems theories does not work. That's what we tried to do with the CENDES/OPS method—solve a social problem based on systems theory. . . . I believe that social problems are problems that can only be solved through political conflict."[43] Later in life, Ferrara would go so far as to say that the WHO definition of health was "the discourse of the colonizer" meant to preserve the status quo, by focusing on individual conditions rather than collective action, avoiding the questions of social injustice and the structural roots of population health crisis.[44] His textbook, *Medicina de la Comunidad*, cowritten with Eduardo Acebal and Jose Paganini, was one of the first to rigorously analyze and compare theories from social sciences (especially anthropology and sociology), going beyond functionalism to understand social relations, permanence, and change in institutional structures in public health and medicine.[45]

But we are possibly getting ahead of ourselves. Eventually these critiques would fit perfectly into the zeitgeist of the 1970s, with its widely felt suspicion of large and powerful systems. But health systems planning was a hegemonic project in the 1960s, the so-called decade of Latin American development, and its influence has been long-lasting. Planning in the health sector has never disappeared; it has only evolved, and arguably taken on even more pretentions as a rational scientific endeavor with the advance of methods in fields like metrics and evaluation.[46] As we will see in chapters 6 and 7, technocratic management of health systems serves as an enduring foil for social medicine advocates. Still, the characterization of health planning as a handmaiden to, or leading edge for, capitalist development also needs to be approached with some caution. Socialist governments, as well, have always had large bureaucracies devoted to central planning. As Eden Medina explains in the book *Cybernetic Revolutionaries*, Salvador Allende sought (and had begun to develop) the most technologically cutting-edge systems for monitoring and manipulating the national economy during his socialist regime from 1970 to 1973.[47] During the 1960s, Cuba took part in the OPS/CENDES planning project—even though the country was outside of the Alliance for Progress—and the legacy of its emphasis on efficient use of resources to target population health problems has helped make Cuba's health system one of the most cost-efficient in the world. In addition, many Latin American health experts were acquainted with the health system of the Soviet Union.[48] Possibly, OPS/CENDES was a perfect fit for the ideological context of the Cold War, where the technocratic and rationalist approaches did at least *seem* apolitical, palatable to an international development apparatus that increased its legitimacy by staying out of geopolitical matters.

Abraham Horwitz: The Consummate International Health Technocrat

Abraham Horwitz was the avatar of the new type of modern international health technocrat in the postwar era. Serving as the director of the PAHO from 1958 to 1974, Horwitz was obviously an astute political actor, but he also sought to isolate public health from the realm of Cold War politics. As a Chilean—and one with a conservative ideology—he was familiar with the chaotic political battles between left and right, and the dangers of mixing politics with the work of the health professions. He chose a new path, one facilitated by the expansion of opportunities in the international development apparatus, but his loyalty to the American-led project of modernization was more than mere opportunism. He shared the values of the Alliance for Progress, in his conviction that rational scientific planning could engineer public health progress and lasting social stability.

Horwitz was part of the generation of Chilean public health experts who attempted to transcend the intense ideological conflicts of the day by concentrating on building the institution of the SNS, which finally came into being in 1952.[49] Horwitz had an early career trajectory similar to other accomplished Chilean *salubristas* of the era, such as Gustavo Molina Guzmán and Benjamin Viel: a medical degree at the University of Chile; graduate study in public health at Johns Hopkins, sponsored by a fellowship from the RF, from 1942 to 1944; teaching and research at the Escuela de Salubridad in Santiago (also accomplished with funding from the RF); and higher administrative posts in the SNS.[50] Horwitz was fully aware that he and his closest allies were attempting to reshape the Chilean public health system according to international standards that were set down in places like Baltimore and Washington, DC: "We were labeled derisively as the '*American Boys*' and the new school [the Escuela de Salubridad] was '*Little Hopkins*'. We were aware that the influence of Anglo-Saxon thought in medicine and health introduced the concept of measuring vital phenomena, which served as the basis for experimental and applied epidemiology, it created an international language and it determined health indicators that the WHO disseminated after 1948. I felt it was an enormous advance."[51] Implicitly, this new orientation in public health was an advance over social medicine, with its theoretical pluralism, lack of systematic methods, and mixing of science and politics. Horwitz, like the RF's Bauer in his assessment of Paz Soldán in Peru, or Bernardo Houssay's judgment of Ramón Carrillo in Argentina, viewed social medicine as antiquated and ideologically driven, as compared with a new public health based on rigorous, positivist scientific research. With his connections to the US-based network of public health technocrats, Horwitz was poised to take on a more powerful role in Pan-American health.

Horwitz's view of the relationship between economic development and health dovetailed with the US view conveyed in the Alliance for Progress. In fact, from the time he succeeded Fred L. Soper as the head of the PAHO, Horwitz was deeply involved with the high-level international meetings that led to the Conference of Punta del Este, where the AFP was created in 1961.[52] While it was obviously a US-sponsored effort, the modernizationist and cepalino camps were united by a devotion to rational economic planning.[53] As the Chilean Hernán Romero, a leader in the field of health planning in Latin America, wrote: "In it [the Charter of Punta del Este] there is the sign of an agreement among the governments of the Americas to simultaneously plan economic growth and social progress."[54] Soon after the Punta del Este meeting, Horwitz wrote: "Today there is a consciousness of the necessity of simultaneously stimulating economic growth and social progress by way of rationally conceived plans that attend to priorities and are oriented towards the use of growing resources."[55] Horwitz had a good relationship with the head of the IADB, Felipe Herrera, also from Chile.[56] Horwitz's major initiative to improve sanitation across the Americas was funded primarily by the IADB, and such sanitation projects would become a regular part of the bank's development portfolio. Horwitz also continued to prioritize Soper's malaria eradication program, while developing new initiatives to reduce childhood malnutrition and infant mortality and to promote immunizations and the control of tuberculosis.[57] But above all this, he promoted *planning*: continuous improvement in gathering and disseminating data, and the incorporation of new planning methodologies, such as those being developed at CEPAL and CENDES.[58]

Horwitz became director of the PAHO in 1958, just before the Cuban Revolution, and managing communist Cuba's relationship to the PAHO was a deft political act. In his own politics, Horwitz was firmly anticommunist. Mario Testa, the Argentine health systems planner who often worked with Horwitz during the 1960s, explained to me that Horwitz was, as "a man of the extreme right wing," his ideological opposite.[59] Horwitz even called himself a *momio*, appropriating the pejorative term used by Chilean leftists to insult their conservative opponents, a play on the Spanish word for "mummy." Given Horwitz's own political orientation, the considerable US influence on the PAHO, and Cuba's expulsion from the Organization of American States in 1962, it would not have been surprising for the PAHO to exclude Cuba. And yet, as Testa observed firsthand, Horwitz worked hard to keep Cuba in the fold, flying the Cuban flag along with those of other PAHO member states at the organization's headquarters, not far from the US State Department.

Was Horwitz simply a political pragmatist? Certainly, but more than anything, he wanted the PAHO to be a technical, specialist organization that transcended geopolitics. As Carlos Montoya Aguilar explained to me, to manage this feat meant, ironically, that Horwitz had to be "more of a politician than a technician."[60] This required "having to create equilibrium" among the many member states of the PAHO. In 1966, in a speech he gave in Chile, he counted as one of his great achievements "achieving consensus over the most antagonistic ideologies," which was possible "when what is sought is devoted exclusively to the welfare of human beings and societies."[61] As Pires-Alves and Chor Maio explain, Horwitz adroitly spoke the language of postwar development; even as he explicitly endorsed Rostow's modernization theory, Horwitz "avoided the themes of political and economic liberties, democracy, and so-called Western values" in the midst of the Cold War, instead focusing on themes of "basic education, housing, scientific and technological cooperation, planning, and, of course, health—in other words, a set of issues more fitting to what were considered eminently technical approaches and thus perhaps constituting a more comfortable array for an intergovernmental, sectoral organization like PAHO."[62]

In 1977, in a speech on the occasion of the PAHO's seventy-fifth anniversary (and now in the role of former director), Horwitz asserted that every society had to find its own way, whatever its political structure, toward guaranteeing the health of the population, and that Latin America, as a region, was better off for the diversity of its political systems.[63] In Testa's view, before the worst of the military dictatorships in the 1970s, there was more "tolerance" of opposing political viewpoints within the world of Pan-American health.[64] Similarly, Giorgio Solimano—who served in the Ministry of Health during Allende's government, went into exile under Pinochet, and later became director of the School of Public Health in Santiago—told me that Allende and Horwitz were friends; when I expressed surprise, Solimano explained that there was broad consensus and ideological pluralism within Chile's health leadership of the postwar generation: "The SNS was created through unanimity in the political world, especially in health, where there were people *de todos colores*." The SNS was an "effort by everyone," even though today the right tries to "discredit" the SNS as a "socialist" idea, and the left denies the involvement of more conservative actors, such as Horwitz.[65] Horwitz showed his ability to set ideology aside again after the 1973 overthrow of Allende. Directly or indirectly, he helped find positions for leftist Chilean doctors in exile, including Solimano and Montoya, but not at the PAHO—their political reputation being too hot an issue for Horwitz.[66]

Josué de Castro: Against the Grain

In a sense, Josué de Castro was both a bridge between two generations of Latin American social medicine and the opposite of Abraham Horwitz. Roughly contemporaries, born two years apart (Castro in 1908, Horwitz in 1910), they confronted the problems of poverty, modernization, and geopolitics in completely different ways. Where Horwitz focused single-mindedly on the organization of public health work, Castro was an interdisciplinary polymath, bridging the realms of social medicine, anthropology, geography, and food and agriculture. While Horwitz was a political conservative who managed to suppress his ideological biases in a technocratic style of leadership, Castro was a leftist politician, representing the Brazilian Labour Party in the national parliament, and moved even farther to the left after his exile at the hands of the military dictatorship in 1964. And whereas Horwitz's alignment with the American project of Third World modernization facilitated his rise in the postwar development technocracy, Castro's radical analysis of the causes of hunger distanced him from the Food and Agriculture Organization of the UN, which he had helped lead in its early days.[67] In a different world, one not shaped by modernization theory, functionalist social sciences, and Cold War geopolitics, Castro might have been a world-renowned figure of social and political change, carrying on the cause of social medicine. But in reality, Castro was mostly forgotten until a recent revival of his thought in fields like geography and food studies.[68]

Castro was born into a well-to-do family in Recife, in northeastern Brazil, and finished his medical degree at the Medical School of the University of Rio de Janeiro in 1929. In his work, he embodied the integrative and eclectic intellectual spirit of early social medicine, crossing boundaries between the biomedical science of nutrition (based in physiology), medicine, geography, and anthropology. Early in his career, he did advanced research with Pedro Escudero, the Argentine nutritionist whose National Institute of Nutrition in Buenos Aires became a model for similar institutions across the continent.[69] Castro's experience with Escudero inspired him to found several national institutes in Brazil for research on nutritional problems.[70] As he became renowned for published works like *The Geography of Hunger*, Castro also participated in the expanding postwar international development apparatus, serving as an adviser to the FAO from its earliest days, and as head of the organization's Executive Committee from 1952 to 1956. All the while, he also cultivated a career in national politics, representing Recife in the national Congress as a member of the Brazilian Labour Party (PTB). Under the Brazilian president João Goulart, also of the PTB, Castro served as Brazil's ambassador to the United Nations agencies in Geneva, from 1962 to 1964.[71] With the 1964 coup that brought down Goulart and ushered in two decades of military rule, Castro was exiled to Paris, where he taught human geography at the University of Vincennes (Paris VIII) and continued to write on international politics and development issues until his death in 1973.[72]

In his most famous work, a book known in English as *The Geography of Hunger*, Castro challenged prevalent neo-Malthusian views of the causes of hunger.[73] Castro's explanation of hunger began with a rich and detailed cultural ecology of malnutrition that linked specific deficiencies in vitamins, proteins, and other nutrients to the widely varying environmental conditions around the world. He then offered a comprehensive history of colonialism and continued economic dependency to explain the political-economic causes of hunger, from Brazil to Mexico to Puerto Rico, where the concentration of landholdings and the emphasis on export of cash crops had curtailed domestic food production, diminished native agricultural know-how, and generated misery for many and wealth for the few. Using this political-economy type of approach, Castro railed against the neo-Malthusians for "blaming the hungry for the fact that there is hunger," for treating demography as governed by natural laws, somehow isolated from questions of power, and for their reactionary and self-serving politics. He concluded with an optimistic agenda for a "geography of abundance," in which agricultural and food system planning would frame food production as a matter of public health and welfare: "The fundamental truth can no longer be concealed from mankind; the world has at its disposal enough resources to provide an adequate diet for everyone, everywhere. And if many of the guests on this earth have not yet been called to the table, it is because all known civilizations, including our own, have been organized on a basis of economic inequality."[74]

Josué de Castro might seem marginal to the story of social medicine in Latin America. It is true that, during the height of Castro's international renown, during the 1950s, his work was rarely cited in social medicine or in public health. At least one exception, a 1956 analysis of the causes of infant mortality in Mendoza province, Argentina, by the physician Juan Maurín Navarro, makes explicit reference to *The Geography of Hunger*.[75] Then again, Castro's analysis builds on the foundations of the international nutritional studies sponsored by the ILO during the interwar period, as discussed briefly in chapter 2. He sought to "denaturalize" the causes of malnutrition, hunger, and famine (in opposition to Malthusian explanations); use a geographical (or human ecology) approach to connect causal mechanisms in a holistic way that foreshadowed political ecology and critical development studies; and apply a historical materialist method to understand the unequal distribution of power and persistent social hierarchies.[76] His ideas were adopted by many "critical" scholars who self-consciously stood outside of, and opposed to, the dominant paradigms in international development, including many protagonists of the next generation of social medicine and collective health (among them Sérgio Arouca, Jaime Breilh, and Naomar Almeida Filho, to be discussed in chapters 6 and 7), geographers like Milton Santos and Ben Wisner, or anthropologists like Nancy Scheper-Hughes. He was, in essence, a bridge between the generations of social medicine—understood as politically conscientious analyses of the biological expression of social inequalities—at a time when the field was out of fashion.

Beyond all that, Castro symbolizes alternatives to desarrollismo and the international development apparatus. He might have had people like Horwitz or Soper in mind when he railed against excessive specialization in the sciences and social sciences in the first pages of *The Geography of Hunger*. Invoking the German intellectual and Weimar-era statesman Walter Rathenau, Castro lamented the steady growth of "a specialists' civilization—directed by men whose scientific outlook is rigorous but who suffer from a deplorable cultural and political myopia. . . . Such men are the dominant type of our cultural elite, representatives of the social dynamic which has brought us to what Rathenau so aptly called 'the vertical invasion of the barbarians.' The narrow specialists, 'men who know more and more about less and less,' are one of the most dangerous elements of our cultural life."[77] Thus, Castro understood, presciently, the limits of the technocratic mindset for engaging in deep, foundational, cross-disciplinary critique. Castro was "explicitly opposed" to the

Alliance for Progress and its model of development as a technical endeavor and as an attempt by the United States to finance counterrevolutionary action.[78] Castro's removal from his UN position and his political exile were also reminders that behind the trappings of officialdom in the liberal international order, geopolitical priorities were dominant, and he still served at the pleasure of the national state, now taken over by authoritarians. For that reason, later in life Castro sought new forms of internationalism outside of these official channels, creating pressure group organizations and engaging in New Left intellectual circles from his base in Paris during the foment of the May Revolution of 1968, until his death in 1973.[79]

Doctors as an Interest Group: Explaining the Resistance to State-Controlled Health Care

Major changes to the health system, in any country, require the consent and cooperation of the organized medical profession. Put another way: "You can't transform a health system without doctors."[80] I heard variations on this notion—possibly attributable to Gastão Wagner de Sousa Campos, the Brazilian sanitarista—many times during my conversations with academics in the social medicine field. They have learned, sometimes through bitter experience, that medical professionals often resist change that might lead toward more equitable and universally accessible health systems.

In the early Cold War era, doctors' unions in both Chile and Argentina shifted gradually away from their social medicine roots toward the protection of their own professional interests and prerogatives. Thinking of doctors as a special interest group adds texture to the study of social medicine's long arc of development and change. Although state intervention in the health sector might be based on the worthy goal of improving equity in access, quality of medical care, and health outcomes, medical professionals, as a group, often stand in the way of those goals. The history of the US case, where the American Medical Association historically stood in the way of socialized medicine, is well known.[81] In general, the political stance of Latin America's doctors also shifted to the right, for a variety of reasons: their middle-class status and a declining sense of noblesse oblige, concerns over state control of the terms of their professional life, worries about socialist revolutions more generally, and a feeling that politics was contaminating a field that values a scientific rationalism.

This purported disconnection between doctors and society at large would become a major theme of study for the emerging second wave of social medicine. Conceptualizing the medical profession as a politically interested group is itself an innovation of critical social scientists of the 1970s, such as Carlos Bloch and Susana Belmartino, of the Centro de Estudio Sanitarios y Sociales (CESS) research group in Rosario, Argentina; Juan César García, the PAHO official who promoted a covert network of social medicine thinkers across the Americas; Mario Testa, the Argentine health planner turned social critic; and Vicente Navarro, the Catalonian sociologist and longtime editor of the *International Journal of Health Services*. As neo-Marxist social scientists, their analytical starting point was that of the class struggle, and they identified a historical process wherein the interests of the medical profession merged with those of the national bourgeoisie in defense of shared class prerogatives. This perspective was a far cry from the self-image of authority, rationality, and political disinterest historically projected by the profession, but circumstances were changing. For the medical profession in Argentina, the post-Perón era, from the mid-1950s into the 1960s, was a time of retrenchment, an anti-Peronist turn, and the protection of class interests in a complex political scene. Around the same time in Chile, the Colegio Médico, the legacy of the radical AMECH, grew increasingly distant ideologically from its leftist social medicine roots.

In Argentina, Peronismo had changed the dynamics of organizing in the medical profession. As discussed in chapter 4, gremialismo médico had ideological roots in European anarchism, carried on in Argentina by figures such as Juan Lazarte. The stance of his COMRA was that the medical profession needed to preserve its autonomy vis-à-vis the state, not just to avoid being reduced to "mere functionaries" but also to construct a system that would better serve a broader public. Ramón Carrillo, as minister of health, attempted to centralize planning of the health system and pull doctors into a large network of state-run hospitals. In response to the recalcitrance of COMRA, the Perón government formed its own series of medical unions, in attempt to bring doctors under the wing of the state, as it had done with other organized labor. Perón also installed loyalists in the Medical School of the University of Buenos Aires, who in turn expelled respected scientists (and anti-Peronists) like Houssay. Perón's ouster in 1955 was greeted with relief, perhaps even glee, by most doctors in Argentina. Although many of Carrillo's most ambitious plans for centralizing the health system never came to fruition, the Peronist decade had fixed the general structure of the health system, in particular the strengthening of what would be called the obras sociales, semiautonomous, well-funded organizations for health insurance and medical care.

In the decade after 1955, the medical profession continued to tilt to the right, even as it adopted radical political tactics, particularly the labor strike.

According to Susana Belmartino, this period saw an "unprecedented flourish-ing of medical union activity."[82] A national doctor's strike—the Huelga Médica—in 1958 was a key moment in the consolidation of the medical profes-sion's power. The motives for the strike are somewhat hazy; Belmartino and Bloch, who led research on medical labor unions in Argentina, and would thus have understood the issue as well as anyone, remarked feeling "disconcerted" because the strike seemed to come out of nowhere.[83] The initial provocation for the strike, apparently, was a clash with the transport workers' union over who should appoint the new director of its health insurance fund: the union leadership, or the doctors who staffed the union's obra social. The COMRA chapter in the Capital Federal began to strike, intermittently, on June 9, 1958, sparking solidarity walkouts in other provinces, and by mid-September the COMRA had negotiated a favorable settlement and gone back to work. All this took place during the first few months of the presidency of Arturo Frondizi, democratically elected but with the backing of the military, whose truncated term was marked by clashes with the militantly Peronista labor unions. The COMRA was itself at odds with the Peronista unions and worried about becom-ing subservient to them. Given that most doctors now worked for the unions' health insurance services, according to the COMRA, "the different labor unions had become the bosses [*patrones*] of the medical union."[84] This was an inversion of the old social order, which many doctors found unacceptable.

While a confusing (and underresearched) episode, the doctor's strike of 1958 was undoubtedly a successful assertion of the medical profession's power. In Juan Librandi's interpretation, the doctors sought freedom from the state—in the relationship between doctors and patients, in the organization of hospitals and clinics, in the regulation of the profession, in determining the price of treat-ments and procedures—but they also wanted to maintain the government as the source of funding for the social security system.[85] This audacious stance— wanting everything, while giving up nothing—was accompanied by the rough tactics of the strike, which included publishing the names, addresses, and phone numbers of "traitors" (that is, doctors who failed to observe the strike) in the magazine *Mundo Hospitalario*.[86] In Bloch and Belmartino's view, the COMRA sought autonomy from Argentina's tumultuous political scene, and separation from the pro-Peronista labor unions. Surely this stance was partially rooted in class resentment, disdain for an empowered working class. The doctors also thought, apparently, that it was unwise to hitch their own fortunes to a broader union movement that was constantly being pulled into conflict and negotiation with the government (and, in 1959, would engage in a series of debilitating strikes). All the while, even as the medical union used its power to intervene in the design of health policy, it maintained strongly "apolitical" rhetoric. As the union leadership put it during the 1958 strike, "The union movement should maintain its distance from all political participation, whether national or international, since politicization compromises our goals and outcomes.... Although maliciously it might be said that [the strike] had a political character, the strike originated precisely in order to prevent, as in the grim past, the return of politics to the hospitals."[87] Doctors emerged from the strike unified and, indeed, mostly above the fray of everyday politics, and with stronger legislation to protect their rights as professionals.

Not long after the strike ended, Floreal Ferrara and Milcíades Peña conducted a survey of over one thousand doctors in Buenos Aires and La Plata, which revealed the conservative tilt of the medical profession. (It is also one of the few published studies that captured the opinions of the rank-and-file Argentine doctors of that era.) By a three to one margin, the doctors surveyed agreed that the health sector should be organized by doctors rather than the state. At the same time, around 70 percent of respondents agreed that in Argentina, "the medical profession was becoming increasingly proletarianized," in other words, becoming like the working class in its rights, protections, and labor conditions. Answers to these and other questions led Ferrara and Peña to conclude that around 86–87 percent of doctors maintained a "conservative" attitude as opposed to the "reformist" stance of the minority; just as importantly, this pattern was largely the same, regardless of age, implying that younger doctors were just as politically conservative, if not more so. Nevertheless, a majority of doctors believed that a compulsory national health insurance program could be made compatible with a system based on private practice of medicine.[88]

Meanwhile, in Chile the Colegio Médico (CM) became a conspicuous drag on efforts to further centralize the state health system.[89] As explained in chapter 3, the constitution of the Colegio Médico in 1948 consolidated the labor-union functions of the AMECH with governance functions of national medical associations (such as designing and enforcing standards on professional conduct and licensing), under the auspices of the state. Indeed, the CM was a prerequisite for the creation of the Chilean National Health Service in 1952 and the legislation was pushed by "political doctors" in the national Congress, from across the ideological spectrum.[90] Since membership in the CM was mandatory for every doctor in Chile, it had, in the words of Hernán Romero, "enormous power."[91] With Salvador Allende at its head from its inception until 1963, even during his active political career, the CM tended to work harmoniously with the SNS. But, as Azun Candina-Polomer writes, "while the Colegio had supported the creation of the SNS as a necessary public instrument of health care, it worried about turning physicians into 'functionaries' whose professional values and prerogatives were subordinated to the interests of the state."[92] As Carlos Molina Bustos described the situation, after the creation of the SNS, "a small medical oligarchy developed, which began to fight against the Service and began to produce class conflict within the interior of the Colegio Médico."[93] Under the leadership of the more conservative Emilio Villarroel González, the CM pushed for a new law, the Ley del Funcionario Médico, in 1964, which gave doctors additional protection in the workplace. "By the end of the 1960s," according to Candina-Polomer, "we find a professional association that embraced its role in the construction of public-sector medicine and defined it as positive for the country but at the same time defended the economic interests of physicians, displaying a wary attitude toward political changes that might impact those interests or their role in determining public health policy."[94] After 1970, this wariness turned to outright hostility against Allende's ambitions to complete the unification of the health system. In 1972, the CM joined a truckers' strike meant to destabilize the Allende government, and in August 1973 joined another strike, this time demanding Allende's resignation.[95] By September 1973, a clear majority of Chile's Colegio Médico was in favor of the military coup that put Pinochet in power, and some in the CM took an active role in persecuting leftist doctors.[96]

So what was happening to the medical profession in Chile and Argentina during the 1950s and 1960s? As I see it, the medical profession sought to create a defensible space around their hospitals, clinics, laboratories, and medical schools. As a counterpart to this move, doctors mostly abandoned personal involvement in leadership roles in the conventional political arena. That space was increasingly seen as poisonous, unstable, unpredictable, and unscientific. Moreover, doctors' unions and associations saw themselves as defending a meritocratic ethos against the dangers of clientelist relations that seemed endemic to populist, democratic politics. In the words of Testa, who lived through this period, doctors increasingly saw themselves as "social subjects" without any common cause with the working class, and "ideology" became a "barrier" to working with the political left.[97] At the same time, doctors were aligned with the ideology of desarrollismo and the new, semiautonomous political spaces of "techno-bureaucracy" within the state that it created.[98] Although more research is needed to generalize about trends across the Latin American region, at least in Argentina and Chile the medical profession emerged by the late 1960s as more powerful, autonomous, focused on its own professional and class interests, and mostly opposed to the program of the political left.

Social Medicine, between the Waves

What happened to "social medicine" during the 1950s and 1960s? Why did this idea mostly disappear from the lexicon of medicine, public health, and health planning during this period? Some of the most important objectives of the first generation of Latin American social medicine were effectively incorporated into new health systems. However, increasingly large and complex health systems required specialized personnel to plan and manage them. As health system planners developed specialized expertise, they inevitably narrowed their scope of action and became more reductionist in their understanding of how to improve population health conditions. As Josué de Castro presciently understood, the growth of a postwar international development apparatus encouraged these habits of mind and ways of thinking: professional survival and advancement depended on engagement with techno-bureaucratic systems. At the same time, the medical profession also found a temporary exit from what could be dispiriting engagements in the political arena, by asserting its autonomy to preserve professional and class interests. In effect, during this period the spirit of idealism that accompanied the early development of welfare state institutions gave way to the hard politics of interest groups making conflicting demands on the state. The geopolitical context of increasingly strident anti-communism also encouraged a retreat to safer epistemological ground defined by functionalism, positivism, and modernization. And yet the successful figures in Latin American health of this era, like Abraham Horwitz, "stayed in their lanes" not just for the sake of professional self-preservation but also because it promised the best chance for success, which they defined as measurable success in population health outcomes.

Here it is also worth considering an unexamined proposition that technical-scientific advances in the field of medicine, whatever the structure of a given nation's health system, made incremental and sometimes tremendous progress in increasing longevity and quality of life. During this period of rapid economic modernization—an uneven process, to be sure—standards of living improved and more disposable income was devoted to health care, a market-driven relation that did not necessarily require state involvement. As demographers would later quantify, in Latin America after 1950, there was a "rapid and massive downturn in mortality," aided by economic growth and technical interventions, like childhood vaccinations.[99] Even representatives of the second wave of social medicine looked back on the period of 1950–70 as one typified by "the increasing use of antibiotics and surgical techniques and the consolidation of confidence in individualized medical care."[100] Rapid population growth across the region indicated success in mortality declines and prompted new concerns over a demographic explosion.[101] If first-wave social medicine flourished as a response to earlier health crisis, that sense of crisis had diminished in much of Latin America.

Leaving aside such conjectures about the larger factors behind the temporary eclipse of social medicine, it is also clear that by the late 1960s pressure was building for more a systematic critique of health planning, preventive medicine, medical education, and other elements of the international health and development apparatus. The initial drivers of second-wave LASM were mostly discontented international health technocrats, people like Juan Cesar García, Mario Testa, and Gustavo Molina Guzmán. They developed an "internal" critique that came from the experience of working within the international development apparatus, and they introduced new ideas, like Marxist and post-structuralist theory, to address the limits of mainstream functionalism and positivism. Unlike previous iterations of social medicine, this new group would grapple with how to construct a socially just and democratic praxis, not just for the health field, but for society at large. And they worked under conditions of political repression, persecution, threats, and exile, as the relatively peaceable era of the Latin American "development decade" and the AFP gave way to a period dominated by brutal right-wing authoritarianism.

CHAPTER SIX

Revival

The Second Wave of Latin American Social Medicine

This chapter explains the rise of a new wave of social medicine ideas, research, and practice in the 1970s and 1980s. In this period, new theoretical currents from the social sciences, including structural Marxism, feminism, post-structuralism, and postcolonialism, reinvigorated social medicine thought. During an era of right-wing authoritarian governments across the region, these ideas could be too radical for open discussion in universities, academic journals, or the media. The political climate of the time, marked by the Cuban Revolution, student protests in Mexico in 1968, and the violent overthrow of Allende's government in 1973, added urgency to social medicine debates, and many left-leaning health professionals from Argentina and Chile were forced into exile by military regimes. New social medicine thought flourished in key nodes in Mexico, Ecuador, and Argentina, along with Brazil, where it came to be known as saúde coletiva or "collective health." From his privileged position in the PAHO, the Argentinean Juan César García coordinated, sometimes covertly, the activity taking place in these nodes, which eventually coalesced in the formation of ALAMES, an international association of professionals in social medicine.

The second wave of Latin American social medicine can be read, in part, as an insurgency from within the international health technocracy. As discussed earlier, the political energy of the first wave of social medicine ebbed in the 1950s and 1960s, as international health institutions expanded and consolidated their power in a larger apparatus of modernization and development. As time went on, however, a small but influential fraction of technical and administrative personnel in the PAHO and other international institutions grew disenchanted with ineffective bureaucratic routines and sterile, uncritical discourses about public health, including the model of "preventive medicine." For a time, this critique was hard to articulate and it was more like the classic "problem that has no name": a sense of disquiet or unease, concern with being out of step with the currents of political change, a craving for new ideas, and the search for an understanding of the historical roots of the public health enterprise. Without question, García was the most impactful of these restive technocrats, skillfully leveraging his high-level position in the PAHO to spread new ideas and, just as importantly, bring together health workers across the hemisphere who were interested in critique of conventional health planning and more radical theories of change to confront persistent social inequality under increasingly authoritarian governments in the region.

The new social medicine emerged during a period of intellectual ferment in critical studies of health care and international development. Overall, these new intellectual influences can be described as leftist, antiauthoritarian, and skeptical of Western modernity. It would be a bit of a stretch to say that the actors involved in the new LASM were part of the international "counterculture," but their efforts were certainly stimulated by these changing times, marked by decolonization, student protests, antiwar demonstrations, church reforms, new musical styles, and other signals of the disintegration of old orthodoxies and the crisis of modernity in the West.[1]

Even though this chapter necessarily focuses on the smaller world of international health experts, it is important to keep the broader cultural and geopolitical context in mind. In the domain of development studies, we see the rise of leftist dependency theorists, often writing in a polemical mode, and specifically about Latin America, such as Andre Gunder Frank or Eduardo Galeano.[2] Relatedly, Paulo Freire, whose *Pedagogy of the Oppressed* was published in Brazil in 1968, explained how Western education tended to reproduce oppressive and hierarchical social structures. Orlando Fals Borja, a Colombian sociologist, not only recognized the need for social theory from the Global South but also began "opening the space to engage in an experiment in which academic researchers and grassroot activists operated on an equal footing," with his innovative method of participatory action research.[3] Older Marxist intellectuals, from Marx and Engels to Gramsci and Mariátegui, were rediscovered, reread, and incorporated into the canon of university courses in politics and sociology in Latin America.[4] Che Guevara was an indirect but potent influence on social medicine, for his ideas of the communist "new man" and the "revolutionary doctor," but more importantly, as a model for turning ideology into decisive, revolutionary action.[5]

Rising suspicion of Western medicine accompanied this critical, countercultural turn. The iconoclastic Ivan Illich, who, like Freire, was a fierce critic of conventional Western education, turned his focus on the health field, observing the "medicalization" of society with alarm. His book *Medical Nemesis* was widely read among the scholars of the new social medicine, even though some—like Juan César García—would criticize it as atheoretical.[6] But, together with Michel Foucault (whose role is discussed in more detail below) and the French thinker Georges Canguilhem (Foucault's teacher), Illich represented a vigorous medical humanism that anticipated a post-structuralist turn in social medicine, which encouraged a less economistic reading of how biomedicine became a dominant approach in Western societies.[7] For the collective health movement in Brazil in particular, Illich's work helped to stimulate a discussion about the power differential between doctors and patients.[8] Illich, a leftist Catholic priest, was also part of the Liberation Theology movement, which had an important, though sometimes latent, influence on the integration of a social justice vision into Latin American health systems.

The new academic social medicine constructed itself in opposition to what it saw as outmoded theories that tended to justify the status quo: functionalism and positivism in sociological studies of the health field; the emphasis on reductionist biomedicine in medical education, which would subsequently be glossed as the "Flexnerian" model; behavioralism, which permeated the conceptual foundations of interventions in preventive medicine; and modernization theory or desarrollismo in the social sciences. Of course, these new theoretical frameworks did not hatch, fully formed, overnight, but emerged from a concentrated academic effort, in seminars and workshops, new research centers and master's programs, and new journals dedicated to critical research in the health social sciences.[9]

The spirit of youthful revolution that marked the late 1960s gave impetus to the second wave of social medicine, but what made it last and become more than just a fleeting relic of that tumultuous era? Put in different terms, how did Latin American social medicine finally become institutionalized, in its own right, as an academic field, something the first wave never really achieved? This process of institutionalization began in the late 1960s and continued for several decades. According to Everardo Duarte Nunes, a veteran of the LASM movement, there are four distinct phases in the process of institutionalization of an academic field.[10] In the beginning, small groups of experts have exploratory conversations about topics of interest across disciplines; next, there is an increasing frequency of meetings and conferences, a "regularization of discourses, practices, and forms of organization," but a lack of sustained financial support; in the third phase, the field of study gains more prominence, articulates its own "distinct identity," and begins to receive more financial support, for example, from universities, state-funded grant programs, or foundations; and in the final phase of "legitimization," there is the "consolidation of a new field or discipline" with its own journals and degree programs that give it some autonomy from other fields. Although I would argue that these phases tend to overlap, rather than having clean breaks between them, Nunes presents a helpful schema for understanding how the social medicine field achieved permanence and stability in the 1970s and 1980s, by constructing and maintaining networks that were resilient in the face of many kinds of challenges, from political turmoil to ideological divisions to the difficulties of international communication in a less globally connected era.

This chapter focuses on how actors, networks, and ideas wove together to construct a distinctive field, social medicine, during the 1970s and 1980s. I prioritize tracing movements of people and ideas through Latin American networks anchored in specific locales, and leave a more focused examination of theoretical debates in social medicine for chapter 7. This chapter begins with a discussion of Juan César García, a PAHO functionary who was the indispensable glue that initially held this network together and helped it expand, operating from his base in Washington, DC, but crisscrossing the continent in routine official travel. I then turn my attention back to Chile, and the consequences of the 1973 coup. The overthrow of Allende not only meant a reversal of hard-won progress in health equity but also scattered a group of health workers into exile across the world, many to be absorbed into the growing network of Latin American social medicine. The experience of political exile and authoritarian regimes is also a theme in the last two sections of the chapter, focused on Argentina and Brazil and their roles in the new LASM. In Argentina a small group of scholars interested in social medicine, based largely in Buenos Aires and Rosario, carried on their work clandestinely or in exile during the notorious Proceso, without having much impact on health policy or even on the teaching of health social sciences, at least not immediately. By contrast, in Brazil a movement that came to be known as saúde coletiva developed rapidly, achieving the most thorough institutionalization of any of the national groups in the new social medicine.

Juan César García: The Restive Technocrat

Juan César García is undoubtedly the pivotal figure in the second wave of Latin American social medicine. Over a career spanning just two decades, from the mid-1960s to the early 1980s, García tried to set a scholarly agenda for social medicine and to rewrite the history of medicine and public health in Latin America from a structural Marxist perspective. From an advantageous position as a PAHO expert on medical education, he fostered networks of academics and health technocrats that sparked new relationships and new lines of critique and action. During a period of intense Cold War geopolitics and rising political repression, García found a way to work within existing institutions, building what was widely accepted as expertise in the health-related social sciences, in order to question, critique, and reorient these institutions ideologically.

García was raised in Necochea, a small town in the province of Buenos Aires, in humble circumstances. He enrolled at the National University of La Plata in 1950 to study pediatric medicine. As with Gandulfo, Allende, Lazarte, and many other prominent figures in social medicine, García became active in university politics, at a time when Argentina's public universities were drawn into the conflict between Peronists and their adversaries. Perón's administration abrogated many of the university reforms of 1918—which had given the universities substantial autonomy, increased student input in decision making, and promoted academic freedom—and instead sought to incorporate the universities into the Peronist patronage system.[11] As a member of several student activist groups, García was an outspoken opponent of Perón and an avid defender of university autonomy. Meanwhile, García did health work in the rural areas of Buenos Aires province and took an interest in journalistic writing and the social sciences.

A scholarship for graduate study in Chile launched García on a trajectory as an international health bureaucrat. As explained in chapter 5, Santiago, as the home of CEPAL, FLACSO, CELADE, and the Escuela de Salud Pública, was something of a central place in the application of "modern" social sciences to the problems of development during the 1960s. Paulo Freire, who wrote the *Pedagogy of the Oppressed* in Santiago while in exile from Brazil in the late 1960s, later recalled: "Santiago was, in itself, at that time, the best center of 'learning' and knowledge in Latin America. We learned of analyses, reactions, and criticisms by Colombians, Venezuelans, Cubans, Mexicans, Bolivians, Argentineans, Paraguayans, Brazilians, Chileans, and Europeans—analyses ranging from an almost unrestricted acceptance of Christian Democracy to its total rejection. There were sectarian, intolerant criticisms, but also open, radical criticisms in the sense that I advocate."[12] Similarly, Mario Testa recalled that health planners, economists, sociologists, and other social scientists had a rich and continuous exchange of ideas in and around CEPAL.[13] García was part of this cosmopolitan milieu, as a student at the Escuela Latinoamericana de Sociología, within FLACSO, from 1960 to 1962. According to his later reflections on the experience, he received the most advanced education in the social sciences available in Latin America at the time, as part of an effort to build a "critical mass" internationally in the health social sciences for application to modernization projects, though he came to question the school's strong positivist and functionalist bent.[14] His own thesis project focused on the authoritarian character of the doctor-patient relationship. This academic background prepared him well for a position in the department of Human Resources at the PAHO, which served primarily to improve education and training for doctors and other health workers across the region. García started at the PAHO in 1966 and worked there until the end of his life, traveling extensively but returning to Argentina only for short visits.

At the PAHO, García developed his intellectual theory of social medicine while constructing and congealing networks of scholars in the social sciences of health. His official, technical research related to medical education, including an exhaustive survey of medical schools in the Americas that was published in 1972.[15] This project, funded in part by the Milbank and Rockefeller Foundations, was intended primarily to take stock of progress in the teaching of preventive medicine. García crisscrossed the Western hemisphere, developed a huge network of expert correspondents, and used these connections to his advantage.[16] García visited around one hundred different schools of medicine while conducting the research for his 1972 report, surely encompassing the vast majority of medical schools in the region at the time.[17] This report—effectively García's first major published work—departed significantly from the narrow agenda of assessing education in preventive medicine. Rather, García took a different angle and launched a structural critique of university medical schools as centers of power, specifically with the power to reproduce the dominant ideologies of medical care in a given country.[18] His goal was more than program evaluation—he wanted to make medical education a means of social transformation. In this way, García was also channeling the energy of the politically charged student movements that sprang up in places like Paris and Mexico City in 1968.[19] Nevertheless, his political agenda was not conspicuous and he focused more on raising the profile of the social sciences within medical education, going beyond the instrumental use of social scientists to conduct surveys for ends predetermined by health officials, to offer the language and methods of rigorous and reflexive critique of the workings of the health field in general.[20]

Through his official work for the PAHO, García began to organize a network of scholars and health workers interested in developing cutting-edge social science research to be applied to the health field. One strategy for building networks was to "develop seminars in various countries with local groups, which meant the only cost was Juan César's travels."[21] Such events were ancillary to his main, official objective, which was to gather information about medical education, but García used these seminars to exchange scholarly materials, in the form of books and mimeographs, and to discuss new theories and methods.[22] A nucleus of key supporters took shape, starting with a meeting of experts in medical education in Cuenca, Ecuador, in May 1972, which is frequently cited as a formative episode in the new so-cial medicine. Participants included Hugo Mercer, a young public health researcher from Argentina who worked with García at the PAHO; Eve-rardo Duarte Nunes of Brazil, who would become a chronicler of Latin American social medicine; Hesio Cordeiro, also of Brazil, who would later lead ABRASCO, a civil society organization that spurred health system reform in Brazil; Miguel Márquez, an Ecuadoran professor of medicine and PAHO consultant; and Claudio Jimeno, a Chilean sociologist who had collaborated with Gustavo Molina on integrating preventive medicine into the clinical set-ting of San Borja Hospital in the 1960s (an Allende loyalist, Jimeno would be disappeared in the military coup of September 1973).[23] One important result of this meeting was the adoption of a concrete definition of social medicine, which had four components: a concern with the social character of illness, advocacy for the role of the state in addressing the causes of illness, the possibility for quantitative (or systematic) analysis of these problems, and the "combative and revolutionary character of the project."[24]

As this small research network grew, and with García offering support from inside the PAHO, the second wave of Latin American social medicine took shape, with new programs and efforts at institutional permanence. For the next ten years, García sought to advance his vision of an education in so-cial medicine, critical of conventional approaches and increasingly defiant of the US-led modernization agenda. As Márquez put it, while some chose to follow García on his mission of how to analyze and transform the systems of medical education in Latin America, others "returned to their ideological po-sitions, defending the status quo of the university, and the conventional wis-dom in medical education derived from the Flexner Report and the American school of thought."[25] Through his influence, García found positions in the PAHO for health workers in exile from authoritarian governments, like María Isabel Rodríguez of El Salvador.[26] García also helped obtain funding for two new masters' programs for social medicine: one in Mexico, at UAM-Xochimilco, in 1974, and the other in Brazil, at the Universidade do Estado do Rio de Janeiro (UERJ; State University of Rio de Janeiro), in 1973. The latter, in addition to PAHO funding, also received "technical and financial support" from the W. K. Kellogg Foundation.[27]

The choice of UAM-Xochimilco for a social medicine program had a lot to do with Ramón Villarreal, the first rector of the new university, created in response to the student protests in Mexico City in 1968. As García's colleague and predecessor as the head of human resources and medical education at the PAHO, Villarreal prioritized innovative research in the health field. The master's program in social medicine had a notably international corps of faculty. Hugo Mercer of Argentina, who had been part of García's seminar in Cuenca in 1972 and worked under Villarreal at the PAHO for a time, became the program's founding director. Once settled in Xochimilco, Mercer invited José Carlos Escudero and Clara Fassler (in exile from authoritarian governments in Argentina and Chile, respectively) to join as instructors, along with Asa Cristina Laurell, originally from Sweden, who would have a profound influence on Latin American social medicine, both as an academic field and a political project.[28] In 1976, Catalina Eibenschutz, a Mexican endocrinologist with years of experience in health work in communist Cuba, joined the program. To showcase their work, the faculty behind the Xochimilco master's program launched the enduring journal *Salud Problema* in 1978. Meanwhile, the journal *Educación Médica y Salud*, published by the PAHO and edited for many years by Carlos Vidal of Peru, continued to serve as a vehicle of diffusion for the new social medicine.[29] It published many of García's own critical studies, along with articles by Michel Foucault (on the history of medicalization, adapted from lectures he gave in Rio de Janeiro in 1974) and Miguel Márquez and Sérgio Arouca (on Foucault's "archaeology" of science approach), to name just a few.[30] Surely, none of the PAHO's journals delved as deeply into social theory as *Educación Médica y Salud*.

As a scholar, García introduced current social science theory to the study of the medical profession and health systems planning. Principally, he questioned and then rejected the "functionalist" premise that dominated sociology (and other social sciences) in Latin America at the time. Instead, García advanced an explicitly structural Marxist approach. From this perspective, the organization of medicine was a reflection of a given mode of production; medicine was neither functionally autonomous from the rest of society nor ideologically neutral.[31] García had diverse intellectual influences, which only proliferated over the span of his career, but his focus on economic structure, social relations, and medicine drew most immediately on the work of Jean-Claude Polack, now a somewhat forgotten figure in French philosophy, who wrote the book *La médecine du capital* in 1971; Bernhard Stern, an American sociologist, who supplied key elements of the historical materialist approach; and Louis Althusser, whose concept of "relative autonomy" helped García explain how medicine was only loosely determined by economic structure and why it had authority in society.[32] He even recommended, in a memo to his PAHO colleagues and outside collaborators, a reading of David Harvey's *Social Justice and the City*—in the same year it was published, 1973—calling the pioneering Marxist geographer's work a means to "travel roads that are different from the functionalist 'highways.'"[33] Drawing on the work of Henry Sigerist, García also explored the history of social medicine, locating the origins of the concept in the European revolutions of 1848 while mostly ignoring social medicine's first wave in Latin America.[34]

García grew increasingly critical of the field of preventive medicine, which was often the principal means to introduce doctors in training to the social sciences (or "behavioral sciences," the ostensibly more neutral term preferred by PAHO). As we have seen, preventive medicine emerged as a more centrist and pragmatic alternative to social medicine in Chile and Argentina in the 1930s and 1940s, as championed by Eduardo Cruz-Coke, Ramón Carrillo, and others. At the start of García's five-year survey of Latin American medical schools, the PAHO expert commission that he led mostly confirmed recommendations of prior international conferences on preventive medicine (including those in Colorado Springs, France, and England in 1952–53, and seminars in Viña del Mar, Chile, and Tehuacán, Mexico, a few years later), while suggesting a pluralistic approach in which each Latin American university would design its own course of preventive medicine according to national needs. In this context, doctors were viewed as leaders in their society, aiding in the process of national development, by studying, managing, and correcting public attitudes and practices, using accepted techniques grounded in epidemiology and biostatistics.[35]

By 1974, this PAHO commission, consisting of many new members, with García the one constant, had changed its tune. Perhaps cognizant of the conservative turn of the medical profession in countries like Argentina and Chile, the commission questioned whether doctors were actually "agents of change" in society, and, taking care to define the proper "object of study" for social medicine, adopted a completely different angle. Whereas preventive medicine had perpetuated the medical gaze—the doctor examining the patient—the new social medicine's object of study was, increasingly, *the field of medicine itself*—its institutions, their historically contingent nature, their place in the structure of society, and medicine's role in reproducing structures of domination and hierarchy.[36]

The Chilean Exiles

The overthrow of Salvador Allende in September 1973 had enormous consequences in Chile and across the region. Within Chile, the coup d'état led to a rollback of the progressive health policies introduced during the Allende government, although some of the more permanent and substantial reforms to the health system under neoliberal principles would not happen until the late 1970s and early 1980s. Doctors and other health workers affiliated with the Unidad Popular (UP) government, along with many other leftist intellectuals and activists, were jailed, tortured, or killed by the new regime. Crucially for Latin American social medicine, some of the most notable Chilean public health leaders fled the country, taking exile in places all over the world, assisted by ad hoc networks and sympathetic academic institutions, and in many cases, joining exiled health workers from other countries, especially Argentina, which was experiencing political turmoil of its own.[37] For many involved in these networks—the exiles and their supporters—the Chilean coup and its bloody aftermath suggested that promoters of social justice and a right to health could not stay politically neutral. And for those who were still able to speak openly, the Chilean coup validated and magnified a key assumption of leftist social medicine: health systems were not just technical and scientific endeavors; they were a reflection, for better or for worse, of the political-economic conditions of the larger societies in which they were embedded.

As explained in chapter 5, health politics in Chile had become increasingly conflict-ridden in the late 1960s. Although the SNS had continued to grow and the Escuela de Salud Pública in Santiago was considered the best in Latin America, the health system remained fragmented, the private sector was absorbing an increasing level of the demand for medical services, and the medical profession itself became more conservative. Before assuming the presidency in 1970, Allende crafted a plan for health sector reforms that included further centralization or unification of government medical services, democratization of health services through community initiatives, and a shift in priority toward preventive or primary health services.[38] In addition, Allende's policies were meant to improve public health by making changes not just in the health sector, but in the entire national political-economic structure.

Forces within and external to Allende's administration, however, worked against the realization of a bold plan for health.[39] In the UP coalition government, responsibility for health policy planning was divided up mainly among members of the Communist, Socialist, and Radical Parties, and the communists advocated a "go-slow" strategy that hinged on executing specific projects to gain a larger share of public support before launching major health system reform initiatives.[40] According to Carlos Montoya Aguilar, whom I interviewed in 2016, the UP leadership chose to emphasize a short list of policies that made for popular slogans, such as the guarantee of "half a liter of milk for every child," a program devised by Juan Carlos Concha, then the minister of health.[41] This program did prove to be popular, but it was a massive undertaking. Carlos Molina Bustos recalled the scope of the milk campaign that he helped organize: "the calculations, the importation, the unloading on the docks, the storage, the transport, in which ports, in which warehouses ... constructing new warehouses ... controlling the rats in the warehouses. ... It was like a wartime operation."[42] According to UP government calculations, Chile required 48 million kilos of milk per year to meet the needs of every child in the country, but produced only 12 million kilos domestically at the time. Thanks mostly to imports of powdered milk from Australia, New Zealand, and the Netherlands, Chile was meeting its supply goals only 40 days after the program had begun, an early moment of success for the new UP government.

Allende enjoyed the loyal support of a (mostly) young group of health workers, who saw themselves at the center of a political revolution. But when the coup arrived, most of the medical profession had already turned against Allende. The Colegio Médico decided to expel Allende—one of its founders—in 1972, as it allied with reactionary forces in Chilean society. In August 1973, the medical association organized a physician's strike to demand Allende's resignation.[43] And leaders of the Colegio Médico sent a congratulatory telegram to Augusto Pinochet following the coup, according to Vicente Navarro, a Catalonian physician and sociologist who served as a health policy consultant with the UP government.[44] In testimony to the US Congress, a delegation sponsored by the Federation of American Scientists found it "probable" that the Colegio Médico of Chile was "involved in preparing lists of physicians considered not only dangerous but also politically unacceptable" for the Pinochet regime.[45] In the days and weeks after the coup, health workers and students, many affiliated with the Ministry of Health, the Medical School of the University of Chile, or the School of Public Health, were rounded up, sometimes tortured or summarily executed, sometimes placed in jail for a longer period of time.[46] For his activity with the Movimiento de Acción Popular Unitaria (MAPU, a smaller party in the UP coalition), Giorgio Solimano was jailed (and tortured) for six months at the notorious Tejas Verdes prison camp near the port city of San Antonio, and then transferred to a detention center designated for health workers, on a property owned by the SNS, in downtown Santiago (at the corner of Agustinas and MacIver).[47] After a show trial, he was released and he went into exile in the United States. Solimano was relatively fortunate; many health workers lost their lives, and over one hundred medical students at the University of Chile were killed or disappeared by Pinochet's government.

Starting in 1973, and for several years after, progressive Chilean doctors fled their country, relying on personal connections, professional networks, and the benevolence of ad hoc aid groups to survive in exile. The military government facilitated exile for its own ends, expelling around 4,000 Chileans, and another 3,500 or so sought refuge through embassy asylum.[48] The exact number of those in the health sector who were exiled is unclear, and may never be known, but table 1 offers a list of some of the higher-level or better-known health workers who went into exile from Chile after the 1973 coup. They were aided by organizations such as the UN High Commissioner for Refugees or the International Red Cross, as well as personal contacts and ad hoc organizations set up specifically for Chilean exiles from the health sector. With the help of sympathetic American doctors like Victor Sidel and Martin Cherkasky of Montefiore Hospital in the Bronx, and Jack Geiger of the American Public Health Association, Roberto Belmar created the Emergency Committee to Help the Chilean Health Workers. To publicize what was happening in Chile, the group took out a full-page advertisement in the *New York Times* in April 1974.[49] A related group, the American Public Health Association (APHA) Task Force on Chile, became active in 1974 and continued to investigate the conditions of health workers and the health system in Chile, at least until the end of that decade.

In their diaspora, Chilean health workers and their families started new lives across the Americas and beyond. Belmar was placed in the Department of Social Medicine of Montefiore, where he spent most of his American career before returning to Chile after the end of Pinochet's regime. Solimano, like many other Chilean academics in exile, was aided by a scholarship from the Ford Foundation, and found a place at MIT (and later Columbia University) where he did research on nutrition and development issues with Peter Hakim.[50] Carlos Montoya Aguilar, the health systems planner, appealed to Abraham Horwitz for help; Horwitz (who, as we have seen, was politically conservative and tried to steer the PAHO clear of geopolitical tensions) could not offer Montoya a place at the PAHO but pulled strings to find him a role in health planning at the WHO in Geneva.[51] Horwitz failed to help Claudio Sepúlveda, who was finishing out a consulting contract with the PAHO in Lima, Peru, when the coup occurred—apparently, because Horwitz was trying to maintain the support of Peru's military government in his upcoming race for reelection to head the PAHO, he did not want to help an Allende ally (Horwitz won their support, but lost the election anyway).[52] Instead, Sepúlveda made his way to Paris, where he found his mentor, Hernán San Martín, an iconoclastic anthropologist and public health expert from Con-

TABLE 1 Partial list of Chilean health professionals in exile
after the overthrow of Allende

Name	Position during Unidad Popular government	Place of exile and activities there
Hugo Behm Rosas	Director, School of Public Health, University of Chile	Costa Rica: researcher affiliated with CELADE
Roberto Belmar	Primary Health Care program; School of Public Health	United States: Montefiore Medical Center, Department of Social Medicine (worked with Victor Sidel)
Juan Carlos Concha	Minister of health	Germany
Victorino Farga Cuesta	Director, National Institute of Pneumonology	United States and Spain: tuberculosis expert
Clara Fassler	General practitioner; Department of Social and Preventive Medicine, University of Chile	Mexico: Master's in social medicine, UAM-Xochimilco; Uruguay: mental health, gender, and health
Alfredo Jadresic	Dean of Medical School, University of Chile	England: NHS and University of London
Arturo Jirón Vargas	Minister of health	Venezuela: instructor at Universidad Central de Venezuela
Patricio Hevia Rivas	Health Promotion Program, Ministry of Health	Mexico
Pablo López Rojas	Hospital San Juan de Dios	Germany
María Isabel Matamala	Pediatrician, Children's Health Program and member of Movimiento de Izquierda Revolucionaria (MIR)	Various, including Uruguay: Women's Health Movement, Red de Salud de las Mujeres Latinoamericanas y del Caribe
Carlos Matus	Minister of economy	Venezuela: CENDES (worked with Mario Testa)

(continued)

TABLE 1 (*continued*)

Name	Position during Unidad Popular government	Place of exile and activities there
Carlos Molina Bustos	Subsecretary, Ministry of Health	Mexico: Instituto Mexicano de Seguridad Social
Gustavo Molina Guzmán	Zonal director, National Health Service	Colombia: National School of Public Health, Medellín, Antioquia
Carlos Montoya Aguilar	School of Public Health, University of Chile	Switzerland: WHO, Health Planning
Hernán San Martín	Ambassador to Zambia (previously, University of Concepción)	France: Université de Paris I, Sorbonne (Institute of Economic and Social Development)
Claudio Schuftan	Pediatrics, Hospital Arriarán, Santiago	United States: Tulane University; Vietnam: People's Health Movement
Claudio Sepúlveda Alvarez	Head of Planning and Budgets, National Health Service and Ministry of Health	Various (mainly Asia and Latin America): UNICEF
Jaime Sepúlveda Salinas	Pediatrician, and director of Consultorio Renca in Santiago	Costa Rica: Central American Program in Social Sciences, *Revista Centroamericana de Ciencias de la Salud*
Jaime Serra Canales	School of Public Health, University of Chile and Hospital Félix Bulnes	Costa Rica: Hospital Sin Paredes, Alajuela
Giorgio Solimano Canutarias	Nutrition Department, National Health Service	United States: MIT and Columbia University

Source: Pieper Mooney, "From Cold War Pressures"; Sepúlveda Alvarez, *De hombres y sombras;* author interviews with Molina Bustos, Montoya Aguilar, Sepúlveda Alvarez, Sepúlveda Salinas, and Solimano; among others.

cepción, who happened to be the Allende government's ambassador in Zambia at the time of the coup.[53] Eventually, Claudio Sepúlveda spent two decades working for UNICEF, in posts mainly in Asia.[54]

While some of the Chilean doctors in exile continued to work inconspicuously in their specialties in new institutions, others intensified their involvement with leftist movements, including the new wave of Latin American social medicine. Gustavo Molina Guzmán was a veteran of Chilean public health, with decades of international activity, before his exile to Colombia. He joined Allende in the Vanguardia Médica in the 1930s; subsequently attended Johns Hopkins University, where he became an avid follower of Sigerist, the medical historian; became a founding member of the faculty at the Escuela de Salud Pública (based on the Johns Hopkins model) in the 1940s; and, with Benjamín Viel, developed community-based health services under a preventive medicine model in the Quinta Normal district of Santiago.[55] He also worked for several years for the PAHO, in the offices of Professional Education and Public Health, during the 1960s. He was directing a regional office of the Chilean SNS when the coup occurred, and, like Solimano and many others, was jailed at Tejas Verdes and the detention center on Agustinas Street. In 1974, Molina was able to flee to Medellín, Colombia. There, he collaborated with Héctor Abad Gómez, the founder of the National School of Public Health, to develop a program called Integración Operacional de Abajo hacia Arriba (IOPAA), a community health project that benefited from Molina's prior experience in Quinta Normal.[56] (Abad Gómez would be assassinated in 1987 by right-wing paramilitaries in Medellín.) While in military custody in Chile, Molina had begun translating Sigerist's work into Spanish, drawing on Milton Terris's compilations of his essays, which Molina published during his time in Colombia.[57] Molina became an outspoken critic of the new Chilean government and its health policies and of US foreign policy. In a speech to the American Public Health Association in 1976, he decried the Alliance for Progress and its health program, calling it the "inspired delusion of President Kennedy"; he continued, "You cannot buy health with the counterfeit money of social security or of the magic national health services operating in a social vacuum. In Latin America, a decade after the Alliance for Progress was launched, the most common health indicators in every nation, except Cuba, either did not change or worsened."[58] He planned to present the IOPAA project at the 1978 Alma Ata conference (known as the birthplace of the Primary Health Care model), but he died of a brain tumor, just weeks before the meeting.

Other Chilean exiles dispersed across the globe and became a part of what have been called "south–south solidarity" networks.[59] Jaime Sepúlveda found a place at the Programa de Ciencias de Salud in Costa Rica, under the auspices of the Confederación Universitaria Centroamericana, which also included schools in Guatemala, Nicaragua, Honduras, and Panama. There, along with a growing team of health planners and social scientists, he grew more critical of the "community medicine" model, sizing it up as merely an accommodation by the medical field to the exigencies of capitalist development, a "second-class" medicine for poor communities. He also began to question the doctor's role as an authority figure, calling instead for more democratic forms of community development.[60] He aired these ideas in the journal that he founded in 1975, the *Revista Centroamericana de Ciencias de Salud*, which published early Spanish translations of Foucault's essays, including "The Birth of Social Medicine," based on a lecture series in Rio de Janeiro in 1974.[61] Hugo Behm Rosas—a widely respected biostatistician, director of the Escuela de Salud Pública in Santiago, and the founder of the journal *Cuadernos Médico Sociales*—also landed in Costa Rica after being held prisoner in Chile for two years after the coup, thanks to the intervention of the APHA group.[62] As a consultant for CELADE, the demographic research center, Behm continued to focus on the social determinants of mortality (especially among infants), bringing a high level of quantitative rigor to the field of social medicine.[63] He died in Costa Rica in 2011. Claudio Schuftan went into exile in 1974, also spending time at MIT working on health and nutrition issues. Eventually, he would become a driving force behind the international People's Health Movement and serve as a consultant in over fifty countries, with long-term stints in Vietnam and Kenya, and as a major advocate for human rights and primary health care.[64] Another group of exiled health planners from the UP government went to Mozambique, and helped establish the health program of its newly independent, communist government after 1975.[65]

Despite their impressive international reach, the Chilean exiles were mostly powerless to affect events back home. In Chile, the conservative counterreaction was fierce and introduced radical reforms to the health sector and the welfare state. Pinochet's government, as we know, became a laboratory for neoliberal reforms under the direction of "the Chicago Boys," a group of Chilean economists trained at the University of Chicago. Although there were some public health achievements during the Pinochet regime, including a notable decline in childhood malnutrition and progress against tuberculosis, the overall effect was to undo the health system that had been crafted over the previous six decades. State investment in the health sector dropped precipitously, and particularly with a series of reform decrees between 1979 and 1985, a free-market orientation was imposed on the health system. Most of the Chilean doctors in exile avoided published commentary on health policy under the Pinochet regime, although Clara Fassler denounced it in the *Revista Latinoamericana de Salud,* published in Mexico.[66] A few people, like Gilda Gnecco, who worked alongside Benjamin Viel in the Quinta Normal community health project, stayed in Chile and worked covertly to maintain solidarity networks in opposition to the dictatorship.[67]

For those involved in the rising new wave of social medicine across the region, events in Chile confirmed their intuitions and reinforced their world-view. In retrospect, the aborted Project Camelot of the early 1960s had presaged the use of counterinsurgency techniques to move Chilean public opinion against Allende's government. Suspicions that the US government, through the CIA or the military, pulled the strings of supposedly neutral social science research now seemed totally plausible. In any case, the techno-cratic institutions of international development mostly stood by and watched the coup and the repression that followed. After the coup, Navarro observed that Allende's analysis of the workings of international political economy was essentially correct. In his view, Allende's demise was a result of the alliance of national and international elites, defending class interests. The geopolitical real-ity of imperialism and dependency was not just a backdrop for national politics, but was integral to it.[68] The medical profession, representing the national elite, the lumpenbourgeoisie, resented the Allende administration's assault on their class privileges and professional prerogatives; as Belmar and Sidel wrote in 1975 (in Navarro's journal, *International Journal of Health Services*), the "Colegio Médico believed that community participation, the democratization of the health system, and the health team approach would lower the prestige of the physician in society."[69] A slow rollout of health reforms, an example of what Navarro called Allende's gradualist approach in all things, left time for the medi-cal profession to mount a resistance and help sabotage reform efforts. The broader lesson was that the Chilean medical profession was antidemocratic and a force for the status quo, using its scientific and professional authority to de-fend class privileges. The Chilean coup, to Navarro and others, vividly rein-forced a central line of argument in social medicine: "We cannot understand the maldistribution of resources in the health sector without analyzing the dis-tribution of economic and political power in these societies, i.e., the question of who controls what and whom, or what usually is referred to in political econ-omy as who controls the means of production and reproduction."[70] It was im-possible now, for doctors and health planners of good conscience, not to take a side in the great ideological battles of the day.

The Argentina Group

In Chile the change of political regime was punctuated by a single turning point, the overthrow of Allende. Argentina, by contrast, was marked by political chaos and a gradual disintegration of civil society from the late 1960s into the mid-1970s. With so many changes of leadership and realignments of political forces, it was a confusing time. The health sector became increasingly politicized, with inexpert ministers and other upper-level administrators appointed purely for partisan reasons, changing policy direction unexpectedly and using government agencies for unintended purposes. From 1973 to 1975, José López Rega—the shadowy, ultra-right-wing adviser to Juan D. Perón during his second presidency, and to his wife Isabel when she succeeded him—ran the notorious "AAA" death squads from his position as minister of social welfare, that is, while he was in command of the country's health system.[71] Although this is a somewhat extreme example, the notion of an apolitical health bureaucracy became completely untenable during that period.

The sanitaristas of Argentina employed various strategies to cope with these disorienting and violent times. As Mario Hamilton described it, some concentrated even more intensely on the technical aspects of health planning, hoping to create "a sort of technocratic island without political-ideological persecution."[72] Everyone had to rely on their friends and social networks, to provide intelligence, warnings, and a way out of difficult situations. As a result of these associations, no one could really avoid politics, and many doctors and health workers who considered themselves apolitical were drawn into unforeseen conflicts (often within the Peronist ranks). Even before the worst of the state violence and persecution began in 1976, many of the best health workers in Argentina used their connections, sometimes established through previous consulting work with the PAHO, to make their escape to other countries. Brazil was a favored destination, not least because its shared border with Argentina facilitated contact with loved ones during exile, and other health workers ended up in places like Mexico, Venezuela, and Switzerland.

Mario Testa illustrates, as well as anyone, that the new social medicine was a product of disillusioned experts who realized that international health planning bureaucracies had gone off the rails, constructing an unrealistic view of how the world worked and failing on their own terms, with scant improvement in population health.[73] Testa's life story also shows that, for some, exile could be a productive experience; it could offer safety, security, critical distance from national problems, and opportunities for learning with like-minded colleagues across the continent. In any case, Testa led the nomadic life of an international health technocrat. As discussed in chapter 5, after starting his career in Argentina, Testa moved into the OPS/CENDES project, a massive health planning endeavor, based in Caracas and Santiago. This project trained hundreds of Latin Americans, mostly from ministries of health, in the intricacies of national health planning. Returning to Argentina in the early 1970s, he became the dean of the Facultad de Medicina at the University of Buenos Aires, during Perón's second, ill-fated regime. Aligned with the Peronist left wing, Testa became embroiled in internecine political conflicts at the school and resigned his post after about a year.

Testa and his family were living in Europe when the March 1976 coup d'état occurred—the beginnings of the notorious Proceso—and he decided to go to Rio de Janeiro, as a lecturer at the UERJ, thanks to an invitation from Hesio Cordeiro, while his family returned to Buenos Aires. The following year, their apartment in the Barrio Norte was fired upon, and the assailants (probably paramilitaries or secret police) entered and ransacked their home, destroying much of Testa's library in the process. Fortunately, the family was unharmed, as they had been moving between friends' apartments, fearing violence.[74] Soon they reunited with Testa in Brazil. As Testa recalled, he had "packed a suitcase for fifteen days [in Brazil] and ended up spending seven years [abroad]." This exile was spent mainly in Brazil with the nascent saúde coletiva group; Venezuela, where they had lived for several years in the 1960s, and which had become a home for many exiles from Allende's Chile, including Carlos Matus and Darío Pavez, economic planners he knew from the OPS/CENDES days; and Mexico, where he taught at the UAM-Xochimilco at the behest of Catalina Eibenschutz. In 1984, he became one of the cofounders of ALAMES, and the following year he returned, at age sixty, to Argentina, more or less permanently.[75]

While working with OPS/CENDES, Testa had initiated the kinds of intellectual engagements that made him a key figure in Latin American social medicine, and his time in exile, for better or for worse, gave him the critical distance he needed to analyze the shortcomings of the health planning apparatus he was embedded in. On his own, he studied economics, political theory, and sociology, while disregarding much of the literature in mainstream public health. He shared García's perspective that "you can't think about health just from inside the health system, you have to go outside of it, to other places." Early in this long period of "reflection," much of which was encapsulated in his book *Pensar en Salud* (Thinking about Health), Testa realized the futility of the OPS/CENDES approach.[76] Typically, a national ministry of health would use the method to set goals for the health sector, fail to meet those goals, and then use the same method to write a new national health plan. Built on the functionalist foundations of scholars like David Easton, the model presented a complex and rigorous approach for solving simple problems, but failed to consider the dynamic social and economic conditions of a given society. In OPS/CENDES, he told me, "We didn't understand anything about how things really worked." Their key conceptual error was to assume that health planning could take place in a politically neutral arena, with political leaders merely executing rationally conceived plans. Testa decided that epidemiology and other quantitative techniques could not resolve social conflicts, "which could only be resolved through politics" (here, Testa echoed his fellow Peronist health leader, Floreal Ferrara, discussed in chapter 5). Moreover, the functionalist models were ill-suited to the conditions of less developed countries. As he told me, "Except for a brief time, I never lived the American life. As I say, I am an 'underdeveloped thinker' [*pensador subdesarrollado*], I think from underdevelopment, I think from here. So, I know how the problems are in [conditions of] underdevelopment, I do not know what it's like to live in a developed country, I do not know it deeply."[77] This positionality as a thinker from the Global South led Testa to reject universal models unequivocally: "First you have to think about the history that you are stuck in" and "to understand the problems you have, you have to be in the environment that includes you, in many different ways: objectively, subjectively, that is, what shapes your own culture, you own way of being and thinking."[78] But due to his travels, voluntary or coerced, Testa's culture transcended that of any one nation—he was a *Latin American* above all else.

During his exile, Testa stayed in close contact with a small but consequential group of scholars in Rosario, Argentina, including Carlos Bloch, who followed in the footsteps of Juan Lazarte (see chapter 4, in particular). A doctor from Rosario, Bloch became involved in gremialismo during the 1960s, through the auspices of the Federación Médica de Santa Fe and the COMRA.[79] During the Proceso, Bloch was driven from his position as a doctor at a provincial hospital due to his leftist views, and joined the CESS of the Asociación Médica de Rosario, a precursor of the present-day Instituto Juan Lazarte in Rosario, in 1978.[80] Bloch was joined by Susana Belmartino, a sociologist and historian who was forced to resign her position at the National University of Rosario under political pressure, and together they founded the journal *Cuadernos Médico Sociales*, a critical health studies journal, independent from, but inspired by its namesake journal in Chile. Later on, Bloch and Belmartino would collaborate with Testa on portions of his book, *Pensar en Salud*.[81]

Belmartino was trained in social sciences and had never worked in the health sector, not even as part of the interdisciplinary community health project "teams" that had become more common in the 1960s (for example, to support family planning interventions). Her generation of sociologists introduced new lines of social theory and operated with a critical distance on the health professions. Belmartino, similar to Vicente Navarro, approached the medical profession from the perspective of Marxist historical materialism, with a focus on doctors as a class of labor within an expanding capitalist economy. Over time, Belmartino adopted an approach based more on regulation theory in sociology to understand the historical development of the health sector in Argentina.[82] Historically, doctors in Argentina sought to represent their interests, differentiate themselves as a class, increase their legitimate authority in society as a whole, gain the upper hand in negotiations and conflicts, and exercise control over the "rules of the game" governing the health sector. This perspective on the health sector—as *self-interested, politically engaged, seeking power*—was not altogether new, but it certainly ran against the grain of the self-image of the medical profession.[83]

The political activities of this group of scholars were conditioned by the intense authoritarianism of the period. Bloch followed Lazarte's path as a gremialista; the CESS was funded and sponsored by the Asociación Médica de Rosario, which experienced a period of growth and stability in the 1970s. The affiliation with the association also offered the CESS some protection from suspicion by the military authorities. While there were surely leftists within the association, it was not seen, on the whole, as a left-wing organization, and certainly not part of the armed, militant left, since it focused its political energy on defending the interests of the medical profession.[84] To avoid retaliation, members of the CESS sometimes took the precaution of writing under pseudonyms: for one article published in the *Revista Centroamericana de Ciencias de la Salud*, Bloch and Belmartino took on the names Carlos Alarcón and Susana Balmaceda, and Testa wrote under the name Paulo Alexandre for the *Cuadernos Médico Sociales* of Rosario.[85] Fear of persecution or state violence was well-founded. Maria del Carmen Troncoso, another founding member of the CESS, was driven out of her position as dean of the School of Medicine at the Universidad Nacional del Litoral (in Rosario), and went into exile, working as a consultant for the PAHO in their Department of Human Resources, probably with the assistance of Juan César García.[86] Another associate of the CESS, Eduardo Menéndez Spina, fled to Mexico during the Proceso and stayed there, focusing his anthropological research on the relationship between patients and doctors in capitalist societies, which he termed the *modelo médico hegemónico*, or hegemonic medical model; he also cofounded the short-lived *Revista Latinoamericana de Salud* along with Laurell, Escudero, Eibenschutz, and Mercer.[87]

In comparison with the saúde coletiva movement in Brazil, the Argentines in the new social medicine took longer to congeal as a group with a focused agenda and institutions at the national level. Via the *Cuadernos Médico Sociales*, the CESS projected itself more strongly abroad than within Argentina; other schools of medicine and public health in Argentina showed little interest in their work, and the severe repressions of the military government made communication and associational life a challenge.[88] Even with the restoration of democracy, schools of public health in Argentina continued to be dominated by the technocratic modernizationist paradigm, marginalizing people like Mario Testa and obligating them to make international connections to nurture the growing field of social medicine.[89]

Brazil and the Rise of Collective Health

The saúde coletiva or collective health movement was naturally opposed to the Brazilian military regime, the same one that had exiled Josué de Castro and so many other leftist thinkers and political figures. However, in comparison with Chile and Argentina around the same time, in Brazil there were more opportunities for progressive health workers and social scientists to find or develop the spaces for their intellectual and political work. As Carlos Nelson Coutinho, the influential Brazilian Marxist political thinker, explained, Brazil's military government was a "classic example" of the sort of "modernizing and non-fascist dictatorial regimes" that "present a fundamental contradiction: they unleash forces which, in the medium term, they can no longer control, or, in more precise terms, develop the foundations of a civil society that is increasingly beyond its control."[90] After 1967, Brazil's military leaders constructed a "technocratic-military" regime.[91] As time went on, the government became more permissive and tried to orchestrate a transition back to democracy. During the period of the Brazilian "economic miracle" (around 1964–73), much of the public had tolerated crackdowns on political expression in exchange for rapid economic growth, but a prolonged recession put that political bargain into question.[92] Under the government of General Geisel, from 1974 to 1979, there was a political "détente" that included financing of social research within the national development plan. The subsequent government of General João Baptista de Oliveira Figueiredo, from 1979, hastened a transition to democracy, with some political liberties restored (greater freedom of the press, habeas corpus, legalization of multiple political parties), even as the regime's leaders provided for their own amnesty from future prosecution.[93]

Throughout the 1970s, the key figures of the growing saúde coletiva movement carried on their activities, sometimes clandestinely, at times more openly, and cautiously exploited political openings when they presented themselves. Their debates, conferences, and lectures, mostly within the confines of academic institutions, eluded the detection of the military leaders (or, possibly, failed to capture their interest). Living under a military regime sharpened the group's critical portrayal of medicine as an institution of discipline, punishment, and social control. This perspective was informed by influences from abroad, such as the pioneering work of Michel Foucault (in books like *Discipline and Punish* or *The Birth of the Clinic*, which found a receptive audience in Brazilian academia); the Italian mental health reform movement led by Franco Basaglia in the 1960s; and the critical humanism of Ivan Illich, the firebrand priest based in Cuernavaca, Mexico.[94] Albeit an ideologically complex field, saúde coletiva had less a socialist agenda than a liberationist one, with an eye toward a radical restructuring and democratization of power relations in the health field.

As Brazil's authoritarian regime pursued political decentralization, saúde coletiva could thrive in municipalities where progressive ideas were tolerated. One of the best examples was a community health project in Montes Claros, in the state of Minas Gerais, which became a virtual "laboratory for the democratization of health."[95] Initiated in 1975 under the direction of Francisco de Assis Machado—widely known as Chicão—along with Arouca, Testa, and Eugenio Vilaça, the project was funded in part by USAID. Hamilton joined the group in 1976, having fled Argentina for Brazil under the protection of Carlyle Guerra Macedo, an established PAHO technocrat who also worked with Juan César García. Hamilton brought needed expertise in epidemiology, statistics, planning, and modeling, which he was eager to employ in a well-conceived health project that would incorporate the community in meaningful ways. As he recalled in his memoir, "In spite of the restrictions imposed by the dictatorship, in Montes Claros an unexpected space opened up to propose a model of health that was clearly from the left."[96] Just like Testa, Hamilton was skeptical of top-down health planning. Vertically oriented programs, he wrote, "induced a functionalist vision of supervision, focused only on the completion of tasks, which did not favor the exchange of information among health workers, nor did it open up space for discussion of the social determination of disease."[97] To remedy this problem, the Montes Claros project was designed to facilitate a flow of information upward and downward in the health bureaucracy. Community members were trained as health workers to staff the large network of clinics, and meetings and workshops were run democratically to give community members a voice in the process.

The Montes Claros project's ambitious goal went far beyond the efficient delivery of health services. Rather, Chicão aimed "to *reclaim the citizenship* of clients and functionaries, and to ensure broader participation to construct a social base that would modify relations of power and disseminate a new consciousness in health."[98] As Testa put it, Chicão taught him that "the important thing is not to dictate norms but to unleash processes," a sentiment that resonated with budding "grassroots development" approaches of the time, such as participatory action research.[99] Montes Claros was the most concrete example, to that time, of how the broad projects of democratization, promotion of human rights, and improving public health dovetailed in the saúde coletiva movement, and many consider the program to have been the wellspring of the Health Reform movement and the SUS (discussed in more detail in chapter 7).

First in fits and starts, and then with considerable momentum, the field of saúde coletiva became progressively institutionalized in the 1970s: small groups of academics with similar interests developed formal academic programs, started journals, and sponsored conferences that helped define the identity, boundaries, and objectives of the field.[100] Predominantly leftist, this expanding group also worked out its political objectives and tactics, with an eye toward restoring democracy and taking charge of reforming the health sector. Through PAHO, some Brazilians were already involved with the international networks García helped nurture, and such connections generated the possibility for the exchange of new ideas in the health social sciences and humanities, as exemplified by a series of lectures given by Foucault in Rio in 1974, at the invitation of the Instituto de Medicina Social of the UERJ.[101] Two years later, the first national organization for collective health, Centro Brasileiro de Estudos de Saude (CEBES), was launched at a national meeting of the Brazilian Society for the Advancement of Science, held at the University of Brasilia. Most of the founders of CEBES, including David Capistrano da Costa Filho and Sérgio Arouca, were members of the Brazilian Communist Party. However, the party had little control over the direction of the health reform movement and CEBES gathered sanitaristas of many party affiliations.[102] Nevertheless, the Communist Party members in CEBES brought a kind of political "know-how" to the health reform movement, including a dedication to political organizing and skills in movement strategy.

One enduring legacy of CEBES was its journal, *Saúde em Debate*. Edited initially by Capistrano, and said to be inspired by the example of Virchow's short-lived *Die Medizinische Reform*, the journal was "strongly influenced" by Juan César García's vision of social medicine, including his version of the field's history and his selection of key texts.[103] Whether with pointed satire, policy briefs, or more scientific papers, the main objectives of *Saúde em Debate* were to serve as a forum for debate on the contours of health system reform and to galvanize a movement of health workers to take the initiative in promoting democratic reform, in order to institute a more socially just model of development. As a member of the journal's editorial board, Sandra Roncali Mafezolli, wrote in the journal's first issue, in 1976: "Deep changes in the health of our people are dependent on significant changes in the model of economic and social development in place, which would allow the majority of Brazilians access to the fruits of productive [economic] growth. Such changes necessarily include favorable conditions for broad popular participation in the definition of the country's direction."[104] Not all the political statements were so overt: political activity for most in CEBES continued to be clandestine, with the kind of organizing that took place at night in bars and cafés, often to discuss how their group could take control of the unions for doctors and other health workers.[105] As the examples of Chile and Argentina demonstrated, medical unions could be either an obstacle to or a force for political change, depending on the ideological orientation of their leadership.

If one person has come to symbolize the Brazilian Health Reform movement, it is Arouca.[106] Hailing from Ribeirão Preto, a city in northern São Paulo state, Arouca specialized in preventive medicine and helped develop a project in community-based health care—Laboratório de Estudos em Medicina Comunitária (LEMC)—at the University of Campinas, starting in 1967. With the support of the US-based Kellogg Foundation, which sponsored a program to strengthen medical education in Latin America, the LEMC put its ideas into action in the Paulínia Health Center project, which was innovative for including a community council to organize the services offered by the clinic.[107] Another driving force behind the Paulínia project, Joaquim Alberto Cardoso de Melo, a public health educator, was an early adopter of Paulo Freire's revolutionary ideas for democratizing education.[108]

While this effort was short-lived, its radicalism having alienated both Kellogg and the Brazilian government, it helped Arouca draw together a small group of critical scholars in the field of preventive medicine in São Paulo state. After García visited Campinas in 1968, he struck up a friendship with Arouca and thus established an important conduit for new information and ideas. As Arouca's colleague Anamaria Tambellini recalled later, "García would send us packages of literature because we had difficulty acquiring these books since they were considered subversive." At this moment of intellectual "effervescence," the connection to García provided "new ideas" to "formulate a new project in various areas of health"—a project that still did not have a name, but a change had begun.[109] With García's backing, Arouca served as a consultant to PAHO from Brazil, visiting Mexico, the United States, and Colombia in 1972 and Peru, Honduras, and Costa Rica in 1973.

As a result of all these "experiences and questions," Arouca wrote a systematic critique of preventive medicine, in his doctoral thesis, titled "O dilema preventivista" (The preventivist dilemma), which is considered a classic of Latin American social medicine.[110] This 1975 work is notable for its theoretical framework, its counterhegemonic argument about preventive medicine, and its definition of the parameters of saúde coletiva. As in García's work of the same period, Arouca derived his overarching framework from Marxian historical materialism, grafted to Foucault's technique of conducting an "archaeology of knowledge."[111] Arouca criticized preventive medicine as a tool of industrial capitalism, which prioritized making workers more productive and exploiting their surplus value. Arouca traced the history of the idea of preventive medicine, or at least its key theoretical underpinnings, to the "natural history of disease" concept of the Americans Hugh Rodman Leavell and Edwin Gurney Clark. Its popularity and legitimacy stemmed from support and diffusion by the United States as an imperial power, through the PAHO, for example.[112] As a result of all this, even though the discourse of preventive medicine seemed to offer a more "socially aware" outlook than clinical medicine, it ended up representing "the social" as a "void," thus reproducing the individualistic focus of biomedicine and privileging the behavioral sciences, disregarding social hierarchy and structure due to a naive assumption of the equality of subjects.[113] Overall, preventive medicine was a strategy ill-suited to the realities of Latin American societies, Arouca argued, which required substantial restructuring, in political-economic terms, in order to bring about change.

In 1976, on the strength of "O dilema preventivista" and his continuing work in CEBES, Arouca was appointed as a researcher in the Programa de Estudos Socioeconômicos em Saúde (PESES) in the Escola Nacional de Saúde Pública—which today bears his name—at the Oswaldo Cruz Institute. From then on, Arouca combined teaching, research, politics, and international health work like few others. As one biography puts it, "In this new phase of his life, Arouca would definitively establish himself as a sort of 'representative/ spokesperson/leader' of an expanding group that was configured around the defense and dissemination of *saúde coletiva*."[114] In addition to Marx and Foucault, Arouca also admired the work of Josué de Castro, Samuel Pessoa (the Brazilian parasitologist with a sociomedical orientation), and Antonio Gramsci, as he searched for a suitable mode of praxis.[115] As recounted by Sonia Fleury, not long after landing at PESES, Arouca announced to a colleague, "I do not want to do research anymore. I don't like it anymore, I'm going to do politics."[116] Working with a smaller group within CEBES that called itself "Project Andromeda," Arouca began to lay out the political strategy for what would become the Health Reform movement. In 1979, members of this group (including Chicão) launched ABRASCO, which became another institutional vehicle for health reform. Arouca himself was not deeply involved with ABRASCO, as he departed Brazil for Nicaragua in 1980, where he helped organize the health-care system for the new Sandinista government, until 1982.

After his return to Brazil, during the transition to democracy, Arouca became the president of the Oswaldo Cruz Institute (aka Fiocruz), the country's leading public health research institution, in 1985. In one of his first acts, he reinstated ten researchers who had been accused of being communists and were driven out the institute by the dictatorship in 1970 (an event known as the "Massacre of Manguinhos," although it is better described as a political purge).[117] With the opening of democracy, he straddled many different political spaces, as an activist in the Communist Party (and, later, in the Partido Popular Socialista [PPS], which broke off from the communists), government official, and, crucially, a representative of the health reform movement at the Constitutional Assembly of 1987, which eventually led to the SUS. Late in his political career, he served in the national congress, representing Rio de Janeiro for the PPS; he died at the age of sixty-one in 2003.

It would be easy to reduce saúde coletiva to the heroic figure of Sérgio Arouca, the archetype of the politically activist academic who resisted authoritarianism in the 1970s and then rose to power after the opening of democracy. Soon after his death, the official journal of Fiocruz remarked that, in the history of Brazilian public health, there are "two different periods: B. A. (before Arouca) and A. A. (after Arouca)."[118] But he can also be approached as the avatar of a movement; as one Brazilian scholar put it, "In fact, when we talk about Sérgio Arouca we are also talking about a group, we're talking about a movement, we're talking about an era, a generation."[119] The intellectual vibrancy of this generation owes much to Maria Cecília Ferro Donnangelo, a sociologist from São Paulo, who is widely cited as laying out the field of a sociology of health in Brazil, in such works as *Medicina e Sociedade,* her doctoral thesis, published as a book in 1975.[120] In her research, Donnangelo "adopted a critical sociological perspective" that moved the physician's own questions (about patients' attitudes and behaviors) to the side, making the field of medicine the object of study, and framing it as "a profession exercised in a market and a practice carried out in a way that is articulated with the historically given social and political structure," a framework she shared with Belmartino, of the CESS group in Argentina.[121] Other notable figures in the saúde coletiva movement included Jairnilson Paim, Guilherme Rodrigues da Silva, Hesio Cordeiro, Naomar de Almeida-Filho, Everardo Duarte Nunes, Carlyle Guerra Macedo, Sonia Fleury, and Sarah Escorel, to name just a few, who developed notable centers for research in the social sciences of health in Rio, São Paulo, Campinas, and Bahia.

In retrospect, the development of saúde coletiva was remarkable. Despite the limitations imposed by the military government, in roughly fifteen years the field had grown from practically nothing, just a small cohort of dissidents from the mainstream field of preventive medicine, into a small set of academic programs nurtured by García's influence in the continental resurgence of social medicine, to a discrete field, called saúde coletiva, which would have a transformative impact on Brazilian health policy. What made "collective health" distinctive from "social medicine" was the commitment of its members to radical forms of democratization and social inclusion, not only to urge along the move toward democracy in Brazil's formal political institutions but also to democratize relations and flatten hierarchies in the health field. This was not just a health project, but a project of education and consciousness raising that embraced newer forms of democratic education in the mold of Paulo Freire.[122] In the vision of saúde coletiva, doctors, other health workers, and health social scientists would no longer just design programs and implement them in a top-down fashion, but instead incorporate communities, in meaningful ways, into the process of evaluating their own needs, articulating the meaning of development, identifying their goals, and determining the place of health within this bigger picture.

The Consolidation of a Critical Field

In 1983, returning to Cuenca, Ecuador, García and his closest colleagues, including Nunes and Miguel Marquez, took stock of the previous decade of development in the health social sciences.[123] This was also the moment when García, already quite ill with cancer, declared his retirement from the scene, and his hope that a new generation would carry on his work. This hope was realized a few months after his death, in November 1984, with the founding of the Asociación Latinoamericana de Medicina Social in Ouro Preto. This organization brought together academics, activists, and health workers from the various working groups and research centers that had developed starting in the early 1970s.[124] As chapter 7 explains, ALAMES would not only foster the continued development of social medicine (and collective health) as an academic field but also play an important role in contesting the neoliberal agenda in the health sector. By the end of the 1990s, many of the key players in ALAMES would no longer be on the outside looking in, but rather take on the roles of political leaders and decision makers, seeking to institute the ALAMES vision of socially just health policy.

What made this second wave of Latin American social medicine distinctive from what had come before? What gave the new social medicine a clear identity and institutional permanence, compared to previous iterations of social medicine in Latin America that we have examined so far? The first difference that stands out is the development of a base in social theory, and the incorporation of social scientists into the field in a meaningful way. Seemingly abstruse academic innovations, particularly a Marxian historical materialism and Foucault's archaeology of knowledge, actually offered historically and geographically grounded ways to trace the development of social relations and discourses in the health field. In contrast, mainstream social scientists, immersed (usually uncritically) in the epistemologies of positivism and functionalism, staked claims to universal knowledge and created abstract model worlds that translated poorly into Latin American reality. LASM evolved, then, in rhythm with trends in Western social science disciplines, like history, anthropology, and geography, starting in the late 1960s. Scholars like E. P. Thompson, Eric Hobsbawm, Marshall Sahlins, David Harvey, Michael Watts, and Arturo Escobar (to name just a few), questioned the mainstream social sciences as handmaidens of ideologically conservative projects and instruments of social control. Many of the leading social scientists of second-wave social medicine, like Belmartino, Donnangelo, and Menéndez, were not vested in the identity of the medical profession, but were outsiders who trained their critical lenses on medicine as a socially powerful institution. In other words, social medicine and collective health were becoming more autonomous intellectually from the medical field.

Complementing these academic explorations, second-wave social medicine was also grounded in the hard-won experience of disaffected health technocrats. Who better than they to know what ailed health policy? When someone like Testa criticized the OPS/CENDES model, or Arouca leveled his aim at preventive medicine programs, it was not just to expose the defects of their internal logic, or their inadequacy in promoting population health, or their underlying (and misplaced) emphasis on economic efficiency. More importantly, they sought to change the prevailing *style of learning* that characterized endeavors in international development. This style of learning depended on the top-down transmission of models created by experts in specific domains. Did the structures of technocratic institutions allow space to articulate a critique? Did most health planners even understand their models and analytic procedures well enough to offer cogent critiques or make adjustments to those models? Second-wave LASM was born of frustration with the intellectual limitations of technocratic routines. And yet, we should recognize the irony that nearly all the institutions and projects central to the new social medicine—graduate programs in Mexico and Brazil, the Cuenca meetings, *Educación Médica y Salud*, the Montes Claros project—received funding and support from the PAHO, USAID, or American philanthropic foundations.

Another factor was the brutality of dictatorship and the experience of exile that forced the leftist-progressive group of Latin American doctors, health workers, and health social scientists to band together. Possibly, without the pressure exerted by right-wing forces, social medicine would not have coalesced as it did. Many of the leftist-progressive ideas could have been assimilated, as in the earlier period, into the structures of national welfare states and international health bureaucracies—tamed, so to speak. But in the 1970s, the group of leftist health workers in exile was too large and too unorthodox ideologically to be digested into the machinery of official international development. Instead, they were forced to form their own identity through their far-flung networks, as a cohesive outsider group. As a whole, the network placed more value on the open exchange of ideas and information and the maintenance of protective friendships than on the enforcement of any one ideological party line. Thus, the many social medicine journals created in that decade—*Saúde em Debate, Cuadernos Médicos Sociales, Salud Problema, International Journal of Health Services*—aired theory from many different quarters, usually leftist but drawing from the many varieties of Marxist theory, post-structuralism, feminism, and phenomenology. The presence of politically vocal researchers like Vicente Navarro in social medicine networks, or the rising advocacy for a primary health-care model in many parts of the world, suggest that the growth of LASM reflected global trends in health social sciences and health policy. More broadly, we could say that LASM became a part of the international civil society milieu that developed starting in the late 1960s, from pro-democracy movements to human rights organizations like Amnesty International that put pressure on military dictatorships and, especially later on, the World Bank, IMF, and multinational corporations.

Within the nodal institutions of the new social medicine and the networks that connected them, everything in the realm of health and medicine was subject to questioning. The spaces they constructed, gradually and with some trepidation, were spaces for exchange, debate, and critical thought, and for airing theories of change and proposals for different futures. These were open academic spaces carved out of societies marked by conservativism, censorship, and political repression. In the case of people like Mario Testa or Gustavo Molina Guzmán, the experience of exile forced reflection and critical thought; academic spaces were, essentially, the only ones they were permitted to occupy. With time to write and think and with a strong impulse toward political change, it is no wonder they moved away from reading the specialized literature in health planning, epidemiology, or health economics—dry research reports that served the everyday functioning and medium-term orientations of international health—and toward the much more incisive and revealing insights of Althusser, Foucault, or Illich, and, increasingly, of Testa, Arouca, Bloch, and Laurell. With the opening of democracy in Argentina, Chile, Brazil, and many other countries of the region in the 1980s, the social medicine group became more politically effective and began to populate higher-level positions in schools of medicine, hospitals, and public health ministries under more sympathetic governments. But the transition to a more public life was not so straightforward: they would have to square off with intransigent forces and deal with the rising, almost hegemonic ideas of neoliberalism, a confrontation that is the main focus of chapter 7.

CHAPTER SEVEN

Resistance

Social Medicine and Its Impact, 1990s–2000s

The creation of ALAMES in 1984 marked the increasing consolidation and maturation of Latin American social medicine. The continued work of this network in research centers across the continent coincided with a return to democracy across most of the region and an easing of Cold War tensions. However, it was also a time of dismal economic conditions, sparked by the Latin American debt crisis of the 1980s. As a result of the response to this crisis, the transition to a post–Cold War order only intensified the hegemony of the neoliberal economic model, which aimed to dismantle the Latin American welfare state. The new generation of LASM rode the wave of democratization that started in the 1980s to develop into an energetic and innovative international academic community, no longer inhibited by authoritarian governments. LASM scholars used their position to critically evaluate the effects of neoliberalism, challenge conventional ways of thinking about the causes of health inequalities and offer alternatives to business as usual in health systems that clearly failed to serve the needs of the poor. Later, as a "Pink Tide" of leftist leaders took power across the region starting in the late 1990s—most notably, Hugo Chávez in Venezuela, Evo Morales in Bolivia, the Kirchners in Argentina, and Lula (Luiz Inácio Lula da Silva) in Brazil—the activist academics of ALAMES were drafted into policymaking roles. The health policies of New Latin American Left governments instituted many of the principles of social medicine but, as in previous generations, met with opposition from conservative forces and vested interests.

This chapter focuses primarily on the translation of second-wave social medicine (and collective health) ideas from the realm of academia into progressive health policy, starting with the Brazilian health reforms of the 1980s. As a secondary focus, I also discuss the expansion and consolidation of social medicine as an academic field: its advances and innovations in terms of theory and method in research, along with its steady institutionalization, to the point where social medicine and collective health are now mature disciplines with clear research agendas and status in Latin American universities.[1] LASM, with its distinctive conceptual vocabulary and theorization of the social production of health and disease, has been increasingly acknowledged and embraced by health social scientists outside of the region, to critically evaluate the discourse and policy recommendations of mainstream international health institutions, such as the WHO's Commission on the Social Determinants of Health.[2]

How to turn theory into practice is always the big question. LASM scholar-activists have organized strategically to influence health and social politics, and in this respect, the work of ALAMES has been crucial. As the first international association to promote social medicine, it brought together like-minded scholar-activists across the hemisphere. Their exchanges helped sharpen the theory and, just as importantly, the political praxis of LASM. Members of the ALAMES group rose to high positions in the health ministries of leftist governments that took public health seriously in the late 1990s and early 2000s. They included María Isabel Rodríguez in El Salvador, Mario Rovere in Argentina, Asa Cristina Laurell in Mexico, Nila Heredia in Bolivia, and María Lourdes Urbaneja in Venezuela. Nevertheless, my goal in this chapter is not to write a comprehensive history of ALAMES, given that many insider and outsider narratives of the organization exist.[3] We should also consider that ALAMES is not synonymous with LASM and that a lot of health "progress" has happened without much influence from ALAMES. This includes two quite different cases, of Cuba and Costa Rica, where the second-wave LASM group has been weak but where public health achievements are impressive, even extraordinary.

This chapter begins with a discussion of the landmark health reform that took place in Brazil during the 1980s and 1990s, which culminated in the creation of the SUS, the country's unified health system. This was perhaps the most noteworthy achievement of the second wave of LASM, and it demonstrates how the transition to democracy enabled progressive reforms in the health sector. But this achievement of saúde coletiva in Brazil was not widely emulated, due to unfavorable conditions produced by the rise of free-market ideologies across the region. As I explain in the next section, the hegemony of the neoliberal economic model and concomitant structural reforms led, in many countries, to a hollowing out of the public sector in health and a vast reduction of state spending on social welfare. The LASM community took notice and mounted a fierce critique of neoliberalism. When the Pink Tide came, starting in the late 1990s, LASM found an opportunity to directly influence health policy, including in Venezuela, Bolivia, and Mexico City, cases that I examine closely. I then turn to discuss the consolidation of social medicine (and collective health) as an academic field with international reach. Finally, I consider Cuba and Costa Rica, two often-cited public health "success stories" from the Global South, which have seen little of the cutting-edge social theory and militant political praxis that have characterized social medicine over the past few decades. Examining these exceptional cases helps clarify why and under what conditions social medicine tends to thrive—a question I return to in the chapter conclusion.

The Brazilian Health Reform Movement

Brazil's health reform movement (*reforma sanitária*) stands out as the biggest success story of the second wave of social medicine in Latin America. Starting in the early 1970s a network of academics, health workers, and technocrats established spaces to envision a health policy that would be more responsive to social demands, increase the equity of access and outcomes, and participate in the reconstruction of Brazilian society on democratic principles. This group, cohering around the idea of saúde coletiva, or collective health, was represented by CEBES and ABRASCO, whose formation was discussed in chapter 6. These organizations introduce a new ethos into Brazilian health policy:

> In place of an authoritarian outlook, Abrasco and Cebes advocated social participation; in place of disease control policies, especially with regard to transmissible diseases, the promotion of health and improvements in the general quality of life; in place of a sector divided between public health and state-insured medicine, a unified and universal health system. Their agenda in this respect was intimately connected with the crisis in the dictatorship and the return of democracy to Brazilian society, because it was understood in these institutions that changes in the field of health meant measures to make the State and its agencies and decision-making processes more democratic.[4]

In turn, these academic/professional organizations formed loose coalitions with grassroots organizations, including neighborhood associations and religious groups. Together, the coalition for health reform not only rode the wave of the democratic transition but also helped shape the substance of Brazil's new democracy and its emphasis on social rights.[5] And almost uniquely in Latin American history, the design of a new health policy was carried out in the open, in a series of conferences and meetings, including the deliberative and participatory process of a constitutional convention. This health reform movement led to the concrete achievements of constitutional guarantees to a right to health, the architecture of a unified national health system, and palpable improvements in health conditions, including a much-lauded state response to the emerging epidemic of HIV/AIDS in the first decade of this new system's existence.

The sanitaristas, as the health activists were known, followed two parallel routes to reforming Brazil's health system. First, they decided to "occupy the state" during the democratic transition, by "assum[ing] positions in the bureaucracy with the aim of dismantling the old health system and advancing their reform objectives."[6] This strategy was not so different from that of progressive doctors elsewhere in Latin America, who frequently occupied national- and international-level health bureaucracies. Well before the return to democracy, in 1979 CEBES presented a report to the Brazilian Congress's health commission titled "Democracy and Health," which criticized the "commodification of medicine" and signaled popular discontent about expensive, inaccessible health care that failed to address basic needs.[7] Second, the sanitaristas intensified their political participation, engaging with other social movements and taking active part in the new institutional and deliberative spaces that were part of the democratic transition. This dual approach embodies the "insider/outsider" tactics used in Brazilian social movements of the time. As the Brazilian political scientist Ana Maria Doimo put it: "Integrative-incorporative" tactics (i.e., "occupying the state" or other official institutions) were complemented by, or alternated with "expressive-disruptive" maneuvers—"direct action and protest [to] disrupt the normal operations of the current system and delegitimize it in favor of radical change."[8] The leaders of ABRASCO—Brazil's national academic-activist organization for collective health—viewed their project as a "microcosm" of "the process of constructing a new society," which required intensified political activism without forsaking the academic identity of their organization.[9]

Although the health reform movement was steered mainly by academics, doctors, and other health workers, it also incorporated genuinely grassroots action to improve health and sanitary conditions.[10] According to Silvia Gerschman, an Argentinian sociologist who fled to Brazil to avoid persecution during the Proceso, one starting point of Brazilian health reform can be found in grassroots mobilization in Novo Iguaçu, a working-class municipality in the Baixada Fluminense area of Rio de Janeiro. Here, during the dictatorship in the early 1970s, a combination of actors—progressive health workers at the local state clinic, Catholic priests in the liberation theology movement, and vocal neighborhood leaders—began to mobilize their resources.[11] Health care was certainly not the only or even the main concern of local citizens, who also organized for better housing, education, and transportation options. Demands for improved sanitation in these neighborhoods that typically lacked clean running water, sewage treatment, and organized garbage collection, became questions of both infrastructure and social justice. The neighborhood association founded in Novo Iguaçu was the prototype for a national Movimento de Amigos de Bairros (MAB), a federation of groups organized to transmit the demands of poor neighborhoods to agents of the state. Around the same time, the influence of Catholic liberation theology and the educational theories of Paulo Freire led to a proliferation of ecclesiastical base communities (*comunidades eclesiais de base*), the nuclei of a popular health movement, the Movimento Popular em Saúde (MOPS), which made similar demands for Brazil's impoverished masses.[12] Epidemics of dengue fever in Brazil in 1986 gave special urgency to these calls for better sanitation and health care. Under the direction of Hésio Cordeiro—one of the principals of the saúde coletiva group—the national social security agency, INAMPS, launched a special health program for the Baixada Fluminense, which featured cooperation between the agency and the progressive, locally respected Catholic charity Caritas Diocesana, and the creation of community-level councils to oversee the expanding network of hospitals and clinics in the area.[13]

Grassroots organizations like the MAB and the MOPS would have a seat at the table in planning the new Brazilian health system at the consequential Eighth National Sanitary Conference, which took place in Brasília in March 1986. These conferences had been staged periodically since the 1940s, from the time of the populist Vargas government, but this one stood out for several reasons. It was the first to take place after the end of the military dictatorship, and it was also the first to call for participation of groups outside of the health sector, "including representatives from the popular health movement, patients groups, health workers unions, clinics and hospitals, health bureaucrats from all levels of government, and members of Congress."[14] Representatives of ABRASCO (via its Commission on Health Policies, led by Sonia Fleury Teixeira) and CEBES helped to steer the discussions. In a stirring speech to the thousands who were gathered in Brasília's national sports arena, Sérgio Arouca, the chair of the conference, explained that health was "not just the absence of disease," but rather, it was

a social well-being that means people have something more than just not being sick: they have a right to a home, to work, to decent wages, to water, to clothing, to education, to information on how to understand the world and transform it. They have a right to an environment that is not harmful to them, and, quite the contrary, one that allows for a dignified and decent life. The right to a political system that respects free expression, the free possibility of organization and self-determination of a people, and which is not subjected to fear of violence.[15]

Though obviously expanding on the WHO's famous definition of health, Arouca went much further, by laying out a set of civil and social rights that new social movements were advocating for, and by framing health system reform as more than a technical-administrative question, but rather as an integral part of the larger, more momentous process of democratization.[16] By the end of that conference, a blueprint for a new health system emerged, based on a set of guiding principles: the declaration of health care as a right of all citizens, with the state having a duty to protect that right; the need for a single, unified health system for all Brazilians; decentralization of management and provision of health care; and mechanisms to ensure public participation in the management of the health system.

With a crucial constitutional convention on the horizon, ABRASCO strategized to broaden its base of support within and outside of the health sector. The prior effort to "occupy the state" facilitated these engagements. As its director, Cordeiro had already made important reforms to INAMPS, the social security agency, such as decentralization and a dramatic increase in the government's contribution to the agency's budget.[17] These prior actions facilitated the sanitarista agenda at the convention, held between 1987 and 1988, but the reformers had to fight hard for their proposal. Aside from the sanitarista plan for a unified health system with popular participation, two other proposals were before the commission charged with health policy in the new constitution: one, backed by much of the medical profession, pushed for a mainly private system; and another represented the "interests of the large bureaucracy" already present in the national ministries of health and social security.[18] In support of their constitutional amendment, the sanitaristas gathered over 54,000 signatures from "representatives of 168 different civil society organizations."[19] A major sticking point was the demand for citizen oversight of the new health system via "health councils," but this element had sufficient popular support to be maintained in the 1988 constitution. Decentralization of oversight to health councils would be jeopardized again in 1990, when President Fernando Collor de Mello used his line-item veto power to eliminate this and other key aspects of the new health law, but popular mobilizations and renewed pressure from the sanitaristas led to a new bill with these features intact, which Collor signed into law just two months later.[20] Although not quite in final form, the essential elements of the SUS were worked out and in place. As Monika Dowbor argues, all of this political action was really homegrown: it "happened without applying international prescriptions that consisted, at that time, of privatisation or cutting public expenditure," that is, against the grain of the structural reforms that the World Bank was advocating at the time.[21]

The SUS has an innovative structure, with elements not found in many other national health systems. Integrated into the federal political structure of Brazil, the SUS has three different levels of financing and service provision, at the federal, state, and municipal levels. At each level of government there are health councils, comprising, in principle, an even mix of citizens and government officials, which are charged with reviewing policy and approving budgets.[22] The permanent role of the councils, along with periodic health conferences, help ensure genuine public participation in the SUS. The SUS is funded by general taxes (again, at different levels of government), as well as some special funds from social security contributions, and every Brazilian citizen may exercise their right to use the system's services, free of charge. The usual point of contact with the system is the primary health care clinic, publicly funded, staffed by family health teams and community health workers, so that there is less reliance on higher-salaried physicians.[23] By 2010, "there were roughly 236,000 community health workers and 33,000 family health-care teams, reaching about 98 million people in 85% (4,737) of municipalities in Brazil."[24] The secondary and higher levels of care have more of a public–private mix, with most services provided by private facilities under contract with the SUS. Despite its name—the Unified Health System—there are, in fact, public and private subsystems; private spending of all kinds accounts for about 60 percent of total health expenditures in Brazil, including private insurance, out-of-pocket costs for care, and spending on pharmaceuticals. About one-quarter of Brazilians have private health insurance, and this proportion is much higher in the relatively affluent Southeast region of the country.[25] Although, in principle, the same medical services should be available to patients whether or not they have private insurance, having such insurance reduces wait times and provides access to better-quality care in private facilities beyond the purview of the SUS.

The AIDS epidemic offered an early critical test of the SUS and, more broadly, of the state's willingness to ensure the right to health. Although the Brazilian response to AIDS was far from perfect, it became a model for a developing-country approach to the epidemic, proving the value of unified structure, a rights-based approach, and democratic action that were built into the SUS. Detection of the first cases of AIDS in Brazil, in the early 1980s, co-incided with the waning days of the dictatorship, the opening of democracy, and the formation of the SUS. The government response to the AIDS crisis balanced the need for centralized authority to coordinate a response to the cri-sis with the opening of diffuse political spaces for advocacy and participation by civil society groups, such as nongovernmental organizations (NGOs). With the opening of democracy, local AIDS NGOs proliferated, with different em-phases: raising awareness about the epidemic, destigmatizing HIV infection, providing hospice care, or acting as pressure groups to compel government ac-tion.[26] Exemplifying this latter area of focus, the Rio-based Brazilian Interdisci-plinary AIDS Association "would consciously reject any direct role in care or treatment for people with HIV/AIDS, arguing that these functions were noth-ing more than the obligation of the state, and would focus their attention on criticizing government policy—or lack of it, particularly at the federal level."[27]

Pressure from these NGOs led to the creation of the National AIDS Pro-gram (NAP). The NGOs united to oppose health ministers who failed to give the AIDS crisis the attention, budget, and personnel that it deserved, and criticized NAP directors for being slow to act. The NAP worked best—most effectively in an epidemiological sense and most harmoniously in a political sense—when it created and sustained partnerships with civil society organizations. Alongside the AIDS NGOs, the progressive wing of the Cath-olic Church, informed by liberation theology, would play an important role in the rising acceptance of people living with HIV and AIDS, and in imple-menting aspects of the National AIDS Program. In its confrontation with the AIDS epidemic, the Brazilian Catholic Church fused old tropes and values (the virtues of the Good Samaritan, compassion for the sick and excluded) with a "solidarity approach, grounded in an understanding of HIV/AIDS as an outcome of structural violence, [which] facilitated the development of multisector alliances between diverse groups of AIDS activists, academics, religious leaders, and health officials."[28]

The year 1996 was a turning point, as the NAP shifted its policy emphasis to making antiretroviral drugs (ARVs) widely available. Again, the advocacy work of AIDS NGOs was crucial. Brazil's government infringed international patent and copyright law, in order to produce cheaper generic versions of extremely expensive ARVs, or to buy generics from other middle-income countries, like India. For this reason, NGO advocacy efforts transcended the domestic scene, leading to internationally newsworthy protests as well as en-gagements in "global health diplomacy," including negotiations at meetings of the WHO and World Trade Organization, and the formation of alliances with civil society groups in other Global South countries affected by the epidemic.[29]

The Brazilian response to AIDS, then, cannot be reduced to the action of the SUS, yet it was perhaps just what the sanitaristas had envisaged in their calls for health reform. The NAP and the national Ministry of Health could not define AIDS solely in epidemiological terms nor construct a purely technocratic policy of surveillance, containment, prevention, and treatment. Instead, in a functioning democracy, social demands from civil society actors such as NGOs could be channeled into the NAP via civil commissions. When those channels failed, other political strategies were available. Health policy became something that the public could engage with and shape continually, and in the process the boundaries between health and other sectors were redrawn. Put another way, the connections between health politics and other social movements became more fully and clearly articulated. As Doimo puts it, this sort of movement interconnectedness was crucial to creating the participatory spaces to advance the objectives of health system reform.[30] And, as Lindsay Mayka has suggested, the action of the health councils and decentralization worked together to limit clientelism, a common Latin American political model that rewards party loyalty over technical expertise and managerial competence, often resulting in unfair distribution of public services. Instead, "Rejecting clientelist dynamics, these activists [the sanitaristas] sought a new mode of engagement with the state via participatory spaces in which they could articulate demands, push for accountability from the state, and shape the implementation of programs."[31]

The SUS is a role model for a different kind of health policy, in which authentic democratic participation contests and balances the technocratic logics that typify most national health systems. At the same time, some observers have pointed out that the Health Reform movement was less successful "in achieving the reforms it hoped for—a transformation not only of health provision but of society itself"; the SUS "was only one part of the health reform agenda."[32] Community interest in participating in health councils waned over time, with a possible generational shift away from a conception of health care as a right to be defended by collective action, toward a neoliberal view of health care as a commodity.[33] Still, on balance, the movement "contributed towards the spread of the idea of the right to health as part of the attributes of citizenship and towards the democratic reform of the State."[34] Popular support for these values has been robust, even in the midst of dramatic political swings in recent years.

Neoliberalism and the Health Sector in Latin America

During the 1980s and 1990s, the far-reaching effects of neoliberal policy models spurred the LASM group to mount a defense of existing welfare institutions and confront the incursion of market forces and corporate actors into the health sector across the region. To many segments of the political left, including the LASM group, neoliberalism appeared as an intensified stage of economic imperialism—the classic pattern of wealthy countries, especially the United States, exerting their economic hegemony to develop new avenues for returns on investment capital.[35] The fact that the earliest adopter of neoliberal reforms in the region, Chile, had only done so after a US-supported military coup encouraged this view. A more sympathetic take on neoliberalism deserves consideration: it offered a framework that translated into specific policies to address persistent structural problems that created a drag on economic growth in the region. The neoliberal recipe of privatization of state-owned industry, deregulation of banking and investment, reduction of government budgets, labor market flexibility, and free trade were supposed to create more dynamic economies. Accompanying a transition from authoritarianism to democracy in many countries, neoliberalism also promoted a new ethos of individual entrepreneurialism and competition, rather than collective action and social solidarity. In any case, in the context of the 1980s debt crisis, many Latin American governments were essentially forced to accept neoliberal reforms as conditions on loans or other funding from the World Bank, IMF, Inter-American Development Bank, and the US government, a process known as structural adjustment.

These same international financial institutions (IFIs) became increasingly powerful actors in health policy, and the relative influence of the WHO and PAHO waned accordingly. These multilateral health organizations had long taken an agnostic view on the question of health system structure, accepting a diversity of national systems with varying degrees of government involvement, while endorsing the PHC model, predicated on a strong state presence to address gaps in basic health care provision. In retrospect, the 1978 Alma-Ata conference was a high-water mark for the universal health equity agenda, as the major institutional players in international health would soon fall in line with the neoliberal agenda. The neoliberal strategy of "sectoral reform" was a component of structural adjustment intended to reduce the state's role in managing, financing, and provisioning health services.[36] The rationale behind and recommendations for sectoral reform were explained in the World Bank's landmark report, *Investing in Health*, which came out in 1993. Two years later, at a meeting in Washington, DC, the USAID, PAHO, World Bank, and other major international institutions worked out a "consensus" for sectoral reform.[37] This was more than just a philosophical and policy disagreement; it was also about who influenced health policymaking in Latin America. Social medicine advocates had always been able to insinuate their ideas into the work of the PAHO, in particular, but they were far from the new centers of power in neoliberalized international health.

The key concept behind sectoral reform was "structured pluralism," a strategy to supersede the segmented and fragmented systems of social protection that developed in Latin American countries in the mid-twentieth century, as an outcome of processes described in earlier chapters.[38] Many people and institutions were behind the development of "structured pluralism," but Julio Frenk of Mexico and Luis Londoño of Colombia coined the term and had the opportunity to put it into practice early. In essence, structured pluralism rests on separating the functions in national health systems (management and regulation, financing, insurance, and provision of medical services); introducing competition between private for-profit, nonprofit, and state-owned entities to improve efficient execution of these functions; and accepting the existence of different subsystems to serve the needs of different market segments, meaning that the state ought to subsidize care for the very poor, but the middle class might need to pay for more of its own care. In the model of structured pluralism, the government's role in the health system was primarily regulatory: to set up and enforce the new "rules of the game" in a semicompetitive market in the health sector. In functional terms these could be considered "quasi-markets"—similar to those developed in the 1980s in the British National Health Service as it went through neoliberal reforms—where the government controls funding but increasingly invites participation from the private sector, by outsourcing specialty services (e.g., radiology), privatizing inefficient entities (like hospitals), or in controlled competition with nonprofit actors.[39] In this way, structured pluralism reflects a "neo-institutional" analysis of what plagues large government systems; from this perspective, the best role for government is to set the rules to optimally balance equity and efficiency, and otherwise stay out of the way.[40] By the early 2000s, structured pluralism would evolve into the model of universal health coverage (UHC) promoted by the World Bank and the WHO.

Colombia, even more than Chile, was the exemplar of the World Bank's health reform agenda.[41] Chile's reforms represented an extreme, almost purist, form of neoliberal doctrine; such a drastic policy shift was only possible under an authoritarian regime that prevented public participation. It is not just that Chile's neoliberal health reforms were an affront to human rights and democracy; even mainstream economists recognized the severe defects of Chile's reform, especially the problematic practice of Instituciónes de Salud Previsional (ISAPREs, newly created private health insurance companies) selecting for lower-risk clientele (young and healthy people) and pushing the higher-risk groups most in need of care into the public system, thus effectively creating a large state subsidy of the private insurers.[42] (This dynamic exemplifies the economic problem of "adverse selection.") By contrast, the Colombian health reform of 1993, led by Londoño, was well conceived at least from the perspective of then-current health economics, particularly theories about the efficiency of competition and risk in insurance markets, using the model that came to be known as structured pluralism.[43] Through a combination of mandates and incentives, of public money and mixed markets for insurance and health-care services, Colombia's health reforms intended to create a competitive atmosphere that would drive down costs and improve quality.[44] Within ten years after the reform, about 80 percent of Colombians had health insurance coverage, which made "Colombia among the very few countries in the developing world reaching near universal health insurance coverage," according to consultants from the World Bank and Brookings Institution—a tendentious assessment that ignored the success of countries like Costa Rica and Cuba in expanding coverage, which had nothing to do with structured pluralism.[45] Mario Hernández, one of the leaders of ALAMES, noted wryly that the WHO ranked Colombia in the top group for health system performance in 2000, more for its adherence to the World Bank recommendations, and in spite of its mediocre health outcomes.[46]

For every neoliberal "role model" like Colombia, there were other countries, like Argentina, where free-market reforms led to a defunding of the public sector and exacerbated social inequalities. Many scholar-activists in the second wave of LASM focused their research on the health impacts of structural adjustment and documented the incursion of neoliberal rationalities and the movement of global investment capital into Latin American health systems. In this context, Argentina is especially important. When democracy was restored in 1983, Argentina already had a fragmented and decentralized health system, for reasons explained in earlier chapters. In the 1980s, attempts to move toward a national system of socialized medicine, after the return of democracy, were thwarted by fiscal problems and the organized opposition of the medical profession.[47] Following an acute crisis of hyperinflation and social unrest in 1989, the administration of President Carlos Menem introduced a series of neoliberal reforms through the 1990s, which had wide-ranging effects on Argentina's economy and society (not least, a massive increase in unemployment and the rise of a large informal sector) and specific consequences for the health system. The obras sociales sector was deregulated, so that individuals and companies had more freedom to choose insurance providers; moreover, these social insurance funds became more like ordinary corporations, which could be bought and sold, invested in, consolidated or split apart according to the logic of investment capital.[48] Meanwhile, the government health sector fell into disrepair, with declining budgets as demands on services increased, particularly with increasing numbers of workers in the informal economy, who could not benefit from the obras sociales. This decline was especially noticeable in large public hospitals and in government public health services, like disease control campaigns.[49]

In the 1990s, the height of neoliberalism in Argentina, multinational firms took advantage of the possibilities created by health system reform and a political climate friendly to foreign investment. They even had a role in designing those reforms, at least indirectly through their allies in the IMF and other IFIs.[50] In a now-classic article from 2001, Celia Iriart (Argentina), Emerson Elías Merhy (Brazil), and Howard Waitzkin (United States)—all active in the ALAMES group—explained how neoliberalism brought the US logic of "managed care," and even some of its major corporate players, to Argentina. US-based insurance and health management companies like Aetna, CIGNA, American International Group (AIG), Principal, and Prudential all began investing in Argentina. The EXXEL Group was a particularly successful example of a multinational investor that adapted its operations to the conditions presented by financial deregulation, structural adjustment, and health sector reform. EXXEL entered the Argentine market in 1994 to manage investment funds for Oppenheimer and Co., a US investment firm, and attracted investment capital from a variety of sources in the United States, ranging from insurance companies to pension funds to universities and private philanthropic trusts. By 2001, it had become one of the ten largest corporations in Argentina, with an array of investments across many sectors, including energy, logistics, and credit card services. In the health sector, EXXEL bought up many of the prepaid health plans, known as *prepagos*, which mainly serve affluent consumers, and came to manage billing for the public hospitals of the province of San Luis (apparently reaping profits from more aggressive and efficient billing procedures). EXXEL also acquired a small obra social called Witcel, which "previously offered coverage to workers of a paper operation that ceased operation." Acquisition of this tiny fund, with just three hundred beneficiaries, offered EXXEL the legal means to enter the deregulated market of the obras sociales, where consumers were no longer tied to the fund they had paid into by virtue of union membership, but could shop around and enroll in the fund of their choice. Within a matter of months, Witcel grew to over ten thousand members.[51]

As the neoliberalization of the health sector proceeded across the region, the LASM group intensified its critique. One comparative study of Mexico, Chile, and Argentina suggested that privatization of health services under a US-style "managed care" model was increasing out-of-pocket costs (in the form of co-payments) to the poorest segments of the population, making health care less accessible than before.[52] As Iriart, Merhy, and Waitzkin observed in 2001: "Gradually 'common sense' is transformed concerning the conceptualization of health, illness, and health care services. In the official pronouncements we have studied, health care no longer remains a universal right for whose fulfillment the state is responsible, but rather is converted into a good of the marketplace that individuals can acquire. This is a fundamental change in meaning, since health stops being a public good and becomes a private good."[53] In the sectoral reforms supported by the World Bank and WHO, the notion of "solidarity" as a guiding principle for the organization of the health system seemed to disappear, as society was reconceptualized as the mass of individuals acting in a market.[54] Susana Belmartino, who always understood the Argentine health system as a historical layering of values, institutions, and regulations, made a subtler point: neoliberal reforms of the 1990s mostly capitalized on the long-established pattern of strong ingroup solidarity undermining universalism, resulting in continued fragmentation and inequality in health care.[55] Nevertheless, across the region neoliberal reforms of the health sector appeared to have led to the "opposite results" of what the IFIs intended—"increased inequity, less efficiency, and higher dissatisfaction, without improving quality of care"—while creating new opportunities for profit taking that benefited multinational corporations, consulting firms, and the IFIs' own personnel.[56]

Thus, the "demystification of the processes of neoliberal health system reform" became one of the "central pillars of the academic work" of the LASM group in the 1990s, building on a longer tradition of critique of the commercialization of health services.[57] But the group was decidedly marginal in health policy decision making during the heyday of neoliberal hegemony. In the 2000s, however, advocates of social medicine would become increasingly prominent as the New Left surged across Latin America. The "Pink Tide" regimes would offer new possibilities for governing the health sector, based on a general skepticism of neoliberalism and a restoration of the welfare state, and such ideas moved from academic circles into the heart of national and international health politics. For a time, and in some places, members of the LASM group would control the levers of power and put their ideas into action.

Social Medicine, ALAMES, and the New Latin American Left

By the 1990s, the excesses of the neoliberal political-economic model produced a strong counterreaction across the region. Sometimes called the "Pink Tide," a new wave of populist, anti- or post-neoliberal governments took power. The social medicine group, still rather small but well connected through ALAMES, supported this political turn and seized the opportunity to influence health policy within the new regimes. Two of the leading lights of the new Latin American left—Hugo Chávez and Evo Morales—made community clinics and neighborhood-level public health projects a symbol of their new, populist regimes. In Bolivia, health reforms under Morales also tried to incorporate, with mixed success, Indigenous health beliefs and practices, manifesting social medicine's concern with the unequal power relations inherent in Western medicine. In both countries, Cuba made important contributions to health care by way of their program of international health solidarity. In Mexico, there was divergence between the health policy directions of the national and local Mexico City governments, with the latter directed by a key figure of ALAMES, Asa Cristina Laurell, under Governor Andrés Manuel López Obrador. The contrast between the Mexican capital city and the country as a whole served as a microcosm of the contrast between the models of single universal health systems (patterned on Brazil's) and the UHC model supported by the major players in international development and finance (like the World Bank).

Founded in 1984, ALAMES became "the organizational expression of social medicine in Latin America."[58] As explained in chapter 6, this group formally connected the vibrant nodes of academic research in social medicine, such as the UAM-Xochimilco in Mexico and various universities in Brazil, and continued to expand, particularly by means of international conferences held every few years. By 2007, ALAMES had around six hundred individual members, organized in national chapters, but with a decentralized structure to allow for transnational connections in thematic networks (for example, around the theme of gender and health).[59] ALAMES is an academic association but with a commitment to political action to promote social justice. As Débora Tajer, of Argentina's chapter of ALAMES, explained in 2004: "The fact of being, at the same time, a social, academic and political movement, confers enormous potential on ALAMES, but simultaneously, places the organization in the face of a series of internal contradictions and challenges. These challenges arise from the different points of view that social, academic, and political movements take on when they approach the reality of the health field."[60] Here, Tajer was pointing to tensions that had always been part of social medicine, including how to reconcile the norms of academic research, which often prioritize a certain critical distance from the objects of inquiry, with political action. In spite of these tensions, by the 1990s, as a collective, ALAMES projected a clear political agenda, against the forces of neoliberalization and with demands for "social policies that affect the structural determinants of health," "the consolidation and construction of universal and free health systems," and "the right to health for everyone without regard to gender, sexual and ethnic origin," among other political objectives.[61] Around the year 2000, a series of articles in the *American Journal of Public Health* publicized the accomplishments and agenda of ALAMES for English-speaking audiences.[62] By that time, LASM was becoming increasingly influential beyond the academic realm.

In Venezuela, Hugo Chávez made health one dimension of a rights-based agenda to narrow economic inequalities and give political voice to the marginalized. The new constitution of 1999 articulated a right to health, among a bundle of newly guaranteed social rights.[63] Chávez's ministers of health— including María Lourdes Urbaneja, who had been president of ALAMES— "attempted to translate LASM principles into policies and practices."[64] Due in part to the recalcitrance of the Venezuelan Medical Association, reforms to national health policy were mostly unsuccessful in the early years of Chávez's regime. In response, the populist government looked to fashion new institutional spaces to carry out its health work. In 2003, the government launched Misión Barrio Adentro, a vast network of community-based clinics providing free health care to the urban poor. This program stressed "pro-poor, rights-oriented principles" and the "'integrative' frame for health care advocated by LASM," as health work was joined to programs for literacy, food security, housing, and employment.[65] Although many Venezuelan health workers participated, the program's success hinged on the action of doctors and other health personnel from Cuba, who numbered over twenty-three thousand by 2006.[66] Cuba's cooperative efforts extended into Misión Milagro, whose ophthalmology clinics "restored the sight of over a million Venezuelans."[67] Misión Barrio Adentro improved health-care services, but just as importantly, seemed to flatten the social hierarchies typical in doctor-patient interactions—a more "egalitarian" view of medical care that derived directly from social medicine and collective health.[68]

But overreliance on revenues from oil exports—which began falling precipitously after the 2008 Global Financial Crisis—coupled with dubious economic policy decisions by Chávez and his successor, Nicolás Maduro, emptied state coffers, limiting the impact of health services, and producing steady deterioration of the economy, leading to malnutrition, hunger, and the reemergence of old scourges, such as malaria. Trained medical personnel left the country in droves while the health system suffered shortages of basic goods.[69] The early failure to enact comprehensive reform created a public health system so deprived of resources that it led, according to one analyst, to an unanticipated reprivatization of health care in Venezuela.[70] However, as ALAMES itself has argued in its official declarations, US military threats, economic embargoes, and disinformation campaigns have also hampered efforts to maintain a responsive and equitable health system in Venezuela.[71]

Evo Morales was one of Chávez's great allies in the new Latin American left. In many ways, the Bolivian and Venezuelan experiences were similar: a socialist-populist government responded to long-neglected social demands after years of neoliberal policy failure, faced opposition from intransigent middle- and upper-class sectors (including most of the medical profession), created new social programs strongly identified with the ruling party, and made use of Cuban physicians and other medical personnel to expand government health services. But the problems of the health sector in Bolivia ran much deeper, due not only to the country's poverty and lack of trained personnel but also to deep cultural divides. Official medicine was a Western knowledge system practiced mainly by the Bolivian elite of European descent. For the Indigenous majority of the country—Aymara, Quechua, Guarani, and many other groups—health care was another institution of colonial domination.[72]

Morales's health reform program was highly ambitious, even radical, because it extended the government's larger philosophy of social transformation into the health arena. As the anthropologist Brian Johnson has explained, Morales sought to embed principles of "decolonization" and "interculturality" into Bolivian life, creating "an experiment in national soul-searching and (re-)creation in a variety of aspects of daily life—from education to law, entertainment, and health."[73] Traditional Indigenous medicine had been outlawed for centuries in Bolivia, just one dimension of the discrimination faced under colonial structures that did not disappear with formal independence. An Indigenous health movement, led by Walter Álvarez Quispe, a *kallawaya* or traditional healer (who was also trained in biomedicine in socialist Cuba in the 1960s), successfully decriminalized Indigenous medical practices by the 1980s.[74] The trajectory of this movement led to "indigenous participation in the new State's health policy" and "the new Constitution [of 2009] incorporated several articles related to health, including the right to health and the valorization of indigenous cosmovision, or spiritual worldview, within the health care system."[75]

With Nila Heredia, another member of ALAMES, leading as the minister of health and sports, the new Bolivian government created the cornerstone program of its new approach to health: Salud Familiar Comunitaria Intercultural (SAFCI; the Family Community Intercultural Health Policy). SAFCI was essentially a PHC program, extending medical care to long underserved populations across the country. Community participation helped identify local needs, and alternative forms of care, such as the incorporation of Indigenous midwives, were adopted, though not without friction.[76] According to the anthropologist Susana Ramírez Hita, SAFCI's positive aspects, such as increased community participation and a discursive shift to incorporate interculturality, while laudable, were insufficient to overcome tangible structural deficiencies in Bolivia's health system, including a lack of human and technological resources to resolve community health problems.[77] With Morales's sudden relinquishing of power under pressure, in 2019, the future of these policy changes has been unclear.[78]

Mexico City offered another example of "what social medicine does when it governs." In 2000, historic elections in Mexico ended the stranglehold of the PRI, the ruling party, in national political life. In the national presidential election, Vicente Fox, the neoliberal candidate for the PAN, was victorious, while in Mexico City, a leftist from the PRD, López Obrador, was elected. They set about employing two quite different models of health policy. Fox appointed Julio Frenk, discussed earlier, to oversee the implementation of the Seguro Popular program, a textbook example of structured pluralism in action. Meanwhile, López Obrador appointed Asa Cristina Laurell, a longtime faculty member in the social medicine program at the UAM-Xochimilco, as his minister of health. They opted out of the national Seguro Popular program and instead introduced a "broadened health care model" intended to "guarantee that all services offered at Mexico City health care facilities will comply with the concept of equal access to services given the same need."[79] Budgets for public hospitals, primary care clinics, and public health services increased, while government health spending declined with efforts to fight waste and corruption. Community involvement with the health system was decentralized to small neighborhood councils, resembling the SUS in Brazil. Such changes went hand in hand with the creation of a universal pension system. According to Laurell, these programs were widely popular and by 2003, López Obrador enjoyed an "unprecedented 80–85% approval rating" in Mexico City.[80]

At the national level, Frenk unveiled the Seguro Popular program in 2003, which was part of a series of neoliberal health reforms. As an exemplar of the Universal Health Coverage model, as in Colombia, Seguro Popular centered on a program of government-subsidized insurance for the poor, to complement existing social security institutes for formal public- and private-sector employees. Laurell remained adamantly opposed to UHC as an expression of neoliberal values.[81] And, she argued, UHC failed on its own terms: by 2010, there were still over thirty-five million Mexicans without any health insurance coverage, compared to thirty-one million enrolled in the Seguro Popular.[82] This disappointing figure said nothing about the quality of care received and the impact on population health. Laurell has also pointed out that the UHC model emphasizes clinical care (and perhaps especially high-cost, high-tech interventions) while ignoring public health and preventive measures.[83] Here, Laurell echoes the primordial view of social medicine, that "liberal" medicine, based on private market relations and clinical interventions, can never adequately serve the health needs of a broad swath of the population in a modern society. When López Obrador became president of Mexico in 2018, he put Laurell in charge of a new reform to the national health system; the Seguro Popular program was summarily eliminated, and replaced with the Instituto de Salud para el Bienestar (INSABI), which took effect in January 2020.[84] In its structure, INSABI embodies the SUS approach, but Frenk—now the president of the University of Miami—has criticized it as unrealistic, underfunded, and ideologically driven.[85]

The dispute between Laurell and Frenk is, in some ways, a microcosm of health politics in much of the region today. Frenk, while no longer active in health policy, is essentially a technocrat who accepts broader political economic conditions and works with the institutions that help set the rules of the game (e.g., the World Bank). The UHC model that he helped to develop may be a pragmatic approach to health equity, in its accommodation of public- and private-sector involvement in the health sector, but it does nothing to change the dominant late capitalist systems and ideologies that produce and reproduce social inequality. Rather, the UHC approach demands that health systems accommodate themselves to "nations' economic and cultural norms."[86] Laurell, in contrast, is an outsider to the global health and development technocracy and finds the broader structural conditions to be intolerable. She also represents the ALAMES consensus view that UHC uses "the 'right to health' as a smokescreen for the privatisation of healthcare."[87] As with so many others in the ALAMES group, Laurell's influence depends on the political fortunes of left-wing politicians like López Obrador; when they are part of the in-party, they play an important role in the construction of health policy, but when they are out of power, their impact is limited (as the four-year presidential term of Mauricio Macri in Argentina, or Brazil under Jair Bolsonaro, also demonstrate). As a result, there is little political consensus around the proper direction for health policy in many Latin American countries, and health may have become an even more politically polarized space than before.[88]

Academic Social Medicine: Trends and Trajectories

As Jaime Breilh points out, social medicine and collective health have always manifested as both a sociopolitical movement and a "critical and interdisciplinary" academic field.[89] As we have seen throughout this book, social medicine seeks to join theory and praxis, becoming a discipline for scholar-activists with a commitment to social justice. Still, it is worth separating out the academic research side of social medicine for deeper consideration. While the political achievements of LASM might be sporadic and contingent on favorable circumstances, its academic production is constant, and continually evolving in its conceptual breadth. As a critical scholarly field, LASM has started to make an impact outside the region, reaching a wider international audience than ever before, which reflects an encouraging trend of greater attention to scholarship emanating from the Global South in discussions of health equity, social and structural determinants of health, and epistemological tensions in the health sector.

To begin this exploration of recent developments in LASM, it is important to recognize, as Breilh and others have suggested, that academia itself is a power-laden space where knowledges and insights from the Global South have been held in disregard by the mainstream of health sciences and social sciences. LASM has usually found its work excluded from the "mainstream" of public health and medical journals, located in the academic centers of the Global North. As Breilh argues, "Their editorial boards and reviewers put up obstacles to publications that fail to conform to the positivist canons of scientific rigor. The dominance of English and the hegemony of acritical paradigms, whether in the spheres of quantitative or qualitative analysis, has caused Latin American books and articles, which have offered fundamental, pioneering approaches, to be utterly ignored by the 'mainstream' of the

North, leading to a vicious circle of relegation and the impossibility of diffusion and gaining status."[90] Without a doubt, many mainstream English-language scientific journals would find much of LASM to be too politically radical, and perhaps just even too place-specific and contextual, to publish in an effort to build "universal scientific knowledge." At the same time, conceptual debates in LASM would not be out of place in such journals as *Social Science and Medicine*, but even these outlets have moved toward publishing less critical and politically pointed research, in favor of studies based on increasingly sophisticated statistical modeling.[91] Additionally, within the world of English-language publication, social medicine concepts are often marginalized, or made invisible, even in the work of fields like social epidemiology or medical anthropology.[92] Thus LASM scholarship has faced multiple challenges to getting wider recognition.

By the early 2000s, though, thanks to influential international bridge figures like Waitzkin, Nancy Krieger, and Jerry Spiegel, the insights of the LASM group were becoming more widely known outside the region. A series of English-language articles in the *American Journal of Public Health* and the *Lancet* in the early 2000s were especially important for showcasing progress in LASM for a wider international audience.[93] New journals based in Latin America appeared, such as *Ciência & Saúde Coletiva*, a Brazil-based publication of ABRASCO, which began in 1996, and *Salud Colectiva*, a publication of the Institute of Collective Health at the Universidad Nacional de Lanús in Argentina, launched in 2005. ALAMES, in conjunction with the Montefiore Medical Center at the Albert Einstein College of Medicine (one of the US institutions most sympathetic to the social medicine orientation, and in solidarity with leftist Latin American health workers since the 1970s), began publishing the bilingual journal *Medicina Social/Social Medicine* in 2006.

These journals have gained traction thanks to some general tendencies in academic publishing in Latin America. The content of most scientific journals is digital, open and accessible, free of charge, and indexed in equally accessible academic databases, such as SciELO. Often, journals present their content in two languages (Spanish or Portuguese, and English). Such openness and accessibility run counter to the practices of major North American or European publishers like Elsevier, Springer, or Taylor and Francis, which commodify their content with expensive subscription models. In all, the conditions for the circulation of knowledge are vastly different from those of the 1970s or 1980s, when Juan César Garcia handed out photocopies of important books and articles to his close-knit network of associates, often surreptitiously.

The potential for LASM insights to find an international audience today has few practical or technological obstacles.

Much of the published research of LASM is theoretical, with the development of core concepts that are intended to address the epistemological shortcomings of the mainstream health sciences. Contesting epistemology in the health social sciences has long been at the core of second-wave LASM, evident in classics like Arouca's *The Preventivist Dilemma* (an early challenge to preventive medicine) and Naomar Almeida-Filho's *Epidemiology without Numbers* (a historically rich critique of modern epidemiology).[94] Along similar lines, LASM scholars, led by Jaime Breilh, have questioned the mainstream concept of "social determinants" of health, countering with a language of "social *determination* of health" that emphasizes attention to historical political-economic processes that produce socially differentiated outcomes in health.[95] As Carolina Morales-Borrero and her colleagues have written, "While the [social determinants of health] understand society in its population sense, as a sum of individuals, [social determination] assumes society as a totality irreducible to individual-level dynamics. While the [social determinants of health] hold a functionalist perspective of society, privileging the idea of homeostasis as a baseline and of any alteration as deviation, the [social determination of health] holds a perspective of society as conflictual, which implies a dialectical relationship between the biological and the social, in a hierarchical structure where the biological is subsumed in the social, through processes of production and social reproduction."[96] Sebastian Fonseca calls the social determination model "*the* epistemological basis of Latin American social medicine."[97]

LASM has been critical of the "social determinants of health" paradigm, especially as articulated by the WHO Commission on the Social Determinants of Health, led by Michael Marmot. In the international health mainstream, that commission's 2008 report, *Closing the Gap in a Generation*, was a remarkable advance in the agenda for health equity, but many LASM scholars have found it wanting. A workshop organized by ALAMES in October 2008 criticized the Marmot Commission for "failing to touch the nature of capitalist society at its core" and for sponsoring a "political agenda [that] does not question or address the oppressive capitalist system that leads to social health inequities and inequalities."[98] The mainstream social-determinants approach, according to the same workshop participants, lacks any explicit theorization of the structure of society, and in consequence elevates "factors" (occupation, income, level of education) to explain health disparities without examining the processes behind the production of social inequality.[99] Another meeting at Harvard in 2009, organized by Nancy Krieger—whose well-known "ecosocial" theory bears the imprint of social medicine—and including many from the LASM group (Almeida-Filho, Franco, Barreto, Laurell), reached a similar conclusion: "Understanding and changing determinants of health inequities requires explicit attention to societies' political, economic, cultural and ecological priorities in historical context and how they become embodied; depoliticising and de-historicising health inequities will compromise evidence, knowledge and action." In closing, they asked: "Would anyone like to argue otherwise?"[100]

As discussed in earlier chapters, such critiques of functionalist sociology, superficial analysis of social inequality, and apolitical technocratic interventions have been integral to the second wave of LASM. Linked to the social "determination" framework, the *proceso salud-enfermedad* (the health-disease process), developed by Laurell in the 1980s, called into question many aspects of the conventional (biomedical) wisdom about illness: that it results from discrete biological pathologies, or comes as an anomalous episode against a backdrop of normally good health, or that it is even mainly a problem of individuals, as opposed to groups within the population.[101] As Roberto Castro explains the concept, "Health and disease cannot be considered as separate entities, but they are two moments (linked in a dialectical way) of the same phenomenon, which mutually constitute one another."[102] In original empirical studies developing the concept, Laurell emphasized that such variables as "income" or "occupation" were insufficient to explain differences in health according to class; a historical-materialist concept of class relations was necessary to situate patterns of illness and fatigue in working conditions and distinctive modes of production.[103] Later, Eduardo Menéndez, an Argentinean in exile in Mexico, integrated sociological aspects of health care into Laurell's formula, leading to the *proceso salud-enfermedad-atención* concept. This innovation went along with Menéndez's equally influential theorization of the *modelo médico hegemónico*—the hegemonic model of medicine—to explain the dominance of Western biomedicine as a result of capitalist processes that lead to the commercialization (*mercantilización*) of medical care, as well as the production of new subjects and subjectivities under late capitalism.[104]

Countless studies have employed these terms and concepts, but summarizing just one article, published in the journal *Salud Colectiva*, might help us understand the application of somewhat abstract analytical tools. In 2005, an interdisciplinary research team—with specializations in sociology, public health nutrition, and nursing—investigated the motivations for seeking PHC services in an impoverished neighborhood of Salta, Argentina. At the time, PHC had become more accessible to Argentines of all socioeconomic strata thanks to reforms of the leftist Kirchner government; however, PHC resources in Salta were underutilized, relative to the levels of preventable illness present in the population. Through a series of interviews in the field, the authors found a normalized lack of what they called a "somatic culture"—meaning the "capacity to be able to feel, to listen to the body"—within the community.[105] The daily struggle to merely survive and scratch out a living caused delays in the seeking of care, except in the case of children, whose problems were the primary motivation for seeking care. Class plays a pivotal role in shaping attitudes and behaviors; for the working class, "health is a means for life, not an end in itself; caring [for health] is something incorporated into everyday life as something natural, not as an object of constant preoccupation."[106]

The Salta study also demonstrates theoretical developments within academic social medicine, which has moved beyond a strictly historical-materialist mode of analysis. While the early writings of Laurell and Menéndez did not ignore the construction of subjectivities, these were perhaps overly determined by class position, understood, in the Marxian fashion, as relations through labor to the modes of production. Under the influence of social theorists like Pierre Bourdieu and his notion of the "habitus," researchers have paid more attention to the complexities of subjectivity, and how perceptions of health and disease become embedded in culture and the habits of daily life.[107] In the structure-agency debate, concepts like the habitus offer a middle ground. In sync with a broader trend in the social sciences of health, a structuralist fixation on class gave way to explorations of other kinds of social identity that conditioned perceptions of health, notions of citizenship and belonging, and power relations in medicine—particularly gender, sexual orientation, and race and ethnicity.

Women's health concerns and feminist theory have been on the rise in the social medicine scholarship of recent decades. Differences in vulnerability to health issues according to gender are seen to arise from the structures (and restructuring) of Latin American economies. The gender division of labor (at least for middle-class women) that prevailed in the mid-twentieth century—based on the "sexual division of labor produced by the requirements of the modern industrial model, which needed women-mothers who care for the domestic space and care for future workers"—no longer prevailed due to the economic restructuring and change in social roles required by neoliberalism.[108] Under the new economic model, women's nonremunerated domestic labor is increasingly piled on top of their wage labor, leading to the problem of the *doble presencia* (double duty) or *síndrome de la supermujer* (superwoman syndrome); moreover, cuts to government social programs in times of neoliberal austerity fall disproportionately on women.[109] In a series of studies on vulnerability to cardiovascular health risks, the Argentine psychologist Débora Tajer and her collaborators sought to define the "specific modes" of the construction of vulnerability according to gender and class. Reflecting a widespread change in the international discourse about gender and heart disease, this group of Argentine researchers interrogated the gender ideology embedded in narratives, or "social imaginaries," of cardiovascular problems, while describing specific ways that subjective class and gender roles lead to minimizing risks, unhealthy behaviors, and delayed care. Rather than conceiving of class and gender as categories of "social determinants," Tajer and her colleagues instead embraced the notion of "social determination," oriented toward analyzing the processes by which differential risk and vulnerability are constructed. The fact that the summary of this multiyear research project was published in an Argentine cardiology journal spoke to the rising appreciation of critical social science research in the medical mainstream.[110]

Another line of research in social medicine explores the right to health, and how it is realized through specific legal instruments. The default normative stance within the social medicine community is that a right to health is fundamental and health care should be universal and provided or managed by the state. Some scholars have moved beyond platitudes to examine the right to health, how it is operationalized, and some contradictions of health citizenship. Sonia Fleury of Brazil has been one of the leading scholars in this area. In her formulation, health citizenship has numerous dimensions—normative, civic or public, legal, and institutional. Fleury, among others, has examined a rising tendency of the "judicialization of health," particularly in Colombia, Costa Rica, and Brazil, where newer legal frameworks offer citizens expansive rights to sue the health-care system to cover needed procedures and medications. Overall, judicialization has led to an unprecedented role for the courts in adjudicating the services offered by national health systems, and such legal procedures may serve to avoid or postpone consideration of fundamental inequities in health coverage.[111]

These legalistic assertions of patients' rights dovetail, perhaps ironically, with the capitalist logics of twenty-first-century health care. As Eduardo Menéndez has argued more recently, multinational pharmaceutical companies, especially, have a financial stake in such cases, since judgments in favor of patients tend to lead to the purchase or subsidy of expensive drugs. More broadly, Menéndez points out that the empowerment of the patient-consumer (with legal rights, discourses of self-care, and more widely accessible information) tends to diminish the status of physicians, even leading to their "proletarianization" within complex biomedical systems; recent advances in genetics and biotechnology portend new biopolitical subjects with hopes of personalized therapies (as opposed to the citizen-subject underlying the endeavor of collective health).[112] The anthropologist Jessica Scott Jerome finds analogous shifts in the conception of rights, citizenship, and consumerism in her study of the local-level engagements with the SUS in Fortaleza, Brazil.[113]

Many LASM scholars have become influential leaders in higher education, viewed as another arena for social transformation. This trend is captured in the trajectory of Naomar Almeida-Filho. Widely known in his native Brazil and across the LASM network for his first book, *Epidemiology without Numbers*, he helped to create (with Mauricio Barreto, Jairnilson Silva Paim, and others) the Instituto de Saúde Coletiva at the Universidade Federal da Bahia (UFBA), after years in its department of preventive medicine, in 1994.[114] His research focused on health inequalities and epistemological questions, leading to the development of his approach to critical social epidemiology, often in productive dialogue with Jaime Breilh.[115] Almeida-Filho, who had received his PhD in epidemiology at the University of North Carolina-Chapel Hill, made the most of international connections, including collaborations with social epidemiologists at North American universities such as Krieger, Ichiro Kawachi, and S. V. Subramanian.[116] These collaborations of the early 2000s helped incorporate the intellectual production of Latin American social epidemiologists into a field dominated internationally by North Americans and Europeans.[117] Like Breilh, who became rector of the Universidad Andina Simón Bolívar in Quito, Almeida-Filho served for two terms as rector of the UFBA, from 2002 to 2010, before working to establish the Universidade Federal do Sul da Bahia, starting in 2013. In this administrative work, Almeida-Filho has applied the same critical lens on higher education as he has on the health field, in the hopes of constructing "new forms of counter-hegemonic knowledge."[118] In a practical sense, this work includes the opening of educational opportunity to wider swaths of the Bahia population and engaging social movement organizations in the planning of the new university. Philosophically, Almeida-Filho cites not only the major figures of social medicine and collective health but also Boaventura de Sousa Santos (the Portuguese theoretician of decolonial epistemologies), Milton Santos (the influential Brazilian geographer), and Paulo Freire. In his career path, Almeida-Filho demonstrates a model of transformative praxis via the education field, rather than, say, deep participation in academic-activist organizations (like ABRASCO) or government health ministries.

As the academic production of LASM garners more attention internationally, often it is the most epistemologically radical theorizations (and politically unactionable proposals) that filter through. Breilh, after a long career, is becoming more widely known to English-language audiences through his theorizing of "critical epidemiology" and his relating of health crises to "planetary environmental crises" that can only be overcome with new "intercultural awakening"—a radical reassessment of the foundations of Western thought.[119] These kinds of transgressive encounters are admired by critical health social scientists who seek a vocabulary for a radical "re-imagining" of global health.[120] However, these representations outside of Latin America of LASM as a radical field may ignore that the "normal" research published in journals like *Salud Colectiva* is somewhat more prosaic and not always so overtly political; these studies engage the same questions, methods, and theories that drive established fields like social epidemiology and medical anthropology. The portrayals of LASM's epistemological radicalism also miss out on more subtle treatments of important issues, like the right to health or power differentials in the health-care field. Scholars like Fleury, Menéndez, and Almeida-Filho, rather than invoking utopias, are grounded in the challenges and contradictions of the health field in complex and dynamic societies.

Health Equity without Social Medicine: The Exceptional Cases of Costa Rica and Cuba

As an academic community with international reach, LASM has had increasing policy influence. Second-wave LASM can take credit for progressive health policy reforms in countries like Brazil, Bolivia, and Venezuela, while slowing the momentum of neoliberalization of health in Mexico, Chile, and Colombia. During this period, the ALAMES group has offered a critical and oppositional voice—though, by no means, a single voice—to counter mainstream thought in international health. Curiously, however, the international LASM network has relatively weak links to two of the Latin American countries most admired and renowned for achieving effective, universal health systems in low- and middle-income settings: Cuba and Costa Rica. Instead, health policy leaders in these two countries have been mostly disconnected, perhaps even aloof, from the theory and praxis of social medicine.

In this section, I examine Cuba and Costa Rica as exceptional cases that exemplify many of the objectives of social medicine (in particular, single, universal health systems), but mostly without the political militancy of doctors, health workers, and academics that seems to define social medicine elsewhere in the region. Although I will briefly discuss the essential aspects of the countries' health systems, it is impossible to do a full analysis of those systems in such a small space. Rather, I focus more on how Cuba and Costa Rica are perceived by members of the LASM community, and how the two countries, currently, have political conditions and cultures in health systems that work against the development of a strong social medicine movement.

At first glance, Cuba and Costa Rica could hardly be more different: Cuba, as a socialist country, has a command economy and a highly centralized health system, and is well-known for the use of health diplomacy, whereby Cuban doctors are sent around the world on humanitarian missions in exchange for needed commodities, hard currency, or favorable trade conditions. The 1959 revolution put Cuba on a distinctive path that has inspired leftists throughout Latin America, including many members of the LASM group. Che Guevara, as an icon of "revolutionary medicine," also has great symbolic value for LASM and influenced the militancy of the movement.[121] That distinctiveness, however, also makes the Cuban model difficult to emulate in practice. Costa Rica, meanwhile, has been an island of peace and political stability in Central America, and since the early 1990s it has followed the neoliberal recipe book (structural reform, privatization, trade liberalization) across most sectors *except* health, where the state remains the dominant player in a social welfare- and solidarity-oriented model that has served the Costa Rican population well. Despite these and other differences, Cuba and Costa Rica are the only countries in Latin America with unified health systems (along with Brazil, since the creation of the SUS).[122] Cuba and Costa Rica also share a strong biomedical or "Flexnerian" tendency in their health practices, lack of critical social science perspectives, and relatively little interest in analyzing the social determination of health.

Even before 1959, Cuba had already made considerable public health progress, despite political repression and extreme income inequality. Wading through historiographical disputes, both statistical and ideological, James McGuire and Laura Frankel found that Cuba had some of the lowest infant mortality rates in Latin America at the start of the revolutionary period. They conclude that, in addition to the health benefits of economic modernization, "factors that contributed to rapid mortality decline in pre-revolutionary Cuba included a bountiful supply of doctors and nurses, fairly good health services for the urban poor, and access to at least some health services for the rural poor."[123] While many doctors fled Cuba for the United States and other destinations after the revolution, the new government built on established success in public health and medicine, and developed numerous initiatives to continuously improve health conditions on the island. These initiatives included a rural health program that built up health infrastructure and sent health personnel to some of the most remote parts of Cuba; successful campaigns for malaria eradication and mass vaccination for smallpox, polio, and measles; making medical school available for free to Cubans of all social classes, which eventually produced a superabundance of health workers on the island; and a unified health system by 1970, which provided health care free of charge for all Cubans.[124] During the 1970s, Cuba oriented its health system to the provision of primary health care, preventive medicine, and community medicine, becoming one of the cited models for the "Health Care for All" PHC model that emerged from the Alma Ata conference in 1978.

Starting as early as 1960, when Cuba sent health personnel to Chile on a humanitarian mission in the aftermath of the Valdivia earthquake, continuing through the Cold War with particular focus on socialist and nonaligned countries, and accelerating in the 1990s during the "special period" after Cuba lost the economic support of the Soviet Union, the Cuban government has engaged in a form of soft diplomacy termed "Cuban medical internationalism."[125] This includes the export of Cuban medical brigades abroad (in recent years, to Venezuela, Bolivia, and other friendly states) and the hosting of medical students from across the region, at the Escuela Latinoamericana de Medicina in Havana.

How does LASM see Cuba? On the one hand, the Cuban health model virtually embodies the wish list of LASM: a unified health system, free health care for all, and equitable outcomes, within a non- or anti-capitalist political economic model. As Howard Waitzkin puts it, "The nature of Cuba's revolution encouraged more dramatic improvements that moved beyond reformism and toward a structurally different health-care system. The rapid transformation of Cuban society permitted a rapid reconstruction of its health-care system, and the consolidation of state power allowed for a remarkable series of reforms and structural modifications."[126] Beyond these material achievements, Cuba also plays a symbolic role for the LASM group: as the geopolitical adversary and ideological antithesis of the United States and its free-market model of health care. Cuba has stubbornly resisted the incursions of US imperialism for six decades, giving hope to those who resist the spread of neoliberalism across the region; in the early 2000s, Cuban health diplomacy seemed to be one dimension of a robust alternative international alliance based on "south–south cooperation" to counter the hegemony of the neoliberal policy apparatus.[127]

In other ways, though, Cuba is a poor fit as a model for Latin American social medicine. Leaders of the Cuban health system have largely opted to pursue a top-down, technocratic model that emphasizes excellence in biomedicine. As Waitzkin and his colleagues contend, there is a "'Flexnerian' overemphasis on biological issues" in Cuba, partly as a side effect revolutionary success. "Within Cuba, the same accomplishments [in public health] led to a questioning of the need for social medicine. The revolution had achieved improved health conditions largely through broad social change. . . . Against this background, the remaining challenges in Cuba seemed to require a focus on technical issues more than the social issues emphasized by social medicine."[128] In my conversations with him, Mario Testa concurred. Reflecting on the period of the late 1960s when he visited Cuba frequently as a consultant on the OPS/CENDES health planning method (which the country avidly adopted), Testa said that "the Cubans were very rigid in their thinking on how to do things, very rigid in the sense that it was very rigorous, but at the same time they were tied to very specific norms." The system that Cuba developed "was very hierarchical, orderly, and particular about what had to be done." In a tour of the country with a Cuban health minister in the early 1970s, Testa observed that hospitals followed the norms laid down by the ministry "to the letter." But he found it hard to convey the value of the Cuban example to PAHO functionaries or to health planners in other countries, for political reasons: to accomplish what they had in Cuba, "first we would need to have a revolution."[129]

Within Cuban medical education, there has been little interest in social medicine thought, deemed "too theoretical" (although ALAMES held its eighth meeting there, in 2000, and a research center, or *ateneo*, honoring Juan César Garcia was set up in Havana around that time).[130] In fact, the social sciences of health are weakly developed in Cuba, having mostly neglected the innovations of the past few decades that provide the critical tools for understanding relations between health and society. Ironically, the models of preventive and community medicine that prevail in Cuba still rely on functionalist/positivist approaches. Mario Rovere put it a different way: "Broadly speaking, Cuba does not contribute much to intellectual production in social medicine. In Cuba, they *do* social medicine, not write about it."[131] Along the same lines, a sympathetic appraisal of Cuban medical education notes the emphasis on international cooperation, recruitment and training of physicians from marginalized groups from across the Americas, and a growing emphasis on complementary and alternative medicine, which make this system a model for the end goal, promoting equity and health as a human right.[132]

Costa Rica is conspicuous in its near absence from the world of contemporary LASM. Since the inception of ALAMES in 1984, Costa Ricans have seldom been represented at the organization's international meetings; Testa told me: "I do not remember anyone from Costa Rica at an ALAMES meeting, or at least the ones I went to." A search of the journals *Social Medicine/Medicina Social* (United States) and *Salud Colectiva* (Lanús, Argentina), both major outlets for the LASM group, yields exactly one article focused principally on Costa Rica (over more than thirty volumes of the journals, combined).

The virtual absence of Costa Rica from the community of LASM is surprising, considering the fame of its universal health-care system and its origins in the first wave of social medicine in the 1930s and 1940s. As noted briefly in previous chapters, the Costa Rican government developed a fruitful collaboration with the Rockefeller Foundation that by the 1930s led to the creation of a network of rural clinics that integrated health care and social work, and the country established the foundations of its modern health system in 1948, with the creation of the Caja Costarricence de Seguridad Social (CCSS), modeled on the Chilean CSO.[133] Following a classically "Bismarckian" model at first, the CCSS—popularly known as La Caja—was funded by tripartite payroll contributions from employer, employee, and the state. As we have seen, one pitfall of social security funding schemes for health insurance, across Latin America, is the tendency to create segmented and fragmented systems, where some groups (e.g., state workers, unionized labor in corporatist regimes) tend to defend their hard-won benefits, leaving the poorest at the mercy of underfunded state-run health systems. Costa Rica instead managed to construct a unified system by covering the least advantaged first, and then expanding coverage into higher income brackets.[134] This has engendered the social solidarity necessary for sustaining the health system; despite complaints about wait times, the vast majority of Costa Ricans pay into the system and get good to excellent health care in return.

Against the neoliberal strategy of "structured pluralism," which prescribes a separation of functions of financing, insurance, and provision, the CCSS has, over time, integrated all these functions together. In stages, the CCSS took over most of the functions of the national Ministry of Health, including ownership and management of the physical assets of the health system (hospitals and the PHC clinics, known as EBAIS), leaving the Ministry of Health with the functions of planning and oversight, and control over some aspects of public health and sanitation. Moreover, Costa Rica stood up to the World Bank at pivotal moments, accepting loans to improve health services while resisting demands for privatization, decentralization, and sectoral reform, which were unpopular among the public and doctors alike.[135] As a result, the CCSS functions as an autonomous, state-owned institution, with considerable independence from the vagaries of electoral politics. There is actually a substantial private medical sector in Costa Rica, but private health insurance is virtually nonexistent, and so is the much-criticized modality of US-style managed care.

Given all this, why does social medicine have so little interest in Costa Rica, and Costa Ricans, apparently, so little interest in social medicine? Possibly, this disconnection comes from the contrasting political styles of Costa Rican health professionals and the LASM group, along with the relatively low position of the health social sciences in Costa Rica. In chapter 5, I discussed the rise of technocracy in the health sector in the 1950s and 1960s, and in chapter 6, how disillusionment with technocratic planning led to a new wave of social medicine. In Costa Rica, apparently that moment of disillusionment never arrived, and the guiding spirit of health policy is more an Abraham Horwitz than a Juan César García type. Technical analysis and incremental reform to a well-functioning but never perfect system, rather than structural critique and radical change, is preferred. As the Brazilian Sonia Fleury argues in a comparative analysis of universal health-care systems in Latin America, political mobilization "from below" may play a role in some countries' moves toward universal health care, but in Costa Rica "societal pressures and preferences played a relatively minor role while governmental leadership and technocrats pushed the reform."[136] For example, Costa Rica's excellent PHC evolved from innovations within the system (such as the "Hospital Sin Paredes" experiment, led by Juan G. Ortiz Guier and Jaime Serra Canales, a Chilean exile), adapted and incorporated into the larger architecture of the CCSS.[137] At junctures of major health policy reform in Costa Rica—all of which tended toward increased universalization and centralization of services—there was neither a strong mobilization of popular or civil society sectors in support of reform, nor powerful organized opposition against them.[138] During the period of the consolidation of Costa Rica's health system in the late Cold War era, the country had a functioning democracy, no military (possibly freeing up resources for social spending), and a political consensus around investing in health and education, unlike most other countries in Latin America. And for whatever reason, still unclear, the Costa Rican government was able to resist the push from the World Bank and other external actors to follow their recipe for health sector reform.

The Counterhegemonic Project of LASM

The success of second-wave Latin American social medicine is, in many ways, impressive. A small group of leftist academics, increasingly from the social sciences of health (rather than or in addition to having been trained in medicine), has risen to prominence and shaped the health policy of countries as varied as Mexico, Brazil, Argentina, and Bolivia. For the most part, they work outside of the mainstream of the international health and development technocracy. Instead, they have created their own, alternative international networks, not just within the health field, but cutting across sectors, to join forces with other social movements. They have taken advantage of the opportunities created by democratization, building up new academic programs in the field, often with a radical-left ideological orientation, and thriving in the new global civil society spaces opened up since the 1980s. The international connections of LASM extend not only to allies in North American and European universities, but into truly global, multifaceted networks like the People's Health Movement, "a global network formed in 2000 which comprises grassroots health activists, other civil society organizations, issue-based networks, academics, researchers and activists from low, middle and high-income countries."[139] With ALAMES as one of its affiliate networks, it continues to advocate for the "Health for All" pledge articulated at the 1978 Alma-Ata meeting, serves as a watchdog organization for institutions like the WHO, and seeks an inclusive politics of health, demanding authentic collective involvement, not just bureaucratic routines, a leitmotif of second-wave LASM.

The LASM group, organized in ALAMES (and national associations like Brazil's ABRASCO), deftly networked its way into health policy planning for the New Left regimes of the Pink Tide, and proved to be effective in pushing back against neoliberal restructuring of the health sector, at least for a time. Democratization has been a vehicle not just for opening up critique, debate, and resistance but also for assessing the effectiveness of policies. Progressive health policies have been embraced because they are responsive to popular demands. And whereas social medicine was once dominated by physicians with a social conscience or a leftist political bent, now it is dominated by social scientists with distinctive scholarly traditions, ways of knowing, and notions of political praxis. Reflecting the increased relevance of social science in the second wave of LASM, even the Oswaldo Cruz Institute in Brazil—Fiocruz, one of the premier medical science research institutes in Latin America—was led by a sociologist, Nisia Trindade Lima, starting in 2017 (and she was appointed as Brazil's Minister of Health by Lula after his re-election in 2022).

Yet a strong network of activist-academics in social medicine is not a prerequisite for equitable and effective health systems. The examples of Cuba and Costa Rica, largely disconnected from such networks, prove that point. Based on this analysis, we can conclude that the second wave of LASM has thrived as a critical and oppositional movement in places where conventional democratic processes were cut off by authoritarian governments (or single-party regimes, as in Mexico); where severe and palpable social inequalities and health inequities existed; where leftist academics and health workers found political space to join other social movements and push for progressive reform; and where capitalist development seemed only to exacerbate inequality and to undermine population health, including the rising infiltration of market logics into the health sector under neoliberalism.

Credit is due LASM for breathing new life into theorizations of health inequality, creating new spaces for contestation of the hegemonic models of Western biomedicine and neoliberal economic development strategies. Social medicine does what a serious academic field should, deploying critical frameworks to understand the workings of society, especially the complicated relationship between the state, the market, the health sector, and different population groups. Still, LASM seems destined to remain an oppositional movement outside the international health policy mainstream. The international development field produces policy frameworks, such as UHC or the social determinants of health, which, many would say, adjust pragmatically to the conditions presented by the hegemonic forces of neoliberal, globalized capitalism. The "counter-hegemonic" project of LASM is, in many ways, quixotic, if the goal is to change business as usual at the WHO, World Bank, or other globally influential institutions. Nevertheless, LASM academics, activists, and policymakers sustain an effective international network that consistently fosters solidarity, mutual support, and ideological consistency, with occasional policy achievements.

Conclusion
Making Sense of Latin American Social Medicine

"What is social medicine?" Early in the course of my research for this book, a close friend in Argentina asked me this question. It's not that he wanted my definition of a well-known but difficult-to-define idea—rather he had never heard the term at all. I should mention that this friend is a practicing physician, and over the years I have received similar questions from people in the health field when I try to explain my research interests. For better or for worse, social medicine remains at the fringes of mainstream medical education and the practices of medicine and public health in Latin America. It would be a mistake to imagine that the strongly held views of a small cohort immersed in social medicine thought—like the ALAMES group, which numbers several hundred members—represents the values or concerns of the millions of people working in the health sector across Latin America.

With a merely numerical assessment of influence, one could dismiss LASM as a minor and marginal movement in the larger scheme of things. But we might instead draw a completely different, more positive conclusion: despite its small numbers, social medicine has had an outsized and lasting influence on health and social policy in many parts of Latin America, thanks to the deep commitment of its proponents, the quality of their analysis of problems in the health sector, and their ability to influence the political process at critical junctures. It is noteworthy and encouraging that health is considered a right protected by the state across Latin America, despite the region having some of the widest inequalities in wealth and income anywhere in the world.[1] Much of the credit for establishing this right and holding governments accountable for protecting it should go to social medicine proponents, past and present. Latin American social medicine has also served as an inspiration for critical social scientists in the health field outside of the region. Progressive academics in fields like social epidemiology increasingly look to their Latin American counterparts for alternative discourses and practices in the health field.

Social medicine began as an offshoot of the hygiene movement, especially as public health policy concerns began to gravitate away from infectious disease and sanitation and toward chronic population health issues amid the construction of Latin American welfare states. The first wave of social medicine, with its integrative, systemic, and holistic perspective, was helped along by support from international players like the League of Nations and the ILO, although they were less impactful than networks of hygienists and health and social policy experts within Latin America. Two countries where social medicine became sufficiently organized and coherent as a movement able to make policy impacts were Chile and Argentina in the 1930s and 1940s. In the former, existing institutions of state medicine (the health insurance funds, or cajas) provided a framework for activist physicians to push for doctors' control of the health system, increased spending on hospitals and clinics, and structural change in Chilean society to address the root causes of population health problems. Alongside this "medical vanguard" were more moderate proposals from factions in social medicine influenced by Catholic social doctrine. In Argentina, social medicine never quite cohered as a movement, but organized doctors' desires for autonomy and the internal conflicts in the Peronist coalition produced the foundations of the country's highly fragmented health system.

During the early Cold War period, social medicine faded both internationally and in Latin America specifically. A growing international health and development apparatus promoted narrowly conceived projects and avoided contentious political questions. Social medicine seemed a relic alongside more scientific and supposedly apolitical approaches like health systems planning, preventive medicine, and disease eradication campaigns. But, disaffected technocrats within this larger apparatus emerged as the nucleus for the second wave of social medicine in Latin America in the early 1970s. The authoritarian regimes of the 1970s sent Chilean, Argentinean, and Brazilian health workers into exile, where they formed solidarity networks, programs of study in social medicine, new journals, and, eventually, associations like ALAMES and ABRASCO. The second wave of social medicine (and "collective health") led directly to major health systems reform in Brazil, resisted the incursions of neoliberalism in the health sector, shaped the health policies of "Pink Tide" governments of the region, and offered imaginative ways of thinking about health, disease, and society.

Throughout, social medicine has changed in response to dynamic political conditions and academic innovations. Like a species that evolves in response to changes in the environment around it, social medicine has shed certain values, concepts, and associations (eugenics, medical paternalism, hygienic moralizing) while gaining new ones (more sophisticated social theories, flattening hierarchies in the health field, stronger connections to other social movements, a commitment to participatory democracy). Despite its internal diversity and fluctuations in broader influence, social medicine nonetheless remains recognizable and consistent over the long run, with its critical perspectives on mainstream medicine, commitment to health equity, and advocacy for strong state involvement in the health sector.

In the rest of this conclusion, I want to return to some of the major themes of the book. I start with an in-depth discussion of two questions raised in the book's introduction, regarding the role of expert networks and the question of political will. Then, I offer some key conclusions about the history of Latin American social medicine that emerge from the narrative I have constructed, which covers several decades across a large region with diverse national experiences. Along the way, I try to point out shortcomings of my analysis and opportunities for further research.

Networks

As a field, LASM emerges and persists in a dynamic network within an international context that is itself constantly changing. These networks consist of individuals and organizations, connected for a variety of reasons, including shared intellectual interests or political objectives, complementary training and skills put to use in specific projects, professional ties, and mentor-student relationships. Binding these networks together are ties of friendship, trust, solidarity, and reciprocity. The broader context also matters. The identity of LASM—the group's shared recognition of common roots, values, and aspirations—is constructed relationally, that is, in opposition to, or at least in dialogue with, the identity of other groups. As Rafael de la Dehesa puts it, social medicine has been developed through "counterhegemonic" transnational knowledge networks, which can "articulate, with varying degrees of formalization, public and private actors at the local, national and supranational levels, potentially including government agencies, international organizations, foundations, research institutes, professional associations, corporations and nongovernmental organizations."[2] Even as it articulates with social movements from other domains—for example, with feminism, as de la Dehesa argues—LASM also takes on an oppositional role in relation to the mainstream international health and development field.[3] It would be hard to conceive of an ALAMES without its foils in, say, the WHO or the World Bank.

At the same time, the accomplishments of social medicine depend on a favorable international context. In the interwar period, two organizations based in Europe, but with international reach, were important. The League of Nations Health Organization, a kind of precursor to the WHO, tended to favor a holistic social medicine framework in its approach to problems such as malaria, tuberculosis, and rural health. The International Labor Organization promoted the social security model as a way to achieve peace between labor and capital, its principal goal, while it also helped to set international standards for working conditions and nutritional requirements. These Geneva-based organizations, although not especially powerful, were important for the setting of norms in social and health policy in Latin America. Later, more robust multilateral health and development institutions—the PAHO and WHO, for instance—had complex effects on the trajectory of LASM. On the one hand, the international health and development apparatus of the early Cold War era followed a politically cautious and technocratic pathway. In this context, those who adopted a social medicine slant found limited opportunities for influence, Josué de Castro being a prime example. Yet, simultaneously, the strength and reach of expert networks with official connections were pivotal to the rise of second-wave social medicine. Notably, this network started to develop among internationally connected technocrats in public health and health planning, such as Juan César García or Mario Testa, who were privileged to circulate through places like Washington, DC, Santiago, and Caracas, which were leading centers in the modernization-oriented social sciences of health in the 1960s and 1970s. The PAHO, especially, created spaces for social medicine to thrive—for example, in human resources and medical education—even though the organization as a whole was not radical in its orientation.

We often think of social medicine consciousness emerging, as a revelation or moral provocation, from direct contact with human suffering. Often-cited paradigmatic cases of the "heroes" of social medicine, like Che Guevara during his South American travels, Sidney and Emily Kark in South Africa, or Paul Farmer in rural Haiti evoke such narratives. However, what spawned the second wave of social medicine in Latin America was not quite so dramatic or romantic: disillusioned technocrats rediscovered social medicine as they confronted the opacity of bureaucracy and the limits of modernization theory, functionalism, and positivism. They approached social medicine obliquely, not so much from clinical experience but from auxiliary fields like health systems planning, preventive medicine, and medical education.

With the repressive action of authoritarian governments intensifying after 1970, these new social medicine groups not only supplied much-needed intellectual oxygen but also served as solidarity networks. In particular, Chilean health workers who survived the overthrow of Allende found crucial lifelines in ad hoc solidarity groups, US and Latin American universities, and international organizations like the PAHO or WHO. Strong international solidarity and the shared experience of political repression throughout the 1970s helped to shape the outlook of ALAMES, formed in 1984. Even today, many of the members of ALAMES have served at one time or another as consultants to the PAHO or WHO. Whatever their outward policy stances, these international health organizations are perhaps more ideologically tolerant and intellectually diverse internally than might appear at first glance.

Tracing expert networks can be a challenge methodologically. When I embarked on this project, I had planned a more formal analysis to understand the contours of networks, strength of connections (linkages), prominence of key actors (nodes), and changes over time. Although I used some network-analysis tools to help visualize networks and keep track of the large cast of characters, formal techniques proved daunting and, ultimately, not in harmony with my larger objectives. I found that formal analysis involving connectivity metrics did not help in understanding the substance of social medicine thought, nor could it capture the contingent and sentimental nature of the relationships between actors. The structure of networks can be analyzed objectively, but such an approach misses the crucial subjectivity of actors within the networks—that is, how participants understand and describe the networks they are embedded in, to construct a movement identity. Other researchers could potentially build on this book with more formal network-analysis methods, to gain more insight into the development of the social medicine field and its relationship to other academic and sociopolitical movements.

Where Does "Political Will" Come From?
The Irreplaceable Role of the Medical Profession

With few exceptions in Latin America's history, developing systems of socialized medicine depended not just on the *acquiescence* of the medical profession, but rather on their *active support* for such systems. Because of its social status, irreplaceable expertise, and control over the production of new doctors in universities, the medical profession in Latin American countries has wielded considerable power, with an enviable measure of autonomy from the fractious realm of normal politics. In terms of health systems reform, not much could get done without them.

Medical union organizing can be unpredictable, its goals contingent on historical circumstance. But doctors historically have organized mainly to protect their professional interests and autonomy. Sometimes those interests align with those of other organized labor sectors or popular social movements, especially in times of extreme economic or political crisis (as in Chile in the mid-1930s) or in windows of accelerated institutional disruption and change (as in Brazil during the 1980s, with the reopening of democracy). At other times, doctors have organized to fend off state incursions into the health sector, as in the activism of COMRA during the first Perón era in Argentina. The medical profession is not ideologically homogeneous; leftist doctors can get pulled into and lead broader political movements. Often, however, the organized medical profession is an obstacle to what many would consider progressive health policy change. That is because professional autonomy is highly cherished and threats to autonomy may prompt a defensive reaction that overrides other considerations. Again, Chile provides a classic example, as the Colegio Médico—originally planned as a formal association of doctors with the National Health Service—became increasingly conservative in the 1960s and 1970s, alarmed by the prospect of a socialist revolution and irritated by the strictures of the state health system. Doctors, when organized, have a lot of power, but it is not always exercised to advance progressive political objectives.

So, when we ask the question, as many scholars have: "Where does the political will for broad-based, equitable, health systems come from?" my answer is that we have to start with the organized interests of the health sector. This position can be seen as rather old-fashioned for the history of public health because it is so focused on the medical profession, rather than on policies and actors external to it, but clearly it plays a significant role in the construction of health systems, and probably will continue to do so. Yet, as Eduardo L. Menéndez has suggested, the development of a "more symmetrical" power relationship between doctors and patients—with rising empowerment of the patient and the relative loss of status and prestige of the doctor—is an ongoing process that aligns with other tendencies in the medical field today, including its focus on individuals rather than the collective and the biological rather than the social.[4] Thus, one of the more complicated challenges for social medicine/collective health today lies in convincing doctors to share power in the health sector—to democratize health—while also moving whole systems toward greater equity and justice.

Leftist political parties in power are much more likely to increase the state's role in the health system. It is also evident that social medicine's goals and values tend to align with the political left. However, from this history it remains unclear whether labor organizing and the effective channeling of working-class demands necessarily lead to more equitable and universal health-care systems. This is an assumption held by many advocates of unitary health systems. Adam Gaffney, borrowing from Vicente Navarro, an important scholar associated with second-wave social medicine, argues that "some of the more uniquely decommodified universal healthcare systems—i.e. those that provide (often free) care to all without tiers or stratification— emerged in part as a result of Left and working-class political power and/or ideological pressure."[5] As Navarro puts it, "In all countries, the major force behind the establishment of an NHP [a national health program] has been the labor movement (and its political instruments—the socialist parties) in its pursuit of the welfare state."[6]

However, I would argue that organized labor activism does not usually lead to universal health care, for a few different reasons. First, there are questions of political priorities: improvements in the health system might be a priority for people close to the system, but the working class might demand other things, like good housing or fair wages. A more significant problem is that organized labor is often an obstacle to health reform, since unions usually want to hold on to hard-won benefits (like health insurance coverage or access to high-quality medical care). Sometimes the social medicine group may be too optimistic about the prospects for building coalitions across social class. In her 2017 analysis of health politics in Mexico, Asa Cristina Laurell writes, "Paradoxically, the large trade unions have also maintained or negotiated private medical insurance and/or services as a labor benefit, although one would expect them to adhere to the ideals of solidarity, equality, redistribution, and the right to health as a citizen's right."[7] However, the history of health politics in Latin America, as I have shown throughout this book, suggests that organized interests are usually intransigent in their defense of group-based benefits, presenting a major obstacle to the conversion of fragmented, segmented systems into genuinely universal health systems. Only rarely, as in the case of the creation of the SUS in Brazil (as described in the introduction and in chapters 6 and 7) do political conditions align for fundamental and long-lasting health systems reforms.

Related to the question of political will is the enigma of solidarity. Returning to Laurell's quotation above, solidarity can be understood as an ideal or a value that must be widely shared to enable pro-poor and egalitarian health policies. However, as Barbara Prainsack and Alena Buyx argue, "Solidarity signifies *shared practices reflecting a collective commitment to carry 'costs' (financial, social, emotional, or otherwise) to assist others.* It is important to note that solidarity is understood here as a *practice* and not as an inner sentiment or an abstract value."[8] A consistent sense and *practice* of solidarity can provide a baseline consensus for expansive, egalitarian social policies. Always looming as a threat to well-established systems of socialized medicine—in Costa Rica, say—is a fracturing of that solidarity, allowing for (or accelerating) the "exit" from the system by wealthier segments of society, and new possibilities for private-sector investment and accumulation.[9]

Solidarity is clearly vital to supporting egalitarian health and social policies, but where does such solidarity come from? Rather tentatively, I observe that during times of crisis or major political change, social medicine leaders have persuasively deployed the rhetoric of nationalism to engender a necessary sense of solidarity. The rhetoric of Salvador Allende, for example, was strongly nationalistic, in part predicated on opposition to US imperialism, a search for economic self-sufficiency (which is a theme of Latin American national development policies in mid-century), and a concern for the quality of the national stock, framed in biological terms—as "bio-power" that needs to be harnessed for national progress. Even with international norms around human rights to support health sector reforms, health citizenship is still mainly understood and effectively realized in relation to the nation-state. Sérgio Arouca, in his address to the 1986 conference that offered a decisive shift toward health systems reform, appealed to this sense of national, democratic citizenship: the new health system must be "built, desired, assembled, and invented by Brazilian society."[10] In a democratic society, well-functioning systems themselves engender solidarity—people are more likely to back systems and structures that work for them. One persistent dilemma, though, is that national identity projects are simultaneously inclusive and exclusive. In any country, national identity projects conceal or silence the diverse communities that might have their own histories of marginalization in the national territorial space, such as Indigenous and Afro-descended peoples, a problem that social medicine, as an academic community, has considered in recent years.

Such questions about political will, solidarity, participatory democracy, and citizenship can be frustratingly abstract. And I do not think my answers are necessarily sufficient or persuasive. However, I believe that social medicine could become more influential by engaging in broader dialogues on such questions, and by finding ways to be politically persuasive beyond its core of like-minded activists.

Key Conclusions

First, *social medicine's influence on health policy must be understood dialectically.* Invariably, social medicine pushes a leftist-radical program for health sector reform. However, when successful it tends to produce technocratic institutions to implement and manage more equitable and far-reaching health policies (like primary health care). This process of institutionalization usually defuses the radical outsider spirit of social medicine. This was certainly the case in Chile. Between the 1930s and the 1950s, a cohort of relatively radicalized doctors (along with more politically conservative actors with sympathy toward social medicine) pushed for a transformation of the health system. This system was inherited by a generation of professionals with more technical training and specific kinds of expertise, ensconced within institutions like the SNS or the Escuela de Salud Pública, people like the archetypal health technocrat Abraham Horwitz. From the 1950s to the 1970s, across the region, social medicine practically faded out of existence, because of the triumph of technocracy, the predominance of international norms-making institutions like the WHO, and pervasive anticommunist sentiment in the early Cold War era. The resurgence of social medicine in the 1970s stems from disillusionment with technocratic modernization, opposition to authoritarianism, and the emergence of new social theories. From there, social medicine consolidated as a response to neoliberal reforms, intensifying in the 1980s, which threatened to undermine national health systems that the earlier generation of social medicine had fought so hard to create. In this long-term dialectic process, militancy leads to policy achievements, which leads to institutionalization—a narrowing of focus and concentration of effort along technical lines. When the institutions are thrown into crisis or fail to respond to the new demands of organized sectors, disillusionment and critique rise and may initiate new cycles of activism.

When we think of social medicine dialectically—as a field of radical critique interacting with the mainstream—we see that this relationship is laden with contradictions that keep social medicine from ever becoming the dominant view. It is a field that offers expansive explanations of the social causes of health inequality, and it resists the straitjacket of reductionist biomedical science.[11] However, the poor and marginalized continue to demand better, higher-quality medical care. It is not that the public at large questions the Western biomedical model; mostly, they just want the benefits of biomedicine to be more available, reliable, effective, and affordable. Another constant dilemma has been the choice between autonomy and incorporation for the medical profession. While most of the social medicine group today supports unified, state-owned health systems, most doctors in most countries do not appear to be behind such a project. That is, in part, because they tend to enjoy the privilege of high levels of autonomy from the state. Even though there are many actors involved in health systems—including "a strong medical-industrial complex" consisting of insurers, private hospitals, pharmaceutical companies, and other elements—doctors, when organized, move the system.[12] And, as this history suggests, it should not be assumed that doctors, even of a progressive bent, will surrender hard-won professional autonomy to state control.

Second, *Latin American social medicine was not derivative of the European school of social medicine.* Leaders in the field were conscious of their peripheral position in the international political economy and aware of social policy advances in other countries, but they did not exist in a state of ideological or intellectual dependency. Characteristically, LASM activists have been engaged in deep analysis of national problems and connected via regional-scale (Latin American) expert networks. Similar to the trajectory of many other regional intellectual and creative movements, from dependency theory in economics to tropical modernism in architecture, the maturing of LASM hinged on recognizing and interrogating dependency on Europe and North America as the twentieth century progressed. As Mario Testa explained his own positionality, "I am an 'underdeveloped thinker' [*pensador subdesarrollado*], I think from underdevelopment, I think from here."[13]

The common overemphasis on European influence derives, in part, from the inertia of received narratives about Latin American social medicine's origins and genealogy—narratives I have tried to complicate throughout this book. But it also has to do with a conflation between social medicine's analysis of causes (of unequal health outcomes) and the project of socialized medicine (state-led health systems). Undoubtedly, Latin Americans have drawn inspiration from European health policy models, from the "Bismarckian" to "Beveridge" types (whose archetypes are found in Germany and the United Kingdom, respectively) to more centralized systems of the former Soviet Union and Eastern Bloc states. In the first sense of social medicine, sensu the academic or analytic lens, there are no doubt influential European theorists (a wide-ranging group of continental philosophers, in particular), but social medicine has always been attuned to the social, political, and economic realities of Latin American countries, and developed its own analytical tools to confront them, as described in chapter 7.

Indeed, a major line of critique in social medicine has been that interventions and strategies that work to improve population health in the Global North may be inappropriate for the circumstances of the Global South.[14] In this way, LASM adopts (and, to some degree, helps to construct) a geopolitical perspective in which Latin America is afflicted by the hegemony of North

America and Europe in its many guises, from Yankee imperialism to the imposition of neoliberal globalization. In this context, it is easy to identify common interests across national boundaries, and a mode of *Latin Americanism* that is not merely an identity construction project, but also a vehicle for promoting alternative development models.[15]

Third, *the history of LASM is part of the history of the social sciences in Latin America.* Reflexively, we might tend to categorize social medicine as part of the culturally dominant realm of health and medicine, and the preponderance, until quite recently, of medical doctors in social medicine helped solidify this association. In the early part of the twentieth century, pioneers of social medicine, such as Carlos Paz Soldán, Salvador Allende, and Ramón Carrillo, used eclectic analytical frames to analyze the roots of public health problems; their arguments were not constrained by the lens of any one social science discipline, since these disciplines themselves were in relative infancy and not widely taught at Latin American universities. Although they did not usually allude directly to Rudolf Virchow, the protagonists of first-wave social medicine in Latin America shared his conviction that the rationality of medical science could be applied to solve the problems of society as a whole.

In the middle of the twentieth century, things began to change. The complexities of managing more expansive welfare states helped promote the development of social sciences like economics and sociology in the region. Under the sway of modernization, international health technocrats used social science concepts and methods steeped in functionalism and positivism for their health systems planning efforts. As LASM matured, starting in the early 1970s, we see the development and influence of Marxist and poststructural theories that offer critical analytical tools to understand the role of health institutions in reproducing inequitable political-economic systems and cultural norms. Even more recently, social medicine has encountered postcolonial and decolonial theories, particularly around the question of incorporating Indigenous ideas and practices into a socially just and inclusive health system. What we find is that, in debates in social medicine, the very definition of society and how it is organized or structured is always up for grabs, itself an unstable object.

The social sciences do not stand outside of history, and more research is needed on the historical development of the social sciences of health in Latin America, to accompany the recent flourishing of scholarship on the history of medicine and public health. A deeper dive into such a history would include more systematic articulation of academic networks in the social sciences, examination of student political activism, and analysis of how new fields emerge, persist, and become institutionalized—and how they articulate with better established and more culturally dominant fields like medicine.

And finally, *the second wave of LASM accompanies a steady process of democratization*. The post-authoritarian openings in political life, especially the development and reinvigoration of democratic institutions in Latin America, are often overlooked in historical accounts of Latin American social medicine. This process of democratization might receive less attention because the same era (from the 1970s to at least the early 2000s) was marked by the growing hegemony of neoliberalism, which led to greater social inequality and the disintegration of older welfare state institutions in many countries. Still, it should be recognized that the ability of academics to articulate politically charged critiques, to form associations, and to influence policy through relatively open processes (demonstrated most dramatically by the Brazilian health reform movement of the 1980s) reflect a flourishing of human freedoms and a growing tolerance of political activism.[16]

I believe that figures like Juan César García, Sérgio Arouca, Salvador Allende, and Gustavo Molina would have celebrated this openness and pluralism, even if many of their political objectives have not been fully realized. And it is my sense that Latin American social medicine will remain a field driven by open exploration of ideas, with a strong ethos of political praxis, while also avoiding the pitfalls of ideologically motivated reasoning. To move toward health equity amid constantly shifting political conditions, as well as the trend toward consumer-driven, individualized medical care, the field of social medicine and collective health will surely continue to evolve.

Notes

Introduction

1. Stonington and Holmes, "Social Medicine"; Porter, "How Did Social Medicine Evolve?"; Gofin, "On 'A Practice of Social Medicine'"; and King, *Social Medicine Reader*.

2. Adams et al., "Re-Imagining Global Health," 2; and Breilh, *Critical Epidemiology*, 21–46.

3. Pieper Mooney, "From Cold War Pressures," 188.

4. The phrase "interventions into the lives of others" paraphrases the subtitle of Packard, *A History of Global Health*.

5. Birn, "Making It Politic(al)," 175.

6. McGuire, "Social Policies in Latin America," 211.

7. McGuire, "Social Policies in Latin America," 203–11.

8. Adams et al., "Re-Imagining Global Health," 10; and Breilh, "Entrevista con Jaime Breilh," 49.

9. Spiegel, Breilh, and Yassi, "Why Language Matters."

10. de Sousa Santos, *End of the Cognitive Empire*; Spiegel, Breilh, and Yassi, "Why Language Matters," 14; Granda Ugalde, *La salud y la vida*, 210; and Breilh, *Critical Epidemiology*, 180–81.

11. Menéndez, "Modelo médico hegemónico"; and Neely, *Reimagining Social Medicine*.

12. Birn, Muntaner, and Afzal, "South-South Cooperation in Health."

13. Taylor and Rieger, "Medicine as Social Science."

14. Waitzkin, *Medicine and Public Health*, 15.

15. Kaufman, "Science Alone Can't Heal a Sick Society."

16. Porter, "How Did Social Medicine Evolve?" 1667; Porter and Porter, "What Was Social Medicine?"; Fee, "Henry E. Sigerist"; and C. Rosenberg, "Erwin H. Ackerknecht," 531.

17. Fee, "Henry E. Sigerist," 127.

18. Fee, "Pleasures and Perils."

19. Borowy, *Coming to Terms*, 21.

20. Galdston, *Social Medicine*.

21. Cueto, Brown, and Fee, *World Health Organization*, 63–64; Packard, *History of Global Health*, 91–104; and Farley, *Brock Chisholm*.

22. Galdston, *Social Medicine*.

23. Gorsky, "British National Health Service."

24. Porter, "Social Medicine," 182.

25. Porter, "Social Medicine," 183; and Krieger, "Theories for Social Epidemiology."

26. Bliss, "Under Surveillance"; and Brickman, "Medical McCarthyism."

27. Cueto, Brown, and Fee, *World Health Organization*; and Packard, *History of Global Health*.

28. Carter and Sánchez Delgado, "Una discusión."

29. Waitzkin et al., "Social Medicine Then and Now," 1594; and Breilh, *Critical Epidemiology*, 25–28.

30. Adams et al., "Re-Imagining Global Health"; Galeano, Trotta, and Spinelli, "Juan César García"; Torres Tovar, "ALAMES"; Porter, "How Did Social Medicine Evolve?"; Waitzkin, "Commentary"; Tajer, "Latin American Social Medicine"; and Krieger, "Latin American Social Medicine."

31. Paiva and Teixera, "Health Reform," 1.

32. Franco et al., *Debates en medicina social*, 21–25.

33. Kapelusz-Poppi, "Rural Health and State Construction"; Labra, "Medicina social en Chile"; and Cueto, "Social Medicine in the Andes."

34. Salvatore, *Disciplinary Conquest*, 14.

35. Fajardo, *World That Latin America Created*, 11.

36. Birn and Necochea Lopez, "Footprints on the Future," 518.

37. Fajardo, *World That Latin America Created*; Salvatore, *Disciplinary Conquest*; and Rappaport, *Cowards Don't Make History*.

38. J. García et al., *Pensamiento social*; J. García, "Las ciencias sociales en medicina"; and Nunes, "Las ciencias sociales en salud."

39. Lemercier, "Formal Network Methods."

40. Galeano, Trotta, and Spinelli, "Juan César García."

41. Herrera León and Herrera González, *América Latina*; and Singleton, "ILO and Social Security."

42. Fonseca, "Latin American Social Medicine"; Rojas Ochoa and Márquez, *ALAMES en la memoria*; and Lima, Paranaguá de Santana, and Paiva, *Saúde coletiva*.

43. Agostoni, "Médicos rurales"; Birn, "Revolution in Rural Health?"; A. Carrillo, "Salud pública y poder"; Kapelusz-Poppi, "Physician Activists"; Kapelusz-Poppi, "Rural Health and State Construction"; and Smith, "Towards a Typology."

44. Carter, *Enemy in the Blood*; Carter, "Malaria Control"; and Carter, "Population Control."

Chapter One

1. Carter and Sánchez Delgado, "Una discusión."

2. Waitzkin, "Commentary," 739; and Fee, "Pleasures and Perils."

3. Porter and Porter, "What Was Social Medicine?" 93.

4. Foucault, "Nacimiento de la medicina social," 91.

5. Stehrenberger and Goltermann, "Disaster Medicine," 318.

6. Stehrenberger and Goltermann, "Disaster Medicine," 318.

7. Falcón, *La Barcelona Argentina*.

8. Ramacciotti and Rayez, "Los ingenieros sanitarios," 126; and Suriano, *La cuestión social*.

9. Grez Toso, "La guerra preventiva."

10. Long, "Informe presentado," 413.

11. *Boletín del Instituto Internacional Americano de Protección a la Infancia (IIPI)* 4 (1931): 415–605.

12. López-Alonso, *Measuring Up*, 193; and Botey, "Los actores sociales," 126.

13. Cueto and Palmer, *Medicine and Public Health*, 65–68; Otero, "Sueños cifrados"; and Carter, "Population Control."

14. Orrego Luco, *La cuestión social*; and Murdock, "Physicians," 566.

15. Cueto and Palmer, *Medicine and Public Health*, 67–68.

16. Illanes, *Cuerpo y sangre*, 14.

17. Illanes, *Cuerpo y sangre*, 21.

18. Zimmermann, "Intellectuals," 200–202, 205.

19. Molyneux, "'Neoliberal Turn,'" 77; Huneeus Madge and Paz Lanas, "Ciencia política e historia"; and Zárate Campos, "Alimentación y previsión biológica," xxii.

20. Guillén and Vale, "Emergence."

21. Acha, "Celia Lapalma de Emery," 35; Grez Toso, *La "Cuestión social" en Chile*, 35; and M. Rosenberg, "Social Security Policymaking," 118.

22. Silva, "State, Politics and the Idea," 466.

23. Huneeus Madge and Paz Lanas, "Ciencia política e historia"; Zárate, "Alimentación y previsión biológica," xxii; Labra, "Medicina social en Chile"; and Toro-Blanco, "La guerra santa."

24. Farmer, "How Liberation Theology Can Inform."

25. Cueto, "Social Medicine in the Andes."

26. Paz Soldán, *La medicina social*.

27. Sand, *Advance to Social Medicine*, 552.

28. Cueto, *Value of Health*, 56.

29. Paz Soldán, *La medicina social*, 11; and Snowden, *The Conquest of Malaria*, 64.

30. Paz Soldán, *La medicina social*, 34–35.

31. Paz Soldán, *La medicina social*, 135.

32. Cueto and Palmer, *Medicine and Public Health*, 70–71; Meade, *"Civilizing" Rio*; and Rodriguez, *Civilizing Argentina*.

33. Lawrence and Weisz, "Medical Holism"; Rosenberg, "Holism in Twentieth-Century Medicine"; Zimmerer, "Ecology as Cornerstone," 161–88; and Carter, "Malaria Control."

34. Carter, "Population Control"; and de la Dehesa, "Social Medicine," 3.

35. Cueto, "Social Medicine in the Andes."

36. Murillo Peña and Franco Paredes, "Nuestra tragedia biológica," 325–26.

37. Cueto, "Social Medicine in the Andes"; and Mendoza and Martínez, "Las ideas eugenésicas."

38. Stepan, *"Hour of Eugenics,"* 78.

39. Stepan, *"Hour of Eugenics,"* 78; and Berro, "La medicina social," 595.

40. Pieper Mooney, *Politics of Motherhood*, 42.

41. Berro, "La medicina social," 595; and Stepan, *"Hour of Eugenics,"* 77.

42. Bettinotti, "El lactario"; Birn, "Doctors on Record," 332; and Huhle, "Transnational Formation," 8.

43. Birn, "Doctors on Record," 349.

44. Pieper Mooney, *Politics of Motherhood*, 13–43.

45. Zaffaroni, "La mala vida," 123.

46. "French Conception of Social Medicine"; and Bard, "Las enfermedades sociales."

47. Gutiérrez and Suriano, "Workers' Housing," 46–48; and Armus, *Ailing City*.

48. Miranda, "La Argentina en el escenario," 45.

49. Bard, "La defensa de la raza."

50. Murillo Peña and Franco Paredes, "Nuestra tragedia biológica," 305.

51. Luisi, "Sobre eugenia"; Birn, "National-International Nexus," 48–49; Lavrín, *Women, Feminism, and Social Change*, 140–41; Ledesma Prietto, *"La revolución sexual,"* 34–35; and Huhle, "Transnational Formation," 9.

52. Lavrín, *Women, Feminism, and Social Change*, 141–42.

53. Ledesma Prietto, *"La revolución sexual."*

54. Ledesma Prietto, *"La revolución sexual,"* 174.

55. Lavrín, *Women, Feminism, and Social Change*, 140.

56. Ramacciotti, "De la culpa al seguro"; and Zylberman, "Fewer Parallels," 83.

57. Zylberman, "Fewer Parallels," 83; and Sand, *Medicina social y progreso nacional*, 108 (emphasis in original).

58. Ramacciotti, "Influencias internacionales"; Yáñez Andrade, "Chile y la Organización Internacional"; and Vergara, "De la higiene industrial."

59. Fuster Sánchez, *El cuerpo como máquina.*

60. Vergara, "Recognition of Silicosis"; and Vergara, "De la higiene industrial."

61. Packard, *History of Global Health*, 84–87.

62. Zylberman, "Fewer Parallels," 83.

63. Paz Soldán, *Demostración de asistencia*, 17.

64. Maradona, *A través de la selva.*

65. Paz Soldán, *Demostración de asistencia*, 15; and Carter, "Malaria Control," 111–27.

66. Paz Soldán, *Las bases médico-sociales*, 2:72.

67. Carter, "Malaria Control," 126.

68. Birn, "Philanthrocapitalism."

69. Hochman, *Sanitation of Brazil*; Botey, "Los actores sociales"; and Palmer, *From Popular Medicine.*

70. Palmer, *Launching Global Health*, 202.

71. Kapelusz-Poppi, "Rural Health and State Construction"; Kapelusz-Poppi, "Physician Activists"; A. Carrillo, "Salud pública y poder"; Smith, "Towards a Typology"; and Agostoni, "Médicos rurales."

72. Birn, "Revolution in Rural Health?" 73, 75.

73. Zabala, *La enfermedad de Chagas.*

74. Maradona, *A través de la selva*; Viñas, *A la sombra de Hipócrates*; and Bosio, *Cartas de un médico rural.*

75. Bengoa, *Sanare*, 52–53.

76. "Esteban Laureano Maradona: Un siglo de amor," *Gente*, 1995. A clipping of this article appears in the front matter of the 2012 edition of Maradona, *A través de la selva.*

77. Kehl, *Eugenía e medicina social*; and Dos Santos, "Intelectuales y redes eugénicas."

78. Cueto and Palmer, *Medicine and Public Health*, 164–68.

79. Serafin Elguin, "Organización científica de la sociedad," *BMC*, March 9, 1935.

80. Armus, "Eugenesia en Buenos Aires," 150.

81. Letelier Carvajal, "Ideas eugenésicas en Chile," 93.

82. Bashford, *Global Population*; and Ledesma Prietto, *"La revolución sexual,"* 119.

83. Stern, *Eugenic Nation*; and Rosemblatt, *Science and Politics of Race.*

84. Wade, *Degrees of Mixture*, 60.

85. Wade, *Degrees of Mixture*, 60.

86. Illanes, *Cuerpo y sangre*, 22.

87. Lazarte, *Chile en la vanguardia*, 19.

88. Wade, *Degrees of Mixture*; and Rosemblatt, *Science and Politics*, 177.

89. Wade, *Degrees of Mixture*, 64.

90. Wade, *Degrees of Mixture*, 55.

91. Wade, *Degrees of Mixture*, 64.

92. Berro, "La medicina social," 598.

93. Letelier Carvajal, "Ideas eugenésicas," 105; and Carter, "Population Control," 96–105.

94. Pohl-Valero, "La raza entra," 474.

95. Miranda and Vallejo, *Una historia de la eugenesia*.

96. Letelier Carvajal, "Ideas eugenésicas," 105.

97. Wade, *Degrees of Mixture*, 55.

98. Letelier Carvajal, "Ideas eugenésicas," 106.

99. Letelier Carvajal, "Ideas eugenésicas," 107.

100. Falcón, *La Barcelona Argentina*.

101. Craib, *Cry of the Renegade*, 171.

102. Craib, *Cry of the Renegade*, 96–97; and Savala, *Beyond Patriotic Phobias*, 86–110.

103. Craib, *Cry of the Renegade*, 54.

104. Alonso Vial, "Nota biográfica," 109; and Craib, *Cry of the Renegade*, 141–44.

105. Zalaquett, "¡Siembra, juventud!"; and Craib, *Cry of the Renegade*, 165.

106. Craib, *Cry of the Renegade*, 19–25, 53; Fuster Sánchez, *El cuerpo como máquina*, 152–54; Grez Toso, "La trayectoria histórica"; and Illanes, "La revolución solidaria."

107. Alonso Vial, "Nota biográfica," 107.

108. "¡Oiga compañero!" *Hoja Sanitaria IWW* (Santiago), February 1925; Muñoz Cortés, *Sin dios ni patrones*, 212; and Fuster Sánchez and Moscoso-Flores, *La Hoja Sanitaria*, 145 (reproductions of all extant editions of the *Hoja Sanitaria* can be found in the 2015 volume edited by Fuster Sánchez and Moscoso-Flores, along with their interpretive essays).

109. Fuster Sánchez, *El cuerpo como máquina*.

110. Alonso Vial, "Nota biográfica," 106.

111. Fuster Sánchez, *El cuerpo como máquina*; and Arias Escobedo, *La prensa obrera en Chile*.

112. Fuster Sánchez and Moscoso-Flores, *La Hoja Sanitaria*.

113. Pavez, "Experiencias autogestionarias en salud," 428.

114. Muñoz Cortés, *Sin dios ni patrones*.

115. "Cartilla de Higiene Personal: Capítulo IV, Elección de los Alimentos," *Hoja Sanitaria IWW*, December 1924.

116. Masjuan and Martinez-Alier, "Conscious Procreation"; and Martinez-Alier, *Environmentalism of the Poor*, 50–52.

117. Ledesma Prietto, *"La revolución sexual,"* 114–16.

118. Craib, *Cry of the Renegade*, 170.

119. Muñoz Cortés, *Sin dios ni patrones*, 44.

120. Adelman, "Political Economy of Labour," 22.

121. Knight, "Great Depression in Latin America," 309.

122. Gutiérrez and Romero, "Barrio Societies," 231.
123. Gutiérrez and Romero, "Barrio Societies," 231.
124. Biernat, Cerdá, and Ramacciotti, *La salud pública*, 170.
125. Huhle, "Transnational Formation," 3–4.

Chapter Two

1. A version of this chapter, which includes more discussion of international networks in nutrition, was previously published as Carter, "Social Medicine and International Expert Networks."
2. Packard, *History of Global Health*, 48; and Weindling, "Social Medicine."
3. Packard, *History of Global Health*, 131; and Stepan, *Eradication*, 105–7.
4. Plata-Stenger, "To Raise Awareness," 108.
5. Krige, "Introduction," 6.
6. Krige, "Introduction," 2.
7. Barany and Krige, "Afterword," 415.
8. Krige, "Introduction," 14.
9. Birn, "National-International Nexus," 57.
10. Birn, "Introduction," 3.
11. Huhle, "Transnational Formation," 3, citing Conrad, "Social Policy History," 223.
12. Compagnon, *América Latina*.
13. Murillo Ramirez, "América Latina," 329.
14. Paz Soldán, *Las bases médico-sociales*, 1:3–5.
15. Ferreras, "La misión de Stephen Lawford Childs," 151.
16. Ferreras, "La misión de Stephen Lawford Childs," 152.
17. Knight, "Great Depression in Latin America," 312.
18. Borowy, "Coming to Terms"; Kott and Droux, *Globalizing Social Rights*; and McPherson and Wehrli, *Beyond Geopolitics*.
19. Guthrie, "ILO."
20. Packard, *History of Global Health*.
21. Dubin, "League of Nations," 59–63.
22. Packard, *History of Global Health*, 57.
23. Packard, *Making of a Tropical Disease*; Packard, *History of Global Health*; and Weindling, "Social Medicine."
24. Cueto, Brown, and Fee, *World Health Organization*, 28; and Zylberman, "Fewer Parallels."
25. Dubin, "League of Nations."
26. International Labour Office, *Report on Social Insurance*, 16.
27. Weindling, "Social Medicine," 138–41.
28. Dubin, "League of Nations"; and Weindling, "League of Nations Health Organization."
29. Birn, "National-International Nexus;" and Scarzanella, "Los Pibes."
30. Wehlri, "Francisco Walker Linares."
31. Cueto and Palmer, *Medicine and Public Health*, 134–35.
32. Zylberman, "Fewer Parallels," 78; and Cueto and Palmer, *Medicine and Public Health*, 134.

33. Zylberman, "Fewer Parallels," 81; and Eilers, "René Sand."

34. Sand, *Medicina social y progreso nacional*.

35. Cueto, "Social Medicine in the Andes," 184; and Sand, *Advance to Social Medicine*, 552.

36. Packard, *History of Global Health*.

37. Plata-Stenger, "'To Raise Awareness,'" 97.

38. Herrera González, "La Primera Conferencia Regional."

39. Cueto and Palmer, *Medicine and Public Health*, 106.

40. Huhle, "Transnational Formation," 14–15.

41. Carter, "Social Medicine and International Expert Networks," 796–99.

42. Singleton, "ILO and Social Security."

43. Cueto and Palmer, *Medicine and Public Health*; and Labra, "Medicina social en Chile."

44. Wehlri, "Francisco Walker Linares."

45. Martínez Franzoni and Sánchez-Ancochea, *Quest for Universal Social Policy*; Pernet, "Developing Nutritional Standards"; and Yáñez Andrade, "La OIT."

46. Wehlri, "Francisco Walker Linares."

47. Singleton, "ILO and Social Security."

48. Herrera González, "El Pacto."

49. Plata-Stegner, "'To Raise Awareness,'" 106.

50. Herrera González, "Beyond Social Legislation."

51. International Labour Office, *Report on Social Insurance*, 50–51.

52. Plata-Stegner, "'To Raise Awareness,'" 107.

53. OIT, *Conferencia del Trabajo*, 245.

54. OIT, *Conferencia del Trabajo*, 64, 255–56.

55. Jensen, "From Geneva"; and Plata-Stegner, "'To Raise Awareness.'"

56. Cueto, *Value of Health*, 49.

57. *Actas Generales de la Novena Conferencia*, 241.

58. *Actas Generales de la Novena Conferencia*, 241–42.

59. Cueto and Palmer, *Medicine and Public Health*, 110–13.

60. Carter, *Enemy in the Blood*.

61. Borowy, "Shifting," 526.

62. J. Garcia, "La enfermedad de la pereza," 157; and J. García, "La medicina estatal."

63. J. García, "La medicina estatal," 95.

64. Cueto and Palmer, *Medicine and Public Health*, 110; Ramacciotti and Rayez, "Los ingenieros sanitarios," 131; and author interview with Mario Rovere, August 11, 2015.

65. Dubin, "League of Nations"; and Huhle, "Transnational Formation," 14.

66. Singleton, "ILO and Social Security," 241.

67. Herrera González, "La Primera Conferencia Regional"; and Singleton, "ILO and Social Security."

68. Birn, "National-International Nexus."

69. Birn, "National-International Nexus."

70. Cohen, "First Inter-American Conference"; Jensen, "From Geneva"; and Singleton, "ILO and Social Security."

71. Oficina Sanitaria Panamericana, "Acta Final, Décima Conferencia," 4.

72. Cueto, Brown, and Fee, *World Health Organization*, 44.

73. "La Actualidad Médico-Social," 7; and "Mensaje al Primer Congreso," 3.

74. I. Elena, "Los Congresos Médico Sociales," 3; and *Primer Congreso Médico Social.*

75. *Boletín Gremial de la AMECH*, February 1947, 7; and "Dr. Harrison H. Shoulders Dies; Surgeon Once Directed A.M.A.," *New York Times*, November 18, 1963.

76. "Primer Congreso Médico Social Panamericano," *Boletín Gremial de la Amech*, 7.

77. Cueto, *Value of Health*; and Jensen, "From Geneva."

78. Selfa, "Mariátegui."

79. Moraga Valle, "El resplandor."

80. Moraga Valle, "El resplandor," 144.

81. Nuccetelli, *Introduction to Latin American Philosophy*, 185.

82. Moraga Valle, "El resplandor"; and Craib, *Cry of the Renegade*, 176.

83. Hernández Toledo, "Apristas en Chile," 81.

84. Nuccetelli, *Introduction to Latin American Philosophy*, 193.

85. García-Bryce, "Transnational Activist."

86. Drinot and Contreras, "Great Depression in Peru," 118.

87. Herrera González, "El pacto," 97.

88. Drinot, "Awaiting the Blood," 88.

89. "Ante las elecciones presidenciales, los intelectuales definen actitud," *BMC*, August 6, 1938.

90. Jeifets and Jeifets, *La Internacional Comunista.*

91. Wehlri, "Francisco Walker Linares."

92. Packard, *History of Global Health.*

93. Weindling, "League of Nations Health Organization"; and Pernet, "Developing Nutritional Standards."

Chapter Three

1. Pieper Mooney, *Politics of Motherhood*, 29.

2. Waitzkin et al., "Social Medicine Then and Now"; Porter, "How Did Social Medicine Evolve?"; and Schuftan, "Una verdadera joya."

3. Waitzkin et al., "Social Medicine Then and Now"; Waitzkin, "Commentary"; Waitzkin, *Medicine and Public Health*; Birn and Nervi, "Political Roots"; and Hartmann, "Postneoliberal Public Health."

4. Mesa-Lago, "Social Security," 358.

5. Illanes, *En el nombre del pueblo.*

6. Carter and Sánchez Delgado, "Una discusión."

7. Rosemblatt, *Gendered Compromises*, 3–4.

8. Molina Bustos, *Institucionalidad sanitaria chilena*, 109–19.

9. Pieper Mooney, "From Cold War Pressures," 188.

10. Silva, "State, Politics and the Idea," 467–68.

11. Illanes, *En el nombre del pueblo*, 224–30; Labra, "Medicina Social en Chile"; Molina Bustos, *Institucionalidad sanitaria chilena*, 60–69; and Romero, "Desarrollo de la medicina," 893–94.

12. Molina Bustos, *Institucionalidad sanitaria chilena*, 64.

13. Allende Gossens, *La realidad médico-social chilena*, 158–59.

14. Labra, "Medicina social en Chile," 209.

15. Illanes, *En el nombre del pueblo*, 226.

16. Illanes, *En el nombre del pueblo*, 227.

17. Molina Bustos, *Institucionalidad sanitaria chilena*, 65.

18. Carter, "Social Medicine and International Expert Networks."

19. Labra, "Medicina social en Chile," 209.

20. Labra, "Medicina social en Chile," 209–10; and "El Dr. Lois defiende al Cuerpo Médico," *Boletín Médico de Chile (BMC)*, December 28, 1935.

21. *Acción Social*, June 1935, 37.

22. *Acción Social*, February 1935, 42.

23. Illanes, *En el nombre del pueblo*, 246–47.

24. "Habla Santiago Labarca, Administrador General," *Acción Social*, June 1935, 37.

25. "Diez años," *Acción Social*, June 1935, 7.

26. *Acción Social*, December 1935, 4–5.

27. *Acción Social*, June 1935, 37.

28. Finer, "Chilean Development Corporation."

29. *Acción Social*, June 1935, 37.

30. Garcia Tello, *Mi experencia*.

31. Rojas Carvajal, "Aplicación"; Allende Gossens, *Realidad financiera*; López Campillay, "Ciencia, médicos y enfermos"; Molina Bustos, "Antecedentes"; and Molina Bustos, *Institucionalidad sanitaria chilena*.

32. Viel, *Conferencias*; Guillermo Padilla Castro, "El Seguro Social: Su fundación y origen," *La Nación* (San José, Costa Rica), December 10, 1966; and Martínez Franzoni and Sánchez-Ancochea, *Quest for Universal Social Policy*.

33. Rosemblatt, *Gendered Compromises*, 3–4.

34. Lazarte, *Chile en la vanguardia*, 61–62.

35. Craib, *Cry of the Renegade*, 62–63.

36. Illanes, *En el nombre del pueblo*, 247; and Molina Bustos, *Institucionalidad sanitaria chilena*, 78.

37. "Insistimos colegas . . . a organizarse!" *BMC*, April 6, 1935.

38. Labra, "Medicina social en Chile," 210.

39. "Trabajadores de la Medicina, que están detenidos en Valparaíso," *BMC*, August 13, 1932; "El profesor Jaime Vidal Oltra detenido en la cárcel pública," *BMC*, September 3, 1932; "Un recurso de amparo," *BMC*, September 3, 1932; and Figueroa Clark, *Salvador Allende*, 25–29.

40. "Vanguardia Médica: Declaración de Principios," *BMC*, September 3, 1932.

41. "Vanguardia Médica: Declaración de Principios," *BMC*, September 3, 1932.

42. Del Campo, "El debate medico," 181; Labra, "Medicina Social en Chile," 211; Molina Bustos, *Institucionalidad sanitaria chilena*, 109; and Lazarte, *Chile en la vanguardia*.

43. Sánchez Delgado, Seiwerth, and Abarzúa, "Las Casas de Limpieza"; and Vergara, "Los trabajadores chilenos."

44. Garcia Tello, *Estructurando*, 18.

45. "Deberes del gremio médico," *BMC*, March 18, 1933.

46. Laval, "Epidemia de tifus exantemático," 314; and Sánchez Delgado, Seiwerth, and Abarzúa, "Las Casas de Limpieza."

47. Guillermo Eliseo Azócar, "Que el país sepa que el Ministro de Hacienda niega los recursos necesarios," *BMC*, January 26, 1935.

48. *BMC*, January 16, 1935.

49. *BMC*, March 16, 1935.

50. Aquiles Machiavello, "Factores económicos y sociales en la epidemia de tifus exantemático," *BMC*, April 20, 1935; and "Sobre el precio de medicamentos," *BMC*, April 1, 1933.

51. *Actas Generales de la Novena Conferencia*, 241–42.

52. Aquiles Machiavello, "Anotaciones sobre tifus exantemático," *BMC*, March 16, 1935; Machiavello, "Factores económicos."

53. "Todo el poder a la AMECH," *BMC*, May 18, 1935.

54. Allende, *La realidad médico-social chilena*, 108.

55. "Nuestra posición: un folleto de la Federación de los médicos," *BMC*, September 22, 1934.

56. Garcia Tello, *Estructurando*, 48–49.

57. *BMC*, January 26, 1935.

58. *BMC*, January 26, 1935.

59. *BMC*, January 26, 1935.

60. Garcia Tello, *Mi experencia*, 17.

61. Garcia Tello, *Estructurando*, 74.

62. *BMC*, January 26, 1935.

63. Ángel Vidal Oltra, "La medicina y el socialismo," *BMC*, July 16, 1932.

64. "Médicos jóvenes de Santiago nos dirigimos a los colegas de todo el país," *BMC*, March 23, 1935.

65. Leonard Guzmán, "Carta abierta a un abogado, Ministro de Salubridad," *BMC*, January 12, 1935; "Obstrucción del Ejecutivo contra la legislación sanitaria," *BMC*, July 6, 1935; and "Todo el poder a la AMECH."

66. "¡Cuidado con la politiquería!" *BMC*, July 9, 1932.

67. Del Campo, "El debate médico."

68. Molina Bustos, *Institucionalidad sanitaria chilena*, 106–19.

69. Silva, "State, Politics and the Idea," 472.

70. Toro-Blanco, "La guerra santa."

71. Zárate Campos, "Alimentación y previsión biológica"; and Pieper Mooney, "From Cold War Pressures," 196.

72. Del Campo, "El debate médico."

73. Cruz-Coke Madrid, *Eduardo Cruz-Coke*, 78–95; and Silva, "State, Politics and the Idea," 467.

74. Cruz-Coke Madrid, *Eduardo Cruz-Coke*, 304.

75. Cruz-Coke Madrid, *Eduardo Cruz-Coke*, 306.

76. Zárate Campos, "Alimentación y previsión biológica."

77. Huneeus Madge and Paz Lanas, "Ciencia política e historia."

78. Dragoni and Burnet, "L'alimentation Populaire au Chili."

79. Rodriguez B., *El Consejo Nacional*; Mardones Restat and Cox, *La alimentación en Chile*; and Zárate Campos, "Alimentación y previsión biológica."

80. Zárate Campos, "Alimentación y previsión biológica," xv.

81. Zárate Campos, "Alimentación y previsión biológica," xlv–xlvii.

82. Cruz-Coke, *Medicina preventiva*, 51; Zárate Campos, "Alimentación y previsión bi-ológica," xlvii; and Cruz-Coke, "Chilean Preventive Medicine Act."

83. "Ante la Ley de Medicina Preventiva," 3–5.

84. "Ante la Ley de Medicina Preventiva," 3–5; Illanes, *En el nombre del pueblo*, 291–311; and Zárate Campos, "Alimentación y previsión biológica."

85. Figueroa Clark, *Salvador Allende*, 21–22; and Craib, *Cry of the Renegade*, 169.

86. Orrego Luco, *La cuestión social*, 48–49.

87. Labra, "Medicina social en Chile," 213.

88. Allende Gossens, *La realidad médico-social chilena*, 81.

89. Dragoni and Burnet, "L'alimentation Populaire au Chili."

90. Allende Gossens, *La realidad médico-social chilena*, 38.

91. Allende Gossens, *La realidad médico-social chilena*, 40.

92. Allende Gossens, *La realidad médico-social chilena*, 196.

93. Paz Soldán, *La medicina social*, 34–35; and Zylberman, "Fewer Parallels," 82.

94. Winn, "Salvador Allende," 132.

95. Salazar Vergara and Altamirano Orrego, *Conversaciones con Carlos Altamirano*; Seo-ane, *Con el ojo izquierdo*, 101; and Drinot, *La seducción*.

96. Mariátegui, "El progreso nacional."

97. Schuftan, "Una verdadera joya," 74.

98. Illanes, *Cuerpo y sangre*, 15.

99. Pieper Mooney, *Politics of Motherhood*, 28–29.

100. Illanes, *En el nombre del pueblo*, 316.

101. Rosemblatt, "Por un hogar bien constituido"; Rosemblatt, *Gendered Compromises*; and Illanes, *Cuerpo y sangre*.

102. Illanes, *En el nombre del pueblo*, 304, 322.

103. Illanes, *En el nombre del pueblo*, 361.

104. Illanes, *En el nombre del pueblo*, 380.

105. Asociación Médica de Chile, "Proyecto de colegio médico"; and Labra, "Medicina social en Chile," 214–17.

106. Pinto and Viel, *Seguridad social chilena*; Labra, "Medicina social en Chile"; Molina Bustos, "Antecedentes"; and Molina Bustos, *Institucionalidad sanitaria chilena*.

107. Labra, "Medicina social en Chile"; and Molina Bustos, *Institucionalidad sanitaria chilena*, 130.

108. Pieper Mooney, "From Cold War Pressures."

109. Illanes, *En el nombre del pueblo*, 316.

110. Labra, "Medicina social en Chile," 219.

Chapter Four

1. Finchelstein, *From Fascism to Populism*, 112.

2. Biernat, Cerdá, and Ramacciotti, *La salud pública*, 26.

3. Finchelstein, *From Fascism to Populism*, 206.

4. Biernat, Cerdá, and Ramacciotti, *La salud pública*, 27.

5. Guy, *Women Build the Welfare State*.

6. Zimmermann, *Los liberales reformistas*; Suriano, *La cuestión social*; González Leandri, "Notas acerca de la profesionalización médica"; Rodriguez, *Civilizing Argentina*; and Biernat, Cerdá, and Ramacciotti, *La salud pública*.

7. Di Liscia and Fernández Marrón, "Sin puerto"; and Rodriguez, *Civilizing Argentina*, 179–99.

8. Armus, *Ailing City*.

9. Carter, *Enemy in the Blood*.

10. Rodriguez, *Civilizing Argentina*, 40; and Zimmermann, *Los liberales reformistas*.

11. Luciani, "La dirección de higiene"; and Bard, *Estampas de una vida*.

12. Biernat, Cerdá, and Ramacciotti, *La salud pública*, 20; and Salvatore, "Burocracias expertas," 24.

13. Adelman, "Political Economy of Labour," 28.

14. Salvatore, "Burocracias expertas," 55; and Carter, *Enemy in the Blood*.

15. Arce, *El sistema de salud*, 78–79; and Guy, *Women Build the Welfare State*.

16. González Bernaldo de Quirós, "El 'momento mutualista,'" 162.

17. Arce, *El sistema de salud*, 81.

18. González Bernaldo de Quirós, "El 'momento mutualista.'"

19. Rayez, "Germinal Rodríguez: entre la higiene," 194.

20. Belmartino, *La atención médica argentina*, 75–76.

21. Belmartino, *La atención médica argentina*, 72–80.

22. Belmartino, *La atención médica argentina*, 86–91.

23. Rayez, "Germinal Rodríguez: entre la higiene," 205.

24. Belmartino, *La atención médica argentina*, 96–102.

25. Lobato, "El Estado en los años treinta," 48; and Biernat, Cerdá, and Ramacciotti, *La salud pública*, 21.

26. "Inauguración de los cursos," 11.

27. Biernat, Cerdá, and Ramacciotti, *La salud pública*, 170.

28. Museo Social Argentino, *Primer Congreso de la Población*.

29. Miranda and Vallejo, *Una historia de la eugenesia*.

30. Armus, "Eugenesia en Buenos Aires."

31. Museo Social Argentino, *Primer Congreso de la Población*, 258.

32. Biernat, Cerdá, and Ramacciotti, *La salud pública*, 169.

33. Palacios and Salomone, *Alfredo L. Palacios*.

34. Carter, *Enemy in the Blood*.

35. Hagood, "Cells in the Body Politic," 113.

36. Lobato, "El Estado en los años treinta," 47; and Hagood, "Cells in the Body Politic."

37. Palacios and Salomone, *Alfredo L. Palacios*, 21.

38. Palacios and Salomone, *Alfredo L. Palacios*, 16.

39. Palacios and Salomone, *Alfredo L. Palacios*, 17–18.

40. P. Escudero, "El cuidado y mejoramiento," 16; and Carter, "Social Medicine and International Expert Networks."

41. P. Escudero, "El cuidado y mejoramiento," 16; and López and Poy, "Historia de la nutrición."

42. P. Escudero and Rothman, "La vivienda en 600 familias"; and Buschini, "La alimentación."

43. Buschini, "La alimentación"; and P. Escudero, "El cuidado y mejoramiento," 49.

44. Landabure, "Pedro Escudero," 1987.

45. Rayez, "Germinal Rodriguez: entre la higiene," 191.

46. Rayez, "Germinal Rodríguez: salud pública."

47. Buschini, "La alimentación," 156–65; and Rayez, "Germinal Rodriguez: entre la higiene," 199.

48. Ledesma Prietto, *"La revolución sexual,"* 37.

49. Pianetto, "Historical Conjuncture," 150–51.

50. Mastrangelo, *Dinámica social,* 59–83; and Cabello, "El gran europeo Georg Friedrich Nicolai."

51. Mastrangelo, *Dinámica social.*

52. Ledesma Prietto, *"La revolución sexual,"* 64; and Gutiérrez and Romero, "Barrio Societies," 224–25.

53. Ledesma Prietto, *"La revolución sexual,"* 165–67.

54. Lazarte, *Chile en la vanguardia,* 138; and Ledesma Prietto, *"La revolución sexual,"* 166.

55. Lazarte, *El contralor;* Ledesma Prietto, *"La revolución sexual,"* 166; Martinez-Alier, *Environmentalism of the Poor;* and Carter, "Population Control," 99–100.

56. Lazarte, *Chile en la vanguardia,* 54–57

57. Ledesma Prietto, *"La revolución sexual,"* 38, 118.

58. Belmartino, *La atención médica argentina,* 86–91.

59. Lazarte, *Problemas de medicina social,* 39.

60. Lazarte, *Problemas de medicina social,* 54.

61. Lazarte, *Problemas de medicina social.*

62. Lazarte, *Problemas de medicina social,* 84.

63. Lazarte, *Problemas de medicina social,* 57.

64. Abad de Santillán, Invaldi, and Capelletti, *Juan Lazarte,* 17–32.

65. Lazarte, *Problemas de medicina social,* 37–38.

66. Lazarte, *Chile en la vanguardia,* 138; and Lazarte, "Asistencia médica."

67. Ledesma Prietto, *"La revolución sexual,"* 47; and Lazarte, *La solución federalista.*

68. Ledesma Prietto, *"La revolución sexual,"* 37–39; Abad de Santillán, Invaldi, and Capelletti, *Juan Lazarte;* and Cano, "Lazarte, Juan."

69. Finchelstein, *From Fascism to Populism.*

70. Ramacciotti, *La política sanitaria,* 50–52; and Carter, *Enemy in the Blood,* 144–49.

71. Ramacciotti, *La política sanitaria,* 49–52; Otero, "Sueños cifrados," 219; and Reggiani, "Depopulation," 288.

72. Ramacciotti, *La política sanitaria,* 52–56.

73. Hurtado and Fernández, "Institutos privados," 10–12.

74. R. Carrillo, "Higiene y medicina social," 30.

75. R. Carrillo, "Higiene y medicina social," 22.

76. L. García, *Los derechos,* 21.

77. Ramacciotti, *La política sanitaria,* 73–74.

78. Ramacciotti, *La política sanitaria,* 73.

79. R. Carrillo, "Política Sanitaria Argentina," 214; and Ramacciotti, *La política sanitaria,* 99.

80. Biernat, Cerdá, and Ramacciotti, *La salud pública,* 125.

81. Ramacciotti, *La política sanitaria,* 105.

82. Armus, *Ailing City*, 48; and Herrero and Carbonetti, "La mortalidad por tuberculosis," 528.

83. Carter, *Enemy in the Blood*.

84. R. Carrillo, *Política Sanitaria Argentina*, 143.

85. Arce, *El sistema de salud*, 113.

86. Lazarte, "Bases," 185; and R. Carrillo, "Higiene y medicina social," 28–30.

87. Partido Peronista, *Manual del peronista*, 74; and Ramacciotti, *La política sanitaria*, 78.

88. Ramacciotti, *La política sanitaria*, 112.

89. Biernat, Cerdá, and Ramacciotti, *La salud pública*, 20–21.

90. L. García, *Los derechos*.

91. Terán, *Historia de las ideas*, 259.

92. Terán, *Historia de las ideas*, 259.

93. R. Carrillo, *Política Sanitaria Argentina*, 222.

94. Hagood, "Cells in the Body Politic," 190.

95. Andrenacci, Falappa, and Lvovich, "Acerca del Estado de Bienestar."

96. Ramacciotti, *La política sanitaria*, 112–13.

97. Ramacciotti, *La política sanitaria*, 116.

98. Carter, "Social Medicine and International Expert Networks."

99. Carter, "Social Medicine and International Expert Networks."

100. E. Elena, *Dignifying Argentina*; Guy, *Women Build the Welfare State*; Pite, *Creating a Common Table*; and Milanesio, *Workers Go Shopping*.

101. Biernat, Cerdá, and Ramacciotti, *La salud pública*, 32.

102. Biernat, Cerdá, and Ramacciotti, *La salud pública*, 29–30; and Belmartino, *La atención médica argentina*.

103. Arce, *El sistema de salud*, 116–17.

104. Arce, *El sistema de salud*, 118.

105. Biernat, Cerdá, and Ramacciotti, *La salud pública*, 34; and Golbert, *De la Sociedad de Beneficencia*, 70.

106. Roemer, *National Health Systems*, 366–67.

107. Biernat, Cerdá, and Ramacciotti, *La salud pública*, 28–29; and Belmartino, "Políticas de salud en Argentina," 16.

108. Biernat, Cerdá, and Ramacciotti, *La salud pública*, 32.

109. Lazarte, "Evolución y destino."

110. Hagood, "Unidad Médica," 88; and Arce, *El sistema de salud*, 177–78.

111. E. Elena, *Dignifying Argentina*.

112. Mesa-Lago, "Social Security," 359.

113. Svampa, *Certezas*, 33.

114. Belmartino, *La atención médica argentina*.

115. Belmartino et al., *Fundamentos históricos*, 249.

116. Arce, *El sistema de salud*, 177–78; Belmartino et al., *Fundamentos históricos*, 249; and Hagood, "Unidad Médica," 89.

117. Rachid, "Perón y Carrillo."

118. Cueto and Palmer, *Medicine and Public Health*, 139.

119. Hagood, "Cells in the Body Politic," 190.

Chapter Five

1. Cueto, "Social Medicine in the Andes," 192.
2. Paz Soldán, "La medicina social al servicio," 545.
3. Cueto and Palmer, *Medicine and Public Health*, 202–3.
4. Pacino, "National Politics and Scientific Pursuits," 55.
5. Bliss, "Under Surveillance"; and Brickman, "Medical McCarthyism."
6. Farley, *Brock Chisholm*; Packard, *History of Global Health*; and Cueto, Brown, and Fee, *World Health Organization*, 70–71.
7. Stepan, *Eradication*.
8. Birn, "Stages."
9. Paim, *Desafíos*, 78.
10. Pires-Alves and Chor Maio, "Health at the Dawn," 4; and Escobar, *Encountering Development*.
11. Pires-Alves and Chor Maio, "Health at the Dawn," 4.
12. Escobar, *Encountering Development*, 86.
13. Escobar, *Encountering Development*, 86.
14. Pires-Alves and Chor Maio, "Health at the Dawn," 10.
15. Frei Montalva, "Alliance," 441.
16. Huntington, "Change to Change," 308.
17. Harrison, *Sociology of Modernization*, 6.
18. Quevedo and Cortés, "El concepto de 'sistema'"; Cross and Albury, "Walter B. Cannon"; and Sturdy, "Biology as Social Theory."
19. Fajardo, *World That Latin America Created*, 13.
20. Fajardo, *World That Latin America Created*, 195.
21. Pieper Mooney, "From Cold War Pressures," 196.
22. Pieper Mooney, "From Cold War Pressures," 195–96.
23. Filerman, "Exploratory Field Study," 128.
24. Horowitz, *Rise and Fall*, 47–49.
25. Filerman, "Exploratory Field Study," 185.
26. Sahlins, "Established Order," 77–78.
27. Pires-Alves and Chor Maio, "Health at the Dawn," 16.
28. Durán, "Enfoque y perspectivas," 50.
29. Fajardo, *World That Latin America Created*, 109–11.
30. Author interview with Mario Testa, Buenos Aires, August 10, 2015.
31. Fassler, "Transformación social," 151.
32. PAHO, "Status of National Health Planning," 7.
33. PAHO, "Status of National Health Planning," 4.
34. Author interview with Testa, August 18, 2015.
35. Chorny, "Planificación en salud," 29.
36. Chorny, "Planificación en salud," 39.
37. Chorny, "Planificación en salud," 39.
38. Fassler, "Transformación social," 159.
39. Author interview with Mario Rovere, La Matanza, Buenos Aires, August 11, 2015.
40. Ferrara, "En torno al concepto de salud," 120.

41. Svampa, *Certezas*, 128.

42. Svampa, *Certezas*, 42.

43. Interview with Testa, August 18, 2015.

44. Svampa, *Certezas*, 44–46.

45. Ferrara, Acebal, and Paganini, *Medicina de la comunidad*.

46. Gorsky and Sirrs, "From 'Planning' to 'Systems Analysis,'" 232.

47. Medina, *Cybernetic Revolutionaries*.

48. Birn, "Introduction," 16.

49. Pieper Mooney, "From Cold War Pressures."

50. Valdivieso, Adriasola, and Horwitz, "Homenaje," 806.

51. Jiménez de la Jara, "Abraham Horwitz," 930.

52. Pires-Alves and Chor Maio, "Health at the Dawn," 7.

53. Pires-Alves and Chor Maio, "Health at the Dawn," 7.

54. Durán, "Enfoque y perspectivas," 41.

55. Horwitz, "Planificación," 379.

56. Ross, "Felipe Herrera."

57. Horwitz, "Planificación."

58. Author interview with Testa, August 10, 2015; Jiménez de la Jara, "Abraham Horwitz"; and Horwitz, "La Organización Panamericana."

59. Author interview with Testa, August 10, 2015.

60. Author interview with Carlos Montoya Aguilar, Santiago, March 7, 2016

61. Valdivieso, Adriasola, and Horwitz, "Homenaje," 811.

62. Pires-Alves and Chor Maio, "Health at the Dawn," 19.

63. Horwitz, "La Organización Panamericana."

64. Author interview with Testa, August 10, 2015.

65. Author interview with Giorgio Solimano, Santiago, March 11, 2016.

66. Interview with Solimano, March 11, 2016, and Montoya, March 7, 2016.

67. Ziegler, *Betting on Famine*, 149.

68. Guedes de Vasconcelos, "Josué de Castro"; Galluzzi Bizzo, "Ação política e pensamento social"; Ferretti, "Rediscovering Other Geographical Traditions"; and Ferretti, "Coffin for Malthusianism."

69. Carter, "Social Medicine and International Expert Networks," 798.

70. Galluzzi Bizzo, "Ação política e pensamento social," 402.

71. Ziegler, *Betting on Famine*, 97.

72. Ziegler, *Betting on Famine*, 97; and Carter, "Population Control."

73. Castro, *Geography of Hunger*.

74. Castro, *Geography of Hunger*.

75. Maurín Navarro, *Esquemas*, 34; and Mastrangelo, "La medicina social."

76. Ferretti, "Coffin for Malthusianism"; and Ferretti, "Rediscovering Other Geographical Traditions."

77. Castro, *Geography of Hunger*, 12.

78. Guedes de Vasconcelos, "Pão ou aço," 488.

79. Horowitz, Castro, and Gerassi, *Latin American Radicalism*; and Ziegler, *Betting on Famine*, 97–101.

80. Testa and Silva Paim, "Memoria e historia," 16.

81. Fee, "Pleasures and Perils," 1643.

82. Belmartino, "Políticas de salud en Argentina," 19.

83. Belmartino et al., *Fundamentos históricos*, 272.

84. Belmartino et al., *Fundamentos históricos*, 276.

85. Juan Martin Librandi, personal communication, April 16, 2019.

86. "Sobre un número."

87. "Huelga médica."

88. Ferrara and Peña, "Qué piensan."

89. Molina Bustos, *Institucionalidad sanitaria chilena*.

90. Candina-Polomer, "Studying Other Memories"; Cruz-Coke, "Síntesis biográfica"; and Molina Bustos, *Institucionalidad sanitaria chilena*.

91. Romero, "El Colegio Médico de Chile," 238.

92. Candina-Polomer, "Studying Other Memories," 77.

93. Author interview with Carlos Molina Bustos, Viña del Mar, Chile, March 8, 2016.

94. Candina-Polomer, "Studying Other Memories," 77–78.

95. Navarro, "What Does Chile Mean," 117; Sagan, Jonsen, and Paredes, *Report of the Recent Mission*, 204; and Belmar and Sidel, "International Perspective," 60.

96. Candina-Polomer, "Studying Other Memories," 79; and author interview with Sergio Sánchez Bustos, Santiago, February 23, 2016.

97. Testa and Silva Paim, "Memoria e historia," 16.

98. Belmartino, "Políticas de salud en Argentina," 20.

99. Palloni, "Fertility and Mortality Decline," 128.

100. Franco et al., *Debates en medicina social*, 98.

101. Carter, "Population Control."

Chapter Six

1. Nunes, "Path Taken by Social Sciences," 66.

2. Fajardo, *World That Latin America Created*.

3. Rappaport, *Cowards Don't Make History*, 13.

4. Nunes, "Las ciencias sociales en salud," 228.

5. Emanuelsson, "Entrevista a Juan Carlos Concha."

6. Hartch, *Prophet of Cuernavaca*; Nogueira, "A segunda crítica social"; and Tabet et al., "Ivan Illich."

7. Caponi, "Canguilhem y el estatuto."

8. Gaudenzi and Ortega, "O estatuto da medicalização"; author interview with Fernando Pires-Alves and Carlos Henrique Paiva, Rio de Janeiro, July 26, 2017.

9. Nunes, "Las ciencias sociales en salud."

10. Nunes, "La salud colectiva en Brasil," 349.

11. Galeano, Trotta, and Spinelli, "Juan César García," 290–91.

12. Holst, "Paulo Freire in Chile," 256.

13. Author interview with Mario and Asia Testa, Buenos Aires, August 10, 2015.

14. J. García, "Juan César García entrevista."

15. J. Garcia, *La educación médica*.

16. Nunes, "O pensamento social."

17. Márquez, "Juan César García," 94.

18. Nunes, "O pensamento social," 1757.

19. Author interview with Mario Rovere, La Matanza, Buenos Aires, August 11, 2015.

20. J. García, "Juan César García entrevista," 6; and Villarreal, "Un hombre," 72.

21. Ferreira, "Un precursor de ideas," 52–53.

22. Ferreira, "Un precursor de ideas," 52–53.

23. OPS/OMS, "Aspectos teóricos"; Molina Guzmán and Jimeno, "Teaching Social Science Concepts"; and Fonseca, "Latin American Social Medicine," 136–39.

24. Márquez, "Juan César García," 109.

25. Márquez, "Juan César García," 94–95.

26. Fonseca, "Latin American Social Medicine," 144.

27. Nunes, "Tendencias y perspectivas," 176; and Cordeiro, "O Instituto de Medicina Social," 344.

28. Mercer, "La incorporación"; Nunes, "Las ciencias sociales"; J. Escudero, "Salud, historia y poder."

29. Vidal, "Veinticinco años," 118.

30. Arouca and Márquez, "La arqueología de la medicina"; and Foucault, "Historia de la medicalización."

31. Nunes, "Salud y sociedad," 198; and author interview with Mario Rovere, August 11, 2015.

32. J. García, "Las ciencias sociales"; and Nunes, "Salud y sociedad," 207.

33. Galeano, Trotta, and Spinelli, "Juan César García," 301.

34. J. García, "Juan César García entrevista," 4–5.

35. Comité de Expertos, "Primer informe sobre la enseñanza."

36. Comité del Programa de Libros, "Enseñanza de la medicina preventiva."

37. Wright and Oñate Zúñiga, "Chilean Political Exile."

38. Navarro, "What Does Chile Mean."

39. Navarro, "What Does Chile Mean"; author interview with Carlos Molina Bustos, Viña del Mar, Chile, March 8, 2016; author interview with Carlos Montoya Aguilar, Santiago, March 7, 2016.

40. Navarro, "What Does Chile Mean," 118.

41. Author interview with Montoya Aguilar, March 7, 2016; and Emanuelsson, "Entrevista a Juan Carlos Concha."

42. Author interview with Molina Bustos, March 8, 2016.

43. Belmar and Sidel, "International Perspective," 58–61.

44. Navarro, "What Does Chile Mean," 94.

45. Sagan, Jonsen, and Paredes, *Report of the Recent Mission to Chile*, 205.

46. UNESCO, "Estudio de los informes de violaciones."

47. Author interview with Giorgio Solimano, Santiago, March 11, 2016.

48. Wright and Oñate Zúñiga, "Chilean Political Exile," 33–34.

49. Jonathan Kandell, "13 Doctors in Chile Reportedly Slain after the Coup," *New York Times*, April 8, 1974.

50. Hakim and Solimano, "Nutrition and National Development"; and Solimano and Hakim, "Nutrition and National Development."

51. Author interview with Montoya Aguilar, March 7, 2016.

52. Sepúlveda Alvarez, *De hombres y sombras*, 113.

53. Sepúlveda Alvarez, *De hombres y sombras*, 113–15; and Conill, "O enfoque ecológico-social."

54. Author interview with Claudio Sepúlveda, Santiago, February 29, 2016.

55. Carter and Sanchez Delgado, "Una discusión"; and Pieper Mooney, "From Cold War Pressures," 195.

56. Muller, *Participación popular*, 86–88; and Juan Carlos Eslava, personal communication, December 5, 2018.

57. Carter and Sánchez Delgado, "Una discusión"; and Sigerist, *Historia y sociología*.

58. Molina Guzman, "Third World Experiences," 143.

59. Birn, Muntaner, and Afzal, "South-South Cooperation in Health."

60. Saborío et al., "Medicina comunitaria."

61. Spinelli, Librandi, and Zábala, "Los Cuadernos Médico Sociales"; and Foucault, "Nacimiento de la medicina social."

62. Molina Martínez, Gamboa De Bernardi, and Novoa, "Dr. Hugo Behm Rosas."

63. Behm, "Determinantes económicos."

64. Schuftan and Narayan, "People's Health Movement."

65. Author interview with Montoya Aguilar, March 7, 2016; Basulto, Conteras, and Glisser, *Chilenos en Mozambique*; and Rovira, "Chilen@s en Mozambique."

66. Fassler, "Política sanitaria."

67. Pieper Mooney, "From Cold War Pressures," 203–4; and author interview with Jaime Sepúlveda Salinas, Santiago-Minnesota (online), August 26, 2021.

68. Navarro, "What Does Chile Mean."

69. Belmar and Sidel, "International Perspective," 61.

70. Navarro, "What Does Chile Mean," 102.

71. Osuna, "La intervención social."

72. Hamilton, *Vida de sanitarista*, 79.

73. Author interviews with Mario and Asia Testa, August 10 and 18, 2015.

74. Author interviews with Mario and Asia Testa, August 10 and 18, 2015; Waitzkin et al., "Social Medicine in Latin America," 317.

75. Testa and Silva Paim, "Memoria e historia."

76. Testa, *Pensar en salud*.

77. Author interviews with Mario and Asia Testa, August 10 and 18, 2015.

78. Testa and Silva Paim, "Memoria e historia," 214.

79. Mastrangelo, *Dinámica social*, 99; and "Morre o médico argentino Carlos Bloch."

80. Spinelli, Librandi, and Zábala, "Los Cuadernos Médico Sociales"; and author interview with Mario Rovere, August 11, 2015.

81. Testa, *Pensar en salud*, 139–79.

82. Belmartino, *La atención médica argentina*.

83. Belmartino, "Políticas de salud en Argentina"; Belmartino, *La atención médica argentina*; and Belmartino et al., *Fundamentos históricos*.

84. Spinelli, Librandi, and Zábala, "Los Cuadernos Médico Sociales."

85. Spinelli, Librandi, and Zábala, "Los Cuadernos Médico Sociales."

86. Author interview with Ernesto Taboada and Sandra Gerlero, Rosario, July 31, 2015; and Comité del Programa de Libros, "Enseñanza de la medicina preventiva."

87. Spinelli, Librandi, and Zábala, "Los Cuadernos Médico Sociales," 881; Menéndez, "Modelo médico hegemónico"; and de Moura Pontes, "Entrevista."

88. Author interview with Ernesto Taboada and Sandra Gerlero, July 31, 2015.

89. Author interview with Mario Rovere, August 11, 2015.

90. Coutinho, *Democracia e socialismo*, 50; and Abreu and Netto, *Projeto memória . . . 1967–1975*, 10.

91. Abreu and Netto, *Projeto memória . . . 1967–1975*, 7–8.

92. Jacobina, "A relação do Cebes."

93. Vieira-da-Silva and Pinell, "Gênese sócio-histórica," 33; Nunes, "La salud colectiva en Brasil," 354.

94. Gaudenzi and Ortega, "O estatuto da medicalização"; author interview with Pires-Alves and Paiva; author interview with Mario Rovere, August 11, 2015; Foot, "Franco Basaglia."

95. Vieira-da-Silva and Pinell, "Gênese sócio-histórica," 36.

96. Hamilton, *Vida de sanitarista*, 111.

97. Hamilton, *Vida de sanitarista*, 114.

98. Hamilton, *Vida de sanitarista*, 112 (emphasis added).

99. Testa and Silva Paim, "Memoria e Historiahistoria," 212; and Rappaport, *Cowards Don't Make History*.

100. Nunes, "La salud colectiva en Brasil."

101. Nunes, "La salud colectiva en Brasil," 353; and Fernández Agis, "La ética y la medicina social."

102. Jacobina, "A relação do Cebes."

103. Spinelli, Librandi, and Zábala, "Los Cuadernos Médico Sociales," 883–84.

104. Roncali Mafezolli, "O cenário depois do golpe"; and Jacobina, "A relação do Cebes," 154.

105. Jacobina, "A relação do Cebes."

106. *Revista de Manguinhos*, "Memoria"; Marques, *Sérgio Arouca*; Dowbor, "Sérgio Arouca"; Abreu and Netto, *Projeto memória . . . 1976–1988*; *Projeto memória . . . 1967–1975*.

107. Testa and Silva Paim, "Memoria e historia," 214; and Dowbor, "Sérgio Arouca."

108. Zancan and Matida, "Trajetórias"; and Abreu and Netto, *Projeto memória . . . 1967–1975*, 73.

109. Abreu and Netto, *Projeto memória . . . 1967–1975*, 17.

110. Arouca, *O dilema preventivista*.

111. Galeano, Trotta, and Spinelli, "Juan César García," 305–6.

112. Comité de Expertos, "Primer informe sobre la enseñanza."

113. Juárez Herrera y Cairo and Castro Vásquez, "El dilema preventivista."

114. Abreu and Netto, *Projeto memória . . . 1967–1975*, 23.

115. Escorel, "Sérgio Arouca," 620.

116. Abreu and Netto, *Projeto memória . . . 1976–1988*, 102.

117. Lent, *O massacre de Manguinhos*.

118. *Revista de Manguinhos*, "Memoria," 30.

119. Abreu and Netto, *Projeto memória . . . 1967–1975*, 26.

120. Schraiber and Mota, "Social in Health"; Abreu and Netto, *Projeto memória . . . 1967–1975*; *Projeto memória . . . 1976–1988*; and Nunes, "La salud colectiva en Brasil."

121. Schraiber and Mota, "Social in Health," 1470.

122. Carlos Henrique Paiva, personal communication, August 24, 2019.

123. Nunes, "Tendencias y perspectivas."

124. The signatories of the "Act of Ouro Preto," the constitution of ALAMES, were Mario Agandoña (Bolivia), Sérgio Arouca (Brazil), Horacio Barri (Argentina), Susana Belmartino (Argentina), Jaime Breilh (Ecuador), Paulo Marchori Buss (Brazil), Francisco Campos (Brazil), Hesio Cordeiro (Brazil), David Capistrano Filho (Brazil), Saúl Franco Agudelo (Colombia), César Ganado C. (Colombia), Guillermo González G. (Nicaragua), Asa Cristina Laurell (México), Francisco de Asís Machado (Brazil), Everardo Duarte Nunes (Brazil), Benedictus Philade de Siqueira (Brazil), Juan S. Yazlle Rocha (Brazil), Ana María Testa Tambellini (Brazil), Mario Testa (Argentina), and Carmen Fontes Texeira (Brazil). Fonseca also includes Edmundo Granda (Ecuador), Sonia Fleury (Brazil), and María Isabel Rodríguez (El Salvador) among the founding members of ALAMES. See Fonseca, "Latin American Social Medicine," 25; and ALAMES, "Acta de Ouro Preto," 264.

Chapter Seven

1. Nunes, "La salud colectiva en Brasil."

2. López Arellano and Saint Martin, "Salud y sociedad"; Hartmann, "Postneoliberal Public Health"; Spiegel, Breilh, and Yassi, "Why Language Matters"; and González Guzmán, "Latin American Social Medicine."

3. Rojas Ochoa and Márquez, *ALAMES en la memoria*; and Fonseca, "Latin American Social Medicine."

4. Paiva and Teixeira, "Health Reform," 22.

5. Fleury, "Política social"; and Fleury, "Brazil's Health-Care Reform."

6. Mayka, "Origins of Strong Institutional Design," 282.

7. Stralen, "O Cebes," 4.

8. Doimo, *A vez e a voz do popular*, 69; and Chappell, *Beginning to End Hunger*, 194.

9. Lima, Paranaguá de Santana, and Paiva, *Saúde coletiva*, 52; and Jairnilson Paim, personal communication, June 15, 2021.

10. Stralen, "O Cebes," 4.

11. Gerschman, *A democracia inconclusa*, 94–106.

12. Jairnilison Paim, personal communication, June 15, 2021.

13. Gerschman, *A democracia inconclusa*; and Pires-Alves, Paiva, and Lima, "Baixada Fluminense."

14. Mayka, "Origins of Strong Institutional Design," 282.

15. Comissão Organizadora da 8ª Conferência Nacional de Saúde, "Democracia é saúde."

16. Lima, Paranaguá de Santana, and Paiva, *Saúde coletiva*, 55.

17. Dowbor, "Origins," 78.

18. Lima, Paranaguá de Santana, and Paiva, *Saúde coletiva*, 58.

19. Mayka, "Origins of Strong Institutional Design," 284.

20. Mayka, "Origins of Strong Institutional Design," 285.

21. Dowbor, "Origins," 78.

22. Fleury, "Brazil's Health-Care Reform," 1724; and Atun et al., "Health-System Reform," 1235.

23. Testa and Paim, "Memoria e historia," 215.

24. Paim et al., "Brazilian Health System," 1788.

25. Paim et al., "Brazilian Health System," 1786.

26. Parker, "Building the Foundations," 157.

27. Parker, "Building the Foundations," 157–58.

28. Murray et al., "Strange Bedfellows," 948.

29. Cueto and Lopes, "AIDS, Antiretrovirals," 6–7.

30. Doimo, *A vez e a voz do popular*, 66–67; and Chappell, *Beginning to End Hunger*, 194.

31. Mayka, "Origins of Strong Institutional Design," 281.

32. Paiva and Teixeira, "Health Reform," 27, 29.

33. Jerome, *Right to Health*, 149–56.

34. Paiva and Teixeira, "Health Reform," 28.

35. Cueto and Palmer, *Medicine and Public Health*, 246.

36. Iriart, Merhy, and Waitzkin, "Managed Care."

37. Cueto and Palmer, *Medicine and Public Health*, 243.

38. Fleury et al., *Right to Health in Latin America*, 18.

39. Sojo, "Reformas"; and Le Grand, "Quasi-Markets and Social Policy."

40. Almeida, "Reforma de sistemas."

41. Homedes and Ugalde, "Why Neoliberal Health Reforms Have Failed."

42. Sojo, "Reformas"; and World Bank, *World Development Report 1993*.

43. Londoño and Frenk, "Structured Pluralism."

44. Giedion and Villar Uribe, "Colombia's Universal Health Insurance," 855.

45. Giedion and Villar Uribe, "Colombia's Universal Health Insurance," 855.

46. Hernández Álvarez, "El enfoque sociopolítico," 490.

47. Rovere, "La salud en la Argentina."

48. Belmartino, "Una década de reforma," 157–58.

49. Katz, *Argentina hospital*; and Rovere, "La salud en la Argentina."

50. Iriart, Merhy, and Waitzkin, "Managed Care."

51. Iriart, Merhy, and Waitzkin, "Managed Care"; "Hubo más de 150.000 cambios de obras sociales," *La Nación*, May 16 1997; and Carlos Manzoni, "El Exxel, un ícono que perdió fuerza," *La Nación*, January 11, 2009.

52. Waitzkin, Jasso-Aguilar, and Iriart, "Privatization of Health Services," 222.

53. Iriart, Merhy, and Waitzkin, "Managed Care."

54. Sojo, "Reformas"; and Almeida, "Reforma de sistemas."

55. Belmartino, "Una década de reforma," 162.

56. Homedes and Ugalde, "Why Neoliberal Health Reforms Have Failed," 92.

57. Tajer, "Latin American Social Medicine," 2025.

58. Torres Tovar, "ALAMES."

59. Torres Tovar, "ALAMES."

60. Tajer, "La medicina social," 23.

61. Torres Tovar, "ALAMES," 126; and Laurell, "Proyectos políticos," 220–21.

62. Waitzkin et al., "Social Medicine Then and Now"; Krieger, "Latin American Social Medicine"; and Tajer, "Latin American Social Medicine."

63. Hartmann, "Postneoliberal Public Health," 2147.

64. Briggs and Mantini-Briggs, "Confronting Health Disparities"; and Tajer, "La medicina social," 31.

65. Briggs and Mantini-Briggs, "Confronting Health Disparities," 552.

66. Briggs and Mantini-Briggs, "Confronting Health Disparities," 552.

67. Kirk, *Healthcare without Borders*, 33.

68. Briggs and Mantini-Briggs, "Confronting Health Disparities," 555.

69. Carrillo Roa, "Sistema de salud."

70. Carrillo Roa, "Sistema de salud."

71. Redsacol/ALAMES. "Declaración."

72. Hartmann, "Postneoliberal Public Health," 2149.

73. Johnson, "Decolonization," 141.

74. Loza, "Medicinas tradicionales."

75. Bernstein, "Personal and Political Histories," 233.

76. Johnson, "Decolonization"; and Bernstein, "Personal and Political Histories."

77. Ramírez Hita, "Aspectos interculturales," 767.

78. Hartmann, "Bolivia's Plurinational Healthcare."

79. Laurell, "What Does Latin American Social Medicine Do?" 2030.

80. Laurell, "What Does Latin American Social Medicine Do?" 2031.

81. Laurell and Giovanella, "Health Policies," 3.

82. Laurell, "Mexican Popular Health Insurance."

83. Laurell, "Social Policy."

84. Reich, "Restructuring," 3.

85. Teresa Moreno, "Insabi es retroceso de 40 años en salud: entrevista con Julio Frenk Mora," *El Universal*, January 15, 2020.

86. Garrett, Chowdhury, and Pablos-Mendez, "All for Universal Health Coverage," 1294.

87. Fonseca, "Latin American Social Medicine," 250.

88. Reich, "Restructuring," 9.

89. Breilh, "Entrevista con Jaime Breilh," 48.

90. Breilh, "Entrevista con Jaime Breilh," 48.

91. Bell, "Whatever Happened?" 164.

92. Adams, "Re-Imagining Global Health," 2.

93. Waitzkin et al., "Social Medicine Then and Now"; Waitzkin et al., "Social Medicine in Latin America"; Krieger, "Latin American Social Medicine"; and Laurell, "What Does Latin American Social Medicine Do?"

94. Arouca, *O dilema preventivista*; and Almeida-Filho, *Epidemiología sin números*.

95. Spiegel, Breilh, and Yassi, "Why Language Matters," 14; and Fonseca, "Latin American Social Medicine," 187.

96. Morales-Borrero et al., "¿Determinación social?" 800.

97. Fonseca, "Latin American Social Medicine," 189, emphasis in original.

98. González Guzmán, "Latin American Social Medicine," 117, 119.

99. López Arellano, Escudero, and Moreno, "Los determinantes sociales," 327–28.

100. Krieger et al., "Who, and What, Causes Health Inequities?" 749.

101. Laurell, "El estudio social."

102. Castro, *Teoría social y salud*, 132.

103. Castro, *Teoría social y salud*, 143; and Laurell, "El estudio social," 5.

104. Menéndez, "Modelo médico hegemónico," 3; and Castro, *Teoría social y salud*, 27–28.

105. Sacchi, Hausberger, and Pereyra, "Percepción del proceso," 276–77.

106. Sacchi, Hausberger, and Pereyra, "Percepción del proceso," 281.

107. Castro, *Teoria social y salud*, 150.

108. Tajer et al., "Investigaciones sobre género," 345.

109. Linardelli, "La salud de las mujeres," 150; and Tajer et al., "Investigaciones sobre género," 346.

110. Tajer et al., "Investigaciones sobre género."

111. Fleury et al., *Right to Health in Latin America*, 13.

112. Menéndez, "Modelo médico hegemónico," 22.

113. Jerome, *Right to Health*.

114. Almeida-Filho, *Epidemiología sin números*.

115. Almeida-Filho, *La ciencia tímida*; and Breilh, *Critical Epidemiology*, 128.

116. Kawachi, Subramanian, and Almeida-Filho, "Glossary for Health Inequalities"; and Krieger et al., "Who, and What, Causes Health Inequities?"

117. Barreto, Almeida-Filho, and Breilh, "Epidemiology."

118. Tavares and Romão, "Emerging Counterhegemonic Models."

119. Breilh, *Critical Epidemiology*.

120. Adams et al., "Re-Imagining Global Health."

121. Fonseca, "Latin American Social Medicine," 116, 137.

122. Atun et al., "Health-System Reform," 1234.

123. McGuire and Frankel, "Mortality Decline," 110.

124. Chaufan, "Desentrañando."

125. Huish and Kirk, "Cuban Medical Internationalism."

126. Waitzkin, *Medicine and Public Health*, 55.

127. Birn, Muntaner, and Afzal, "South-South Cooperation in Health."

128. Waitzkin et al., "Social Medicine in Latin America," 320.

129. Author interview with Mario Testa, Buenos Aires, August 10, 2015; and Testa and Paim, "Memoria e historia," 221.

130. Waitzkin et al., "Social Medicine in Latin America," 320.

131. Author interview with Mario Rovere, La Matanza, Buenos Aires, August 11, 2015.

132. Remen and Holloway, "Student Perspective," 164.

133. Martínez Franzoni and Sánchez-Ancochea, *Quest for Universal Social Policy*, ch. 5.

134. Martínez Franzoni and Sánchez-Ancochea, *Quest for Universal Social Policy*, ch. 5.

135. Homedes and Ugalde, "Why Neoliberal Health Reforms Have Failed," 94; and Martínez Franzoni and Sánchez-Ancochea, *Quest for Universal Social Policy*, ch. 6.

136. Fleury et al., *Right to Health in Latin America*, 18.

137. Serra Canales and Ramírez Guier, "La experiencia"; and Atul Gawande, "Costa Ricans Live Longer Than We Do: What's the Secret?" *New Yorker*, August 30, 2021.

138. Vargas and Muiser, "Promoting Universal Financial Protection," 8.

139. Baum, Sanders, and Narayan, "Global People's Health Movement," 11.

Conclusion

1. Hartmann, "Postneoliberal Public Health," 2149; and Laurell and Giovanella, "Health Policies," 1.

2. de la Dehesa, "Social Medicine," 803.

3. de la Dehesa, "Social Medicine."

4. Menendez, "Modelo médico hegemónico," 22.

5. Gaffney, *To Heal Humankind*, 218.

6. Navarro, *Politics of Health Policy*, xii–xiii; and Gaffney, *To Heal Humankind*.

7. Laurell, "Social Policy," 2.

8. Prainsack and Buyx, "Solidarity," 346 (emphasis in the original).

9. Laurell and Giovanella, "Health Policies," 1.

10. Dowbor, "Sergio Arouca," 1437.

11. Hartmann, "Postneoliberal Public Health," 2146.

12. Laurell and Giovanella, "Health Policies," 23.

13. Author interviews with Mario and Asia Testa, August 10 and 18, 2015.

14. Krieger et al., "Who, and What, Causes Health Inequities?" 747.

15. Hartmann, "Postneoliberal Public Health," 2150.

16. My rhetoric here is inspired by Amartya Sen's capabilities approach, which, for whatever reason, has not been embraced or even discussed among LASM scholars. See Sen, *Development as Freedom*.

Bibliography

Periodicals Surveyed

Acción Social (Chile)
AMECH, Revista Mensual
Anales, Asociación Argentina de Biotipología, Eugenesia y Medicina Social (AAABEMS)
Boletín de la OPS
Boletín del IIPI (Instituto Internacional Americano de Protección de la Infancia)
Boletín Gremial de la AMECH
Boletín Médico de Chile (BMC)
Boletín Médico-Social (Chile)
Cuadernos Médico-Sociales (Rosario, Argentina)
Cuadernos Médico-Sociales (Santiago, Chile)

Educación Medica y Salud
La Hoja Sanitaria (Chile)
La Reforma Médica (Peru)
Revista Centroamericana de Ciencias de la Salud
Revista Chilena de Higiene y Medicina Preventiva
Revista del Servicio Nacional de Salud (Chile)
Revista de Salud Pública (La Plata, Argentina)
Revista Médica de Chile
Salud Colectiva (Lanús, Argentina)
Vida Médica (Chile)

Primary and Secondary Sources

Abad de Santillán, Diego, Ángel Invaldi, and Ángel Capelletti. *Juan Lazarte, militante social, médico, humanista.* Rosario: Grupo Editor de Estudios Sociales, 1964.

Abreu, Regina, and Guilherme Franco Netto, eds. *Projeto memória e patrimônio da saúde pública no Brasil: a trajetória de Sérgio Arouca; Relatório de atividades Sérgio Arouca 1967–1975.* Rio de Janeiro: FIOTEC–Fundação para o Desenvolvimento Científico e Tecnológico em Saúde, 2005.

———. *Projeto memória e patrimônio da saúde pública no Brasil: a trajetória de Sérgio Arouca; Relatório de atividades Sérgio Arouca 1976–1988.* Rio de Janeiro: FIOTEC–Fundação para o Desenvolvimento Científico e Tecnológico em Saúde, 2005.

Acha, Omar. "Celia Lapalma de Emery y la cuestión social desde una perspectiva católica en el temprano siglo XX argentino." *Revista Brasileira de História das Religiões* 7, no. 19 (2014): 31–45.

Actas generales de la Novena Conferencia Sanitaria Panamericana: celebrada en Buenos Aires del 12 al 22 de noviembre de 1934. Baltimore: Reese Press, 1935.

Adams, Vincanne, Dominique Behague, Carlo Caduff, Ilana Löwy, and Francisco Ortega. "Re-imagining Global Health through Social Medicine." *Global Public Health* (2019): 1–18.

Adelman, Jeremy, ed. *Essays in Argentine Labour History, 1870–1930.* London: Macmillan Press, 1992.

————. "Political Economy of Labour, 1870–1930." In Adelman, *Essays in Argentine Labour History*, 1–34.

Agostoni, Claudia. "Médicos rurales y medicina social en el México posrevolucionario." *Historia Mexicana* 63, no. 2 (2013): 745–801.

ALAMES. "Acta de Ouro Preto: Constitución de la Asociación Latinoamericana de Medicina Social (1984)." *Medicina Social* 4, no. 4 (2009): 263–64.

Allende Gossens, Salvador. *La realidad médico-social chilena.* Providencia, Santiago: Editorial Cuarto Propio, 1999 [1939].

————. *Realidad financiera de la Caja de Seguro Obligatorio y modificaciones propuestas por el Senador Dr. Salvador Allende G.* Santiago: Talleres Gráficos "La Nación," 1947.

Almeida, Celia. "Reforma de sistemas de servicios de salud y equidad en América Latina y el Caribe: algunas lecciones de los años 80 y 90." *Cadernos de Saúde Pública* 18 (2002): 905–25.

Almeida-Filho, Naomar de. *Epidemiología sin números: una introducción crítica a la ciencia epidemiológica.* Translated by Jorge Daniel Lemus. Washington, DC: OPS, 1992.

————. *La ciencia tímida: ensayos de deconstrucción de la epidemiología.* Buenos Aires: Lugar Editorial, 2000.

Alonso Vial, Armando. "Nota biográfica sobre Juan Gandulfo." *Revista Médica de Chile* 60, no. 2 (1932): 99–114.

Andrenacci, Luciano, Fernando Falappa, and Daniel Lvovich. "Acerca del Estado de Bienestar en el peronismo clásico (1943–1955)." In *En el país del no me acuerdo: (des) memoria institucional e historia de la política social en la Argentina*, edited by Julián Bertranou, Juan Manuel Palacio and Gerardo M. Serrano, 83–116. Buenos Aires: Prometeo, 2004.

"Ante la Ley de Medicina Preventiva." *AMECH* 1, no. 8 (June–July–August 1938): 3–5.

Arce, Hugo E. *El sistema de salud: de dónde viene y hacia dónde va.* Buenos Aires: Prometeo Libros, 2010.

Arias Escobedo, Osvaldo. *La prensa obrera en Chile, 1900–1930.* Chillán: Universidad de Chile-Chillán, 1970.

Armus, Diego. *The Ailing City: Health, Tuberculosis, and Culture in Buenos Aires, 1870–1950.* Durham, NC: Duke University Press, 2011.

————. "Eugenesia en Buenos Aires: discursos, prácticas, historiografía." *História, Ciências, Saúde-Manguinhos* 23 (2016): 149–70.

Arouca, Sérgio. *O dilema preventivista: contribuição para a compreensão e crítica da medicina preventiva.* São Paulo: Editora UNESP, 2003.

Arouca, Sérgio, and Miguel Márquez. "La arqueología de la medicina." *Educación Médica y Salud* 8, no. 4 (1974): 331–46.

Asociación Médica de Chile. "Proyecto de colegio médico." *Revista Médica de Chile* 60, no. 2 (1932): 153–66.

Atun, Rifat, Luiz Odorico Monteiro De Andrade, Gisele Almeida, Daniel Cotlear, Tania Dmytraczenko, Patricia Frenz, Patrícia Garcia et al. "Health-System Reform and Universal Health Coverage in Latin America." *Lancet* 385, no. 9974 (2015): 1230–47.

Barany, Michael J., and John Krige. "Afterword: Reflections on Writing the Transnational History of Science and Technology." In Krige, *How Knowledge Moves*, 411–18.

Bard, Leopoldo. "La defensa de la raza." *Crónica Médico-Quirúrgica de La Habana* 57 (1931): 401–7.

———. "Las enfermedades sociales." *La Semana Médica* 47 (1925).

———. *Estampas de una vida: la fe puesta en un ideal "llegar a ser algo."* Buenos Aires: J. Perrotti, 1957.

Barreto, Mauricio L., Naomar De Almeida-Filho, and Jaime Breilh. "Epidemiology Is More Than Discourse: Critical Thoughts from Latin America." *Journal of Epidemiology & Community Health* 55, no. 3 (2001): 158–59.

Bashford, Alison. *Global Population: History, Geopolitics, and Life on Earth.* New York: Columbia University Press, 2014.

Basulto, Sergio, Dalmiro Conteras, and Mario Glisser. *Chilenos en Mozambique: experiencias de solidaridad y amistad entre dos pueblos.* Santiago: CEIBO, 2013.

Baum, Fran, David Sanders, and Ravi Narayan. "The Global People's Health Movement: What Is the People's Health Movement?" *Saúde em Debate* 44 (2020): 11–23.

Behm, Hugo. "Determinantes económicos y sociales de la mortalidad en América Latina." *Revista Centroamericana de Ciencias de la Salud* 12 (1979): 69–102.

Bell, Kirsten. "Whatever Happened to the 'Social' Science in *Social Science & Medicine*? On Golden Anniversaries and Gold Standards." *Social Science & Medicine* 214 (2018): 162–66.

Belmar, Roberto, and Victor W. Sidel. "An International Perspective on Strikes and Strike Threats by Physicians: The Case of Chile." *International Journal of Health Services* 5, no. 1 (1975): 53–64.

Belmartino, Susana. *La atención médica argentina en el siglo XX: instituciones y procesos.* Buenos Aires: Siglo Veintiuno Editores Argentina, 2005.

———. "Políticas de salud en Argentina: perspectiva histórica." *Cuadernos Médico Sociales (Rosario)* 55 (March 1991): 13–33.

———. "Una década de reforma de la atención médica en Argentina." *Salud Colectiva* 1 (2005): 155–71.

Belmartino, Susana, Carlos Bloch, María Isabel Carnino, and Ana Virginia Persello. *Fundamentos históricos de la construcción de relaciones de poder en el sector salud: Argentina, 1940–1960.* Buenos Aires: Oficina Panamericana de la Salud, 1991.

Bengoa, José María. *Sanare—hace 50 años: medicina social en el medio rural venezolano.* Caracas: Ediciones CAVENDES, 1992 [1940].

Bernstein, Alissa. "Personal and Political Histories in the Designing of Health Reform Policy in Bolivia." *Social Science & Medicine* 177 (2017): 231–38.

Berro, Roberto. "La medicina social de la infancia." *Boletín del IIPI* 9 (1935–36): 594–609.

Bettinotti, Saúl I. "El lactario: su funcionamiento y resultados." *Boletín del IIPI* 9 (1935–36): 64–72.

Biernat, Carolina, Juan Manuel Cerdá, and Karina Ramacciotti. *La salud pública y la enfermería en la Argentina.* Bernal: Universidad Nacional de Quilmes, 2015.

Birn, Anne-Emanuelle. "Doctors on Record: Uruguay's Infant Mortality Stagnation and Its Remedies, 1895–1945." *Bulletin of the History of Medicine* 82, no. 2 (2008): 311–54.

———. "Introduction: Alternative Destinies and Solidarities for Health and Medicine in Cold War Latin America." In Birn and Necochea López, *Peripheral Nerve*, 1–30.

———. "Making It Politic(al): Closing the Gap in a Generation; Health Equity through Action on the Social Determinants of Health." *Social Medicine* 4, no. 3 (2009): 166–82.

———. "The National-International Nexus in Public Health: Uruguay and the Circulation of Child Health and Welfare Policies, 1890–1940." *História, Ciências, Saúde-Manguinhos* 13, no. 3 (2006): 33–64.

———. "Philanthrocapitalism, Past and Present: The Rockefeller Foundation, the Gates Foundation, and the Setting(s) of the International/Global Health Agenda." *Hypothesis* 12 (2014).

———. "A Revolution in Rural Health? The Struggle over Local Health Units in Mexico, 1928–1940." *Journal of the History of Medicine and Allied Sciences* 53, no. 1 (1998): 43–76.

———. "The Stages of International (Global) Health: Histories of Success or Successes of History?" *Global Public Health* 4, no. 1 (2009): 50–68.

Birn, Anne-Emanuelle, Carles Muntaner, and Zabia Afzal. "South-South Cooperation in Health: Bringing in Theory, Politics, History, and Social Justice." Supplement. *Cadernos de Saúde Pública* 33, no. 2 (2017): S37–S52.

Birn, Anne-Emanuelle, and Raúl Necochea López. "Footprints on the Future: Looking Forward to the History of Health and Medicine in Latin America in the Twenty-First Century." *Hispanic American Historical Review* 91, no. 3 (2011): 503–27.

Birn, Anne-Emanuelle, and Raúl Necochea López, eds. *Peripheral Nerve: Health and Medicine in Cold War Latin America*. Durham, NC: Duke University Press, 2020.

Birn, Anne-Emanuelle, and Laura Nervi. "Political Roots of the Struggle for Health Justice in Latin America." *Lancet* 385, no. 9974 (2015): 1174–75.

Bliss, Katherine E. "Under Surveillance: Public Health, the FBI, and Exile in Cold War Mexico." In Birn and Necochea López, *Peripheral Nerve*, 31–54.

Borowy, Iris. *Coming to Terms with World Health: The League of Nations Health Organisation 1921–1946*. Frankfurt am Main: Peter Lang, 2009.

———. "Shifting between Biomedical and Social Medicine: International Health Organizations in the 20th Century." *History Compass* 12, no. 6 (2014): 517–30.

Bosio, Bartolomé. *Cartas de un médico rural: médicos, medicina y enfermos*. Buenos Aires: Colección Claridad, 1936.

Botey, Ana María. "Los actores sociales y la construcción de las políticas de salud del estado liberal en Costa Rica (1850–1940)." PhD diss., Universidad de Costa Rica, 2013.

Breilh, Jaime. *Critical Epidemiology and the People's Health*. New York: Oxford University Press, USA, 2021.

———. "Entrevista con Jaime Breilh: medicina social (salud colectiva) y medio ambiente." *Ecología Política* 37 (2009).

Brickman, Jane Pacht. "Medical McCarthyism and the Punishment of Internationalist Physicians in the United States." In *Comrades in Health: U.S. Health Internationalists, Abroad and at Home*, edited by Anne-Emanuelle Birn and Theodore M. Brown, 82–100. New Brunswick, NJ: Rutgers University Press, 2013.

Briggs, Charles L., and Clara Mantini-Briggs. "Confronting Health Disparities: Latin American Social Medicine in Venezuela." *American Journal of Public Health* 99, no. 3 (2009): 549–55.

Buschini, José D. "La alimentación como problema científico y objeto de políticas públicas en la Argentina: Pedro Escudero y el Instituto Nacional de la Nutrición, 1928–1946." *Apuntes* 43, no. 79 (2016): 129–56.

Cabello, Felipe. "El gran europeo Georg Friedrich Nicolai: médico y pacifista; Berlín, Alemania, 1874–Santiago, Chile, 1964." *Revista Médica de Chile* 141, no. 4 (2013): 535–39.

Candina-Polomer, Azun. "Studying Other Memories: The Colegio Médico de Chile under Socialism, Dictatorship, and Democracy, 1970–1990." *Latin American Perspectives* 43, no. 6 (2016): 75–87.

Cano, Hipólito Roque. "Lazarte, Juan." *Archivos de la Historia de la Medicina Argentina* 2, no. 7–8 (1973): 19–21.

Caponi, Sandra. "Canguilhem y el estatuto epistemológico del concepto de salud." *História, Ciências, Saúde–Manguinhos* 4, no. 2 (1997): 287–307.

Carrillo, Ana María. "Salud pública y poder en México durante el Cardenismo, 1934–1940." *Dynamis* 25 (2005): 145–78.

Carrillo, Ramón. "Higiene y medicina social (discurso pronunciado al declarar inaugurado el Primer Congreso de Higiene y Medicina Social)." *Archivos de la Secretaría de Salud Pública de la Nación* 3, no. 19 (1948): 22–34.

———. "Política Sanitaria Argentina." *Archivos de la Secretaría de Salud Pública de la Nación* 4, no. 3 (1948): 198–220.

———. *Política Sanitaria Argentina*. Remedios de Escalada: Universidad Nacional de Lanús, 2018 [1949].

Carrillo Roa, Alejandra "Sistema de salud en Venezuela: ¿un paciente sin remedio?" *Cadernos de Saúde Pública* 34 (2018): e00058517.

Carter, Eric D. *Enemy in the Blood: Malaria, Environment, and Development in Argentina*. Tuscaloosa: University of Alabama Press, 2012.

———. "Malaria Control in the Tennessee Valley Authority: Health, Ecology, and Metanarratives of Development." *Journal of Historical Geography* 43 (2014): 111–27.

———. "Population Control, Public Health, and Development in Mid Twentieth Century Latin America." *Journal of Historical Geography* 62 (2018): 96–105.

———. "Social Medicine and International Expert Networks in Latin America, 1930–1945." *Global Public Health* 14, no. 6–7 (2019): 791–802.

Carter, Eric D., and Marcelo Sánchez Delgado. "Una discusión sobre el vínculo entre Salvador Allende, Max Westenhöfer y Rudolf Virchow: aportes a la historia de la medicina social chilena e internacional." *História, Ciências, Saúde–Manguinhos* 27 (2020): 899–917.

Castro, Josué de. *The Geography of Hunger*. Boston: Little, Brown, 1952.

Castro, Roberto. *Teoría social y salud*. Mexico City: Universidad Nacional Autónoma de México/Centro Regional de Investigaciones Multidisciplinarias/El Lugar Editorial, 2010.

Chappell, M. Jahi. *Beginning to End Hunger: Food and the Environment in Belo Horizonte, Brazil, and Beyond*. Berkeley: University of California Press, 2018.

Chaufan, Claudia. "Desentrañando el "milagro cubano": una conversación con el Dr. Enrique Beldarrain Chaple." *Medicina Social* 8, no. 2 (2014): 93–99.

Chorny, Adolfo H. "Planificación en salud: viejas ideas en nuevos ropajes." *Cuadernos Médico-Sociales (Rosario)*, no. 73 (1998): 23–44.

Cohen, Wilbur J. "The First Inter-American Conference on Social Security." *Social Security* 5, no. 10 (1942): 4–7.

Comissão Organizadora da 8ª Conferência Nacional de Saúde. "Democracia é saúde." Rio de Janeiro: VideoSaúde–Distribuidora da Fiocruz, 1986. www.youtube.com/watch?v=-_HmqWCTEeQ&t=28s.

Comité de Expertos de la OPS/OMS. "Primer informe sobre la enseñanza de la medicina preventiva y social en las escuelas de medicina de la América Latina." *Educación Médica y Salud* 3, no. 2 (1969): 132–55.

Comité del Programa de Libros de Texto de la OPS/OMS para la Enseñanza de la Medicina Preventiva y Social en las Escuelas de Medicina de la América Latina. "Enseñanza de la medicina preventiva y social en las escuelas de medicina de la América Latina." In *Serie de Desarrollo de Recursos Humanos.* Washington, DC: PAHO, 1974.

Compagnon, Olivier. *América Latina y la Gran Guerra: el adiós a Europa (Argentina y Brasil, 1914–1939).* Buenos Aires: Crítica, 2014.

Conill, Eleonor Minho. "O enfoque ecológico-social e a atenção primária na construção de sistemas universais na trajetória de Hernán San Martin." *Ciência & Saúde Coletiva* 21 (2016): 173–78.

Conrad, Christoph. "Social Policy History after the Transnational Turn." In *Beyond Welfare State Models: Transnational Historical Perspectives on Social Policy,* edited by Pauli Kettunen and Klaus Petersen, 218–40. Cheltenham: Edward Elgar, 2011.

Cordeiro, Hésio. "O Instituto de Medicina Social e a luta pela Reforma Sanitária: Contribuição à história do SUS." *Physis: Revista de Saúde Coletiva* 14, no. 2 (2004): 343–62.

Coutinho, Carlos Nelson. *Democracia e socialismo.* São Paulo: Cortez, 1992.

Craib, Raymond B. *The Cry of the Renegade: Politics and Poetry in Interwar Chile.* New York: Oxford University Press, 2016.

Cross, Stephen J., and William R. Albury. "Walter B. Cannon, L. J. Henderson, and the Organic Analogy." *Osiris* 3, no. 1 (1987): 165–92.

Cruz-Coke, Eduardo. "The Chilean Preventive Medicine Act." *International Labour Review* 38 (1938): 161–89.

———. *Medicina preventiva y medicina dirigida.* Santiago: Nascimento, 1938.

Cruz-Coke, Ricardo. "Síntesis biográfica del doctor Salvador Allende G." *Revista Médica de Chile* 131, no. 7 (2003): 809–14.

———. "Síntesis biográfica del doctor Salvador Allende G." *Revista Médica de Chile* 131, no. 7 (2003): 809–14.

Cruz-Coke Madrid, Marta. *Eduardo Cruz-Coke: Testimonios.* Santiago: Procultura Fundación, 2015.

Cueto, Marcos. "Social Medicine in the Andes, 1920–1950." In *The Politics of the Healthy Life: An International Perspective,* edited by Esteban Rodríguez Ocaña. European Association for the History of Medicine and Health Publications, 2002.

———. *The Value of Health: A History of the Pan American Health Organization.* Rochester, NY: University of Rochester Press, 2007.

Cueto, Marcos, Theodore M. Brown, and Elizabeth Fee. *The World Health Organization: A History.* Cambridge: Cambridge University Press, 2019.

Cueto, Marcos, and Gabriel Lopes. "AIDS, Antiretrovirals, Brazil and the International Politics of Global Health, 1996–2008." *Social History of Medicine* (2019).

Cueto, Marcos, and Steven Palmer. *Medicine and Public Health in Latin America: A History.* New York: Cambridge University Press, 2015.

de la Dehesa, Rafael. "Social Medicine, Feminism and the Politics of Population: From Transnational Knowledge Networks to National Social Movements in Brazil and Mexico." *Global Public Health* 14, no. 6–7 (2019): 803–16.

Del Campo P., Andrea. "El debate médico sobre el aborto en Chile en la década de 1930."
In *Por la salud del cuerpo: historia y políticas sanitarias en Chile*, edited by María Soledad
Zarate C., 131–88. Santiago: Ediciones Universidad Alberto Hurtado, 2008.

de Moura Pontes, Ana Lúcia. "Entrevista: Eduardo Luis Menéndez Spina." *Trabalho,
Educação e Saúde* 10, no. 2 (2012): 335–45.

de Sousa Santos, Boaventura. *The End of the Cognitive Empire*. Durham, NC: Duke
University Press, 2018.

Di Liscia, María Silvia, and Melisa Fernández Marrón. "Sin puerto para el sueño
americano: Políticas de exclusión, inmigración y tracoma en Argentina (1908–1930)."
Nuevo Mundo Mundos Nuevos (2009).

Doimo, Ana Maria. *A vez e a voz do popular: movimentos sociais e participação política no
Brasil pós-70*. Rio de Janeiro: Relume-Dumará, 1995.

Dos Santos, Ricardo Augusto. "Intelectuales y redes eugénicas de América Latina:
relaciones entre Brasil y Argentina a través de Renato Kehl y Víctor Delfino." In *Una
historia de la eugenesia argentina y las redes biopolíticas internacionales, 1912–1945*, edited
by Marisa Miranda and Gustavo Vallejo, 65–95. Buenos Aires: Editorial Biblos, 2012.

Dowbor, Monika. "Origins of Successful Health Sector Reform: Public Health
Professionals and Institutional Opportunities in Brazil." *IDS Bulletin* 38, no. 6 (2007):
73–80.

———. "Sérgio Arouca, construtor de instituições e inovador democrático." *Ciência &
Saúde Coletiva* 24 (2019): 1431–38.

Dragoni, Carlos, and Etienne Burnet, "L'alimentation Populaire au Chili." *Revista Chilena
de Higiene y Medicina Preventiva* 1, no. 10–12 (1938): 407–611.

Drinot, Paulo. "Awaiting the Blood of a Truly Emancipating Revolution: Che Guevara in
1950s Peru." In *Che's Travels: The Making of a Revolutionary in 1950s Latin America*,
edited by Paulo Drinot, 88–126. Durham, NC: Duke University Press, 2010.

———. *La seducción de la clase obrera*. Lima: Instituto de Estudios Peruanos, 2016.

Drinot, Paulo, and Carlos Contreras. "The Great Depression in Peru." In Drinot and
Knight, *Great Depression in Latin America*, 102–28.

Drinot, Paulo, and Alan Knight, eds. *The Great Depression in Latin America*. Durham, NC:
Duke University Press, 2014.

Dubin, Martin David. "The League of Nations Health Organisation." In Weindling,
International Health Organisations, 56–80.

Durán, Hernán. "Enfoque y perspectivas de la planificación de la salud como parte del
desarrollo en América Latina." *Boletín de la Oficina Panamericana Sanitaria* 68 (1970):
41–52.

Eilers, Kerstin. "René Sand (1877–1953) and His Contribution to International Social
Work, IASSW-President 1946–1953." *Social Work and Society International Online Journal*
5, no. 1 (2007).

Elena, Eduardo. *Dignifying Argentina: Peronism, Citizenship, and Mass Consumption*.
Pittsburgh, PA: University of Pittsburgh Press, 2011.

Elena, Italo V. "Los Congresos Médico Sociales argentinos." *Cuadernos Médico Sociales*
26 (1983): 1–8.

Emanuelsson, Dick. "Entrevista a Juan Carlos Concha, ex Ministro de Salud del gobierno
de Salvador Allende." 2013. www.youtube.com/watch?v=3VBnYUb-cWo.

Escobar, Arturo. *Encountering Development: The Making and Unmaking of the Third World.* Princeton, NJ: Princeton University Press, 1995.

Escorel, Sarah. "Sérgio Arouca: Democracia e Reforma Sanitária." In Hochman and Lima, *Médicos intérpretes do Brasil,* 614–36.

Escudero, José Carlos. "Salud, historia y poder en la América Latina: entrevista con José Carlos Escudero." Buenos Aires: CeDoPS, 2015. www.youtube.com/watch?v =Mg1DdPyjveQ&t=2736s.

Escudero, Pedro. "El cuidado y mejoramiento de la salud en la población sana del país." Buenos Aires: Instituto Nacional de la Nutrición, 1943.

Escudero, Pedro, and Boris Rothman. "La vivienda en 600 familias de obreros y empleados de la Ciudad de Buenos Aires." *Trabajos y Publicaciones del Instituto Nacional de la Nutrición* 2, no. 1 (1938): 190–237.

Fajardo, Margarita. *The World That Latin America Created: The United Nations Economic Commission for Latin America in the Development Era.* Cambridge, MA: Harvard University Press, 2022.

Falcón, Ricardo. *La Barcelona Argentina: migrantes, obreros y militantes en Rosario, 1870–1912.* Buenos Aires: Laborde Editor, 2005.

Farley, John. *Brock Chisholm, the World Health Organization, and the Cold War.* Vancouver: UBC Press, 2008.

Farmer, Paul. "How Liberation Theology Can Inform Public Health." Partners in Health online. Accessed July 20, 2018. www.pih.org/article/dr.-paul-farmer-how-liberation -theology-can-inform-public-health.

Fassler, Clara. "Política sanitaria de la Junta Militar chilena (1973–1980)." *Revista Latinoamericana de Salud (Mexico, DF)* 2 (1982): 26–48.

———. "Transformación social y planificación de salud en América Latina." *Revista Centroamericana de Ciencias de la Salud,* no. 13 (1979): 133–60.

Fee, Elizabeth. "Henry E. Sigerist: From the Social Production of Disease to Medical Management and Scientific Socialism." *Milbank Quarterly* 67 (1989): 127–50.

———. "The Pleasures and Perils of Prophetic Advocacy: Henry E. Sigerist and the Politics of Medical Reform." *American Journal of Public Health* 86, no. 11 (1996): 1637–47.

Fernández Agis, Domingo. "La ética y la medicina social: la perspectiva de Michel Foucault." *História, Ciências, Saúde–Manguinhos* 27 (2020): 171–80.

Ferrara, Floreal A. "En torno al concepto de salud." *Revista de Salud Publica* 8 (1965): 115–20.

Ferrara, Floreal A., Eduardo Acebal, and Jose M. Paganini. *Medicina de la comunidad: medicina preventiva, medicina social, medicina administrativa.* Buenos Aires: Inter-Médica Editorial, 1972.

Ferrara, Floreal, and Milcíades Peña. "¿Qué piensan los médicos argentinos sobre los problemas de su profesión?" *Revista de Salud Pública (La Plata)* 1 (1961): 110–28.

Ferreira, José Roberto. "Un precursor de ideas y acciones de dimensión internacional." In Márquez and Rojas Ochoa, *Juan César García,* 51–54.

Ferreras, Norberto Osvaldo. "La misión de Stephen Lawford Childs de 1934: La relación entre la OIT y el Cono Sur." In Herrera León and Herrera González, *América Latina y la Organización Internacional,* 145–78.

Ferretti, Federico. "A Coffin for Malthusianism: Josué de Castro's Subaltern Geopolitics." *Geopolitics* (2019): 1–26.

———. "Rediscovering Other Geographical Traditions." *Geography Compass* 13 (2019): e12421.

Figueroa Clark, Victor. *Salvador Allende, Revolutionary Democrat*. London: Pluto Press, 2013.

Filerman, Gary Lewis. "An Exploratory Field Study of the National Health Service of Chile: Health Services Organization in Two Communities." PhD diss., University of Minnesota, 1970.

Finchelstein, Federico. *From Fascism to Populism in History*. Oakland: University of California Press, 2017.

Finer, Herman. "The Chilean Development Corporation: A Study in National Planning to Raise Living Standards; Studies and Report, New Series No. 5." Montreal: International Labour Office, 1947.

Fleury, Sonia. "Brazil's Health-Care Reform: Social Movements and Civil Society." *Lancet* 377, no. 9779 (2011): 1724–25.

———. "Política social, exclusión y equidad en América Latina en los 90." *Nueva Sociedad* 156 (1998): 72–94.

Fleury, Sonia, Mariana Faria, Juanita Durán, Hernán Sandoval, Pablo Yanes, Víctor Penchaszadeh, and Víctor Abramovich. *Right to Health in Latin America: Beyond Universalization*. Financing for Development series, no. 249. Santiago: United Nations/ECLAC, 2013.

Fonseca, Sebastian. "Latin American Social Medicine: The Making of a Thought Style." PhD diss., King's College London, 2020.

Foot, John. "Franco Basaglia and the Radical Psychiatry Movement in Italy, 1961–78." *Critical and Radical Social Work* 2, no. 2 (2014): 235–49.

Foucault, Michel. "Historia de la medicalización." *Educación Médica y Salud* 11, no. 1 (1977): 3–25.

———. "Nacimiento de la medicina social." *Revista Centroamericana de Ciencias de la Salud* 6 (1977): 89–108.

Franco, Saúl, Everardo Duarte Nunes, Jaime Breilh, Edmundo Granda, Jose Yépez, Patricia Costales, and Asa Cristina Laurell. *Debates en medicina social*. Quito: OPS, 1991.

Frei Montalva, Eduardo. "The Alliance That Lost Its Way." *Foreign Affairs* 45, no. 3 (1967): 437–48.

"A French Conception of Social Medicine." *Lancet* (December 25, 1920): 1316.

Fuster Sánchez, Nicolás. *El cuerpo como máquina: la medicalización de la fuerza de trabajo en Chile*. Santiago: Ceibo Ediciones, 2013.

Fuster Sánchez, Nicolás, and Pedro Moscoso-Flores, eds. *La Hoja Sanitaria: Archivo del Policlínico Obrero de la I. W. W. Chile, 1924–1927*. Santiago: Ceibo, 2015.

Gaffney, Adam. *To Heal Humankind: The Right to Health in History*. New York: Routledge, 2018.

Galdston, Iago, ed. *Social Medicine: Its Derivations and Objectives; The New York Academy of Medicine Institute on Social Medicine*. New York: Commonwealth Fund, 1949.

Galeano, Diego, Lucia Trotta, and Hugo Spinelli. "Juan César García and the Latin American Social Medicine Movement: Notes on a Life Trajectory." *Salud Colectiva* 7, no. 3 (2011): 285–315.

Galluzzi Bizzo, Maria Letícia. "Ação política e pensamento social em Josué de Castro." *Boletim do Museu Paraense Emílio Goeldi. Ciências Humanas* 4 (2009): 401–20.

García, Juan César. "Juan César García entrevista a Juan César García." In Márquez and Rojas Ochoa, *Juan César García*, 3–14.

———. *La educación médica en América Latina.* Washington, DC: OPS/OMS, 1972.

———. "La enfermedad de la pereza." In García, et al., *Pensamiento social en salud,* 150–71.

———. "La medicina estatal en América Latina." In García, et al., *Pensamiento social en salud,* 95–143.

———. "Las ciencias sociales en medicina." *Revista Cubana de Salud Pública* 34, no. 4 (2008 [1972]): 1–13.

García, Juan César, Everardo Duarte Nunes, María Isabel Rodríquez, and Saúl Franco, eds. *Pensamiento social en salud en America Latina.* Mexico: McGraw-Hill Interamericana, 1994.

García, Lorenzo. *Los derechos a la salud en la nueva Constitución de la Nación Argentina.* Santa Fe, NM: Universidad Nacional del Litoral, 1948.

García-Bryce, Iñigo. "Transnational Activist: Magda Mortal and the American Popular Revolutionary Alliance (Apra), 1926–1950." *The Americas* 70, no. 4 (2014): 677–706.

García Tello, José. *Estructurando la medicina del futuro.* Santiago: Imp. Universitaria, 1933.

———. *Mi experiencia en el policlínico de la Caja de Seguro Obrero de Viña del Mar: memoria del año 1931.* Valparaíso: Droguería del Pacífico, 1931.

Garrett, L., A. M. R. Chowdhury, and A. Pablos-Mendez. "All for Universal Health Coverage." *Lancet* 374 (2009): 1294–99.

Gaudenzi, Paula, and Francisco Ortega. "O estatuto da medicalização e as interpretações de Ivan Illich e Michel Foucault como ferramentas conceituais para o estudo da desmedicalização." *Interface-Comunicação, Saúde, Educação* 16 (2012): 21–34.

Gerschman, Sílvia. *A democracia inconclusa: um estudo da reforma sanitária brasileira.* Rio de Janiero: Editora FIOCRUZ, 2004.

Giedion, Ursula, and Manuela Villar Uribe. "Colombia's Universal Health Insurance System." *Health Affairs* 28, no. 3 (2009): 853–63.

Gofin, Jaime. "On 'A Practice of Social Medicine' by Sidney and Emily Kark." *Social Medicine* 1, no. 2 (2006): 107–15.

Golbert, Laura. *De la Sociedad de Beneficencia a los Derechos Sociales.* Buenos Aires: Ministerio de Trabajo, Empleo y Seguridad Social, 2010.

González Bernaldo de Quirós, Pilar. "El 'momento mutualista' en la formulación de un sistema de protección social en Argentina: socorro mutuo y prevención subsidiada a comienzos del siglo XX." *Revista de Indias* 73, no. 257 (2013): 157–92.

González Guzmán, Rafael. "Latin American Social Medicine and the Report of the WHO Commission on Social Determinants of Health." *Social Medicine* 4, no. 2 (2009): 113–20.

González Leandri, Ricardo. "Notas acerca de la profesionalización médica en Buenos Aires durante la segunda mitad del siglo XIX." In Suriano, *La cuestión social,* 217–43.

Gorsky, Martin. "The British National Health Service 1948–2008: A Review of the Historiography." *Social History of Medicine* 21, no. 3 (2008): 437–60.

Gorsky, Martin, and Christopher Sirrs. "From 'Planning' to 'Systems Analysis': Health Services Strengthening at the World Health Organisation, 1952–1975." *Dynamis* 39, no. 1 (2019): 205–33.

Granda Ugalde, Edmundo. *La salud y la vida.* Quito: OPS, 2009.

Grez Toso, Sergio. *La "Cuestión social" en Chile: ideas y debates precursores, 1804–1902.* Santiago: Dirección de Biblioteca Archivos y Museos, 1995.

———. "La guerra preventiva: Escuela Santa María de Iquique; Las razones del poder." *Diálogo Andino-Revista de Historia, Geografía y Cultura Andina* 31 (2008): 81–89.

———. "La trayectoria histórica del mutualismo en Chile (1853–1990): Apuntes para su estudio." *Revista Mapocho*, no. 35 (1994): 293–316.

Guedes de Vasconcelos, Francisco de Assis. "Josué de Castro and the Geography of Hunger in Brazil." *Cadernos de Saúde Pública* 24, no. 11 (2008): 2710–17.

———. "Pão ou aço: Conflitos e contradições do desenvolvimento econômico brasileiro na obra de Josué de Castro." In Hochman and Lima, *Médicos intérpretes do Brasil*, 476–501.

Guillén, Ana, and Michel Vale. "The Emergence of the Spanish Welfare State: The Role of Ideas in the Policy Process." *International Journal of Political Economy* 20, no. 2 (1990): 82–96.

Guthrie, Jason. "The ILO and the International Technocratic Class." In Kott and Droux, *Globalizing Social Rights*, 115–34.

Gutiérrez, Leandro H., and Luis Alberto Romero. "Barrio Societies, Libraries and Culture." In Adelman, *Essays in Argentine Labour History*, 217–34.

Gutiérrez, Leandro H., and Juan Suriano. "Workers' Housing in Buenos Aires, 1800–1930." In Adelman, *Essays in Argentine Labour History*, 35–51.

Guy, Donna J. *Women Build the Welfare State: Performing Charity and Creating Rights in Argentina, 1880–1955.* Durham, NC: Duke University Press, 2009.

Hagood, Jonathan. "Cells in the Body Politic: Physicians, Social Medicine, and Public Health in Peronist Argentina." Phd Diss., University of California-Davis, 2008.

———. "Unidad Médica: Physicians' Unions and the Rise of Peronism in 1930s–1950s Buenos Aires." *Labor: Studies in Working-Class History of the Americas* 9, no. 3 (2012): 69–90.

Hakim, Peter, and Giorgio Solimano. "Nutrition and National Development: Establishing the Connection." *Food Policy* 1, no. 3 (1976): 249–59.

Hamilton, Mario. *Vida de sanitarista.* Buenos Aires: Lugar Editorial, 2010.

Harrison, David. *The Sociology of Modernization and Development.* London: Routledge, 2003.

Hartch, Todd. *The Prophet of Cuernavaca: Ivan Illich and the Crisis of the West.* New York: Oxford University Press, 2015.

Hartmann, Christopher. "Bolivia's Plurinational Healthcare Revolution Will Not Be Defeated." *NACLA Report on the Americas* (December 19, 2019).

———. "Postneoliberal Public Health Care Reforms: Neoliberalism, Social Medicine, and Persistent Health Inequalities in Latin America." *American Journal of Public Health* 106, no. 12 (2016): 2145–51.

Hernández Álvarez, Mario. "El enfoque sociopolítico para el análisis de las reformas sanitarias en América Latina." In Rojas Ochoa and Márquez, *ALAMES en la memoria*, 490–507.

Hernández Toledo, Sebastián. "Apristas en Chile: circuitos intelectuales y redes políticas durante los años 1930." *Revista de Historia y Geografía* 31 (2014): 77–94.

Herrera González, Patricio. "Beyond Social Legislation: Worker Unity in Latin America and Its Links to the International Labour Organization, 1936–1938." In McPherson and Wehrli, *Beyond Geopolitics*, 115–34.

———. "El pacto por la unidad obrera continental: sus antecedentes en Chile y México, 1936." *Estudios de Historia Moderna y Contemporánea de México* 46 (2013): 87–119.

———. "La Primera Conferencia Regional del Trabajo en América: su influencia en el movimiento obrero (1936)." In Herrera León and Herrera González, *América Latina y la Organización Internacional*, 175–213.

Herrera León, Fabián, and Patricio Herrera González, eds. *América Latina y la Organización Internacional del Trabajo: Redes, cooperación técnica e institucionalidad social (1919–1950)*. Morelia, Mexico: Instituto de Investigaciones Históricas, Universidad Michoacana de San Nicolás de Hidalgo, 2013.

Herrero, María Belén, and Adrián Carbonetti. "La mortalidad por tuberculosis en Argentina a lo largo del siglo XX." *História, Ciências, Saúde–Manguinhos* 20, no. 2 (2013): 521–36.

Hochman, Gilberto. *The Sanitation of Brazil: Nation, State, and Public Health, 1889–1930*. Champaign: University of Illinois Press, 2016.

Hochman, Gilberto, and Nísia Trindade Lima, eds. *Médicos intérpretes do Brasil*. São Paulo: Editora Hucitec, 2015.

Holst, John. "Paulo Freire in Chile, 1964–1969: Pedagogy of the Oppressed in Its Sociopolitical Economic Context." *Harvard Educational Review* 76, no. 2 (2006): 243–70.

Homedes, Núria, and Antonio Ugalde. "Why Neoliberal Health Reforms Have Failed in Latin America." *Health Policy* 71, no. 1 (2005): 83–96.

Horowitz, Irving Louis, ed. *The Rise and Fall of Project Camelot: Studies in the Relationship between Social Science and Practical Politics*. Cambridge, MA: MIT Press, 1974.

Horowitz, Irving Louis, Josue De Castro, and John Gerassi, eds. *Latin American Radicalism*. New York: Vintage, 1969.

Horwitz, Abraham. "La Organización Panamericana de la Salud en su 75o aniversario." *Revista Médica de Chile* 106, no. 2 (1978): 138–43.

———. "Planificación del desarrollo económico y social en la América Latina." *Boletín de la Oficina Sanitaria Panamericana* 51, no. 5 (1961): 379–86.

"Huelga médica: principios gremiales mantenidos en su desarrollo." *Mundo Hospitalario* 182 (July 1959): 11.

Huhle, Teresa. "The Transnational Formation of a Healthy Nation: Uruguayan Travelling Reformers in the Early Twentieth Century (1905–1931)." *Revista Ciencias de la Salud (Universidad del Rosario, Colombia)* 19, no. 3 (2021): 1–22.

Huish, Robert, and John M. Kirk. "Cuban Medical Internationalism and the Development of the Latin American School of Medicine." *Latin American Perspectives* 34, no. 6 (2007): 77–92.

Huneeus Madge, Carlos, and María Paz Lanas. "Ciencia política e historia: Eduardo Cruz-Coke y el estado de bienestar en Chile: 1937–1938." *Historia (Santiago)* 35 (2002): 151–86.

Huntington, Samuel P. "The Change to Change: Modernization, Development, and Politics." *Comparative Politics* 3, no. 3 (1971): 283–322.

Hurtado, Diego, and María José Fernández. "Institutos privados de investigación 'pura' versus políticas públicas de ciencia y tecnología en la Argentina (1943–1955)." *Asclepio* 65, no. 1 (2013): 1–17.

Illanes, Maria Angélica. *Cuerpo y sangre de la política: la construcción histórica de las visitadoras sociales, Chile, 1887–1940*. Santiago: LOM Ediciones, 2006.

———. *"En el nombre del pueblo, del estado y de la ciencia": historia social de la salud pública, Chile 1880–1973; hacia una historia social del siglo XX*. Santiago: Ministerio de Salud, 2010 [1993].

———. "La revolución solidaria: las sociedades de socorros mutuos de artesanos y obreros: un proyecto popular democrático, 1840–1910." In *Chile des-centrado: formación socio-cultural republicana y transición capitalista 1810–1910*. Santiago: LOM Ediciones, 2003.

"Inauguración de los cursos de la escuela politécnica," *AAABEMS* 2, no. 24 (1934): 11.

International Labour Office. *Report on Social Insurance: First Item on the Agenda, Conference of American States Members of the International Labour Organisation, Santiago de Chile, December 1935–January 1936*. Geneva, 1935.

Iriart, Celia, Emerson Elías Merhy, and Howard Waitzkin. "Managed Care in Latin America: The New Common Sense in Health Policy Reform." *Social Science & Medicine* 52, no. 8 (2001): 1243–53.

Jacobina, André Teixeira. "A relação do Cebes com o PCB na emergência do movimento sanitário." *Saúde em Debate* 40 (2016): 148–62.

Jeifets, Víctor, and Lazar Jeifets. *La Internacional Comunista y América Latina, 1919–1943: Diccionario biográfico*. Santiago: Ariadna Ediciones, 2015.

Jensen, Jill. "From Geneva to the Americas: The International Labor Organization and Inter-American Social Security Standards, 1936–1948." *International Labor and Working-Class History* 80 (2011): 215–40.

Jerome, Jessica Scott. *A Right to Health: Medicine, Marginality, and Health Care Reform in Northeastern Brazil*. Austin: University of Texas Press, 2015.

Jiménez de la Jara, Jorge. "Abraham Horwitz (1910–2000) padre de la salud pública panamericana." *Revista Médica de Chile* 131, no. 8 (2003): 929–34.

Johnson, Brian B. "Decolonization and Its Paradoxes The (Re)envisioning of Health Policy in Bolivia." *Latin American Perspectives* 37, no. 3 (2010): 139–59.

Juárez Herrera y Cairo, Lucero Aída, and María del Carmen Castro Vásquez. "El dilema preventivista: contribuciones a la comprensión y crítica de la medicina preventiva." *Región y Sociedad* 24 (2012): 299–307.

Kapelusz-Poppi, Ana María. "Physician Activists and the Development of Rural Health in Postrevolutionary Mexico." *Radical History Review* 80, no. 1 (2001): 35–50.

———. "Rural Health and State Construction in Post-Revolutionary Mexico: The Nicolaita Project for Rural Medical Services." *The Americas* 58, no. 2 (2001): 261–83.

Katz, Ignacio. *Argentina hospital: el rostro oscuro de la salud*. Buenos Aires: Edhasa, 2004.

Kaufman, Jay S. "Science Alone Can't Heal a Sick Society." *New York Times*, September 10, 2021.

Kawachi, Ichiro, S.V. Subramanian, and Naomar Almeida-Filho. "A Glossary for Health Inequalities." *Journal of Epidemiology & Community Health* 56, no. 9 (2002): 647–52.

Kehl, Renato. *Eugenia e medicina social (problemas da vida)*. Rio de Janeiro: Francisco Alves, 1920.

King, Nancy. *The Social Medicine Reader: Patients, Doctors, and Illness*. 2nd ed. Durham, NC: Duke University Press, 2005.

Kirk, John M. *Healthcare without Borders: Understanding Cuban Medical Internationalism.* Gainesville: University Press of Florida, 2015.

Knight, Alan. "The Great Depression in Latin America: An Overview." In Drinot and Knight, *Great Depression in Latin America,* 276–339.

Kott, Sandrine, and Joelle Droux, eds. *Globalizing Social Rights: The International Labour Organization and Beyond.* New York: Palgrave Macmillan, 2013.

Krieger, Nancy. "Latin American Social Medicine: The Quest for Social Justice and Public Health." *American Journal of Public Health* 93, no. 12 (2003): 1989–91.

———. "Theories for Social Epidemiology in the 21st Century: An Ecosocial Perspective." *International Journal of Epidemiology* 30, no. 4 (2001): 668–77.

Krieger, Nancy, Margarita Alegría, Naomar Almeida-Filho, Jarbas Barbosa da Silva, Maurício L Barreto, Jason Beckfield, Lisa Berkman, Anne-Emanuelle Birn et al. "Who, and What, Causes Health Inequities? Reflections on Emerging Debates from an Exploratory Latin American/North American Workshop." *Journal of Epidemiology and Community Health.* 64, no. 9 (2010): 747–49.

Krige, John, ed. *How Knowledge Moves: Writing the Transnational History of Science and Technology.* Chicago: University of Chicago Press, 2019.

Krige, John. "Introduction: Writing the Transnational History of Science and Technology." In Krige, *How Knowledge Moves,* 1–34.

"La Actualidad Médico-Social: Primer Congreso Médico-Social Panamericano." *La Reforma Médica (Lima, Peru)* 33, no. 490 (1947): 7.

Labra, María Eliana. "Medicina social en Chile: Propuestas y debates (1920–1950)." *Cuadernos Médico Sociales (Chile)* 44, no. 4 (2004): 207–19.

Landabure, Pedro B. "Pedro Escudero; su pensamiento, su doctrina y su obra." *La Prensa Médica Argentina* 55, no. 41–42 (1968): 1983–89.

Laurell, Asa Cristina. "El estudio social del proceso salud-enfermedad en América Latina." *Cuadernos Médico Sociales (Argentina)* 37 (1986): 3–18.

———. "The Mexican Popular Health Insurance: Myths and Realities." *International Journal of Health Services* 45, no. 1 (2015): 105–25.

———. "Proyectos políticos y opciones de salud en la América Latina." In Rojas Ochoa and Márquez, *ALAMES en la memoria,* 220–41.

———. "Social Policy and Health Policy in Latin America: A Field of Political Struggle." *Cadernos de Saúde Pública* 33 (2017): e00043916.

———. "What Does Latin American Social Medicine Do When It Governs? The Case of the Mexico City Government." *American Journal of Public Health* 93, no. 12 (2003): 2028–31.

Laurell, Asa Cristina, and Ligia Giovanella. "Health Policies and Systems in Latin America." In *Oxford Research Encyclopedia of Global Public Health.* Oxford: Oxford University Press, 2018.

Laval, Enrique. "Epidemia de tifus exantemático en Chile (1932–1939)." *Revista Chilena de Infectología* 30, no. 3 (2013): 313–16.

Lavrin, Asunción. *Women, Feminism, and Social Change in Argentina, Chile, and Uruguay, 1890–1940.* Lincoln: University of Nebraska Press, 1998.

Lawrence, Christopher, and George Weisz, eds. *Greater Than the Parts: Holism in Biomedicine, 1920–1950.* New York: Oxford University Press, 1998.

————. "Medical Holism: The Context." In Lawrence and Weisz, *Greater Than the Parts*, 1–22.

Lazarte, Juan. "Asistencia médica, gremios y seguros sociales (Chile)." *El Médico Práctico* 11, no. 121 (1955): 8–9.

————. "Bases para una organización de los servicios médicos en los seguros de salud." In *Primer Congreso Nacional de Higiene y Medicina Social*, vol 2, 170–94. Buenos Aires: Asociación Argentina de Higiene, 1948.

————. *Chile en la vanguardia: impresiones.* Valparaiso: Editorial Médica Chilena, 1936.

————. *El contralor de los nacimientos.* Rosario: Librería Ruiz, 1936.

————. "Evolución y destino de la profesión médica." *Revista de la Confederación Médica de la República Argentina* 8, no. 67 (1954): 18–19.

————. *La solución federalista en la crisis histórica argentina.* Buenos Aires: Editorial Reconstruir, 1957.

————. *Problemas de medicina social.* Buenos Aires: Editorial Americalee, 1943.

Ledesma Prietto, Nadia Florencia. *"La revolución sexual de nuestro tiempo": el discurso médico anarquista sobre el control de la natalidad, la maternidad y el placer sexual; Argentina, 1931–1951.* Buenos Aires: Biblos, 2016.

Le Grand, Julian. "Quasi-Markets and Social Policy." *Economic Journal* 101, no. 408 (1991): 1256–67.

Lemercier, Claire. "Formal Network Methods in History: Why and How?" In *Social Networks, Political Institutions, and Rural Societies*, 281–310. Turnhout: Brepols, 2015.

Lent, Herman. *O massacre de Manguinhos.* Rio de Janeiro: Editora FIOCRUZ, 2019.

Letelier Carvajal, Javiera. "Ideas eugenésicas en Chile 1925–1941: una mirada hacia los intentos por mejorar la 'raza chilena.'" In *Control social y objetivación: escrituras y tránsitos de las ciencias en Chile*, edited by Grupo de Estudios en Historia de las Ciencias, 92–110. Santiago: Universidad de Chile, 2012.

Lima, Nísia Trindade, José Paranaguá de Santana, and Carlos Henrique Assuncao Paiva, eds. *Saúde coletiva: a Abrasco em 35 anos de história.* Rio de Janeiro: Fiocruz, 2015.

Linardelli, María Florencia. "La salud de las mujeres y sus trabajos: Convergencias entre la medicina social latinoamericana y la teoría feminista." *RevIISE-Revista de Ciencias Sociales y Humanas* 11, no. 11 (2018): 147–61.

Lobato, Mirta Zaida. "El Estado en los años treinta y el avance desigual de los derechos y la ciudadanía." *Estudios Sociales* 12, no. 1 (1997): 41–58.

Londoño, Juan-Luis, and Julio Frenk. "Structured Pluralism: Towards an Innovative Model for Health System Reform in Latin America." *Health Policy* 41, no. 1 (1997): 1–36.

Long, J. D. "Informe presentado al Gobierno de Chile, a la terminación de sus funciones como Asesor Técnico del Servicio Nacional de Salubridad de ese país." *Boletín de la Oficina Sanitaria Panamericana* 6, no. 5 (1927): 409–14.

López, Laura B., and Susana Poy. "Historia de la nutrición en la Argentina: nacimiento, esplendor y ocaso del Instituto Nacional de la Nutrición." *Diaeta* 30 (2012): 39–46.

López-Alonso, Moramay. *Measuring Up: A History of Living Standards in Mexico, 1850–1950.* Stanford, CA: Stanford University Press, 2012.

López Arellano, Oliva, José Carlos Escudero, and Luz Dary Carmona Moreno. "Los determinantes sociales de la salud: una perspectiva desde el Taller Latinoamericano de

Determinantes Sociales Sobre la Salud, ALAMES." *Medicina Social* 3, no. 4 (2008): 323–35.

López Arellano, Oliva, and Florencia Peña Saint Martin. "Salud y sociedad: aportaciones del pensamiento latinoamericano." *Medicina Social* 1, no. 3 (2006): 82–102.

López Campillay, Marcelo. "Ciencia, médicos y enfermos en el siglo XX: la Caja del Seguro Obligatorio y la lucha antituberculosa en Chile." *Estudios* (May 2012): 53–68.

Loza, Carmen Beatriz. "Medicinas tradicionales andinas y su despenalización: entrevista con Walter Álvarez Quispe." *História, Ciências, Saúde–Manguinhos* 21, no. 4 (2014): 1475–86.

Luciani, María Paula. "La dirección de higiene y seguridad del trabajo: en torno a las tensiones por la delimitación de su función en el Estado Peronista." *Dynamis* 39, no. 2 (2019): 335–55.

Luisi, Paulina. "Sobre eugenia: trabajo presentado al Congreso del Niño." *Revista de Filosofía—Cultura, Ciencias, Educación* 2 (1916): 435–51.

Maradona, Esteban Laureano. *A través de la selva.* La Plata: ProBiota, 2012 [1937].

Mardones Restat, Jorge, and Ricardo Cox. *La alimentación en Chile: estudios del Consejo Nacional de Alimentación.* Santiago: Imprenta Universitaria, 1942.

Mariátegui, José. "El progreso nacional y el capital humano." *Mundial* (Lima), October 9, 1923. www.marxists.org/espanol/mariateg/oc/peruanicemos_al_peru/paginas /progreso.htm.

Marques, Marília Bernardes. *Sérgio Arouca: um cara sedutor.* São Paulo: Editora Brasiliense, 2007.

Márquez, Miguel. "Juan César García, educador médico de proyección multifacética." In Márquez and Rojas Ochoa, *Juan César García,* 83–100.

Márquez, Miguel, and Francisco Rojas Ochoa, eds. *Juan César García: su pensamiento en el tiempo, 1984–2007.* Havana: Sociedad Cubana de Salud Publica, Sección de Medicina Social Ateneo Juan César García, 2007.

Martinez-Alier, Joan. *The Environmentalism of the Poor: A Study of Ecological Conflicts and Valuation.* Cheltenham: Edward Elgar, 2003.

Martínez Franzoni, Juliana, and Diego Sánchez-Ancochea. *The Quest for Universal Social Policy in the South: Actors, Ideas and Architectures.* Cambridge: Cambridge University Press, 2016.

Masjuan, Eduard, and Joan Martinez-Alier. "'Conscious Procreation': Neo-Malthusianism in Southern Europe and Latin America in around 1900." Paper presented at International Society for Ecological Economics, Montreal, July 11–15, 2004.

Mastrangelo, Fabiana. *Dinámica social de la esperanza: vida y obra del doctor Juan Lazarte.* Buenos Aires: Victorioso Ediciones, 2012.

———. "La medicina social," *La Capital* (Rosario), July 22, 2020.

Maurín Navarro, Juan S. *Esquemas de pediatría sanitaria y social.* Mendoza: Talleres Gráficos d'Accurzio, 1956.

Mayka, Lindsay. "The Origins of Strong Institutional Design: Policy Reform and Participatory Institutions in Brazil's Health Sector." *Comparative Politics* 51, no. 2 (2019): 275–94.

McGuire, James W. "Social Policies in Latin America: Causes, Characteristics, and Consequences." In *Routledge Handbook of Latin American Politics,* edited by Peter Kingstone and Deborah J. Yashar, 200–23. New York: Routledge, 2012.

McGuire, James W., and Laura B. Frankel. "Mortality Decline in Cuba, 1900–1959: Patterns, Comparisons, and Causes." *Latin American Research Review* 40, no. 2 (2005): 83–116.

McPherson, Alan, and Yannick Wehrli. *Beyond Geopolitics: New Histories of Latin America at the League of Nations.* Albuquerque: University of New Mexico Press, 2015.

Meade, Teresa A. *"Civilizing" Rio: Reform and Resistance in a Brazilian City, 1889–1930.* University Park: Pennsylvania State University Press, 1999.

Medina, Eden. *Cybernetic Revolutionaries: Technology and Politics in Allende's Chile.* Cambridge, MA: MIT Press, 2011.

Mendoza, Walter, and Oscar Martínez. "Las ideas eugenésicas en la creación del Instituto de Medicina Social." *Anales de la Facultad de Medicina* (Universidad Nacional Mayor de San Marcos) 60, no. 1 (1999): 55–60.

Menéndez, Eduardo L. "Modelo médico hegemónico: tendencias posibles y tendencias más o menos imaginarias." *Salud Colectiva* 16 (2020): e2615.

"Mensaje al Primer Congreso Médico Social Panamericano de La Habana." *Boletín Gremial de la AMECH* 1 (December 1946): 3.

Mercer, Hugo. "La incorporación de las ciencias sociales a la medicina social" (video). Buenos Aires: CeDoPS, 2015. www.youtube.com/watch?v=at77qTvI910.

Mesa-Lago, Carmelo. "Social Security in Latin America and the Caribbean: A Comparative Assessment." In *Social Security in Developing Countries,* edited by Ehtisham Ahmad, Jean Dreze, John Hills and Amartya Sen, 356–94. Oxford: Clarendon, 1991.

Milanesio, Natalia. *Workers Go Shopping in Argentina: The Rise of Popular Consumer Culture.* Albuquerque: University of New Mexico Press, 2013.

Miranda, Marisa. "La Argentina en el escenario eugénico internacional." In Miranda and Vallejo, *Una historia de la eugenesia,* 19–64.

Miranda, Marisa, and Gustavo Vallejo, eds. *Una historia de la eugenesia: Argentina y las redes biopolíticas internacionales, 1912–1945.* Buenos Aires: Editorial Biblos, 2012.

Molina Bustos, Carlos Antonio. "Antecedentes del Servicio Nacional de Salud. Historia de debates y contradicciones, Chile: 1932–1952." *Cuadernos Médico Sociales (Chile)* 46, no. 4 (2006): 284–304.

Molina Bustos, Carlos Antonio. *Institucionalidad sanitaria chilena, 1889–1989.* Santiago: LOM Ediciones, 2010.

Molina Guzmán, Gustavo. "Third World Experiences in Health Planning." *International Journal of Health Services* 9, no. 1 (1979): 139–50.

Molina Guzmán, Gustavo, and Claudio Jimeno. "Teaching Social Science Concepts in a Clinical Setting in Preventive Medicine." *Milbank Memorial Fund Quarterly* 44, no. 2 (1966): 211–25.

Molina Martínez, Gloria, Rubén Gamboa De Bernardi, and Jocelyn Novoa. "Dr. Hugo Behm Rosas: un pionero de la medicina social (Santiago 1913–San José 2011)." *Salud Colectiva* 7, no. 2 (2011): 255–58.

Molyneux, Maxine. "The 'Neoliberal Turn' and the New Social Policy in Latin America: How Neoliberal, How New?" *Development and Change* 39, no. 5 (2008): 775–97.

Moraga Valle, Fabio. "El resplandor en el abismo: el movimiento Clarté y el pacifismo en América Latina (1918–1941)." *Anuario Colombiano de Historia Social y de la Cultura* 42 (2015): 127–59.

Morales-Borrero, Carolina, Elis Borde, Juan C Eslava-Castañeda, and Sonia C. Concha-Sánchez. "¿Determinación social o determinantes sociales? diferencias conceptuales e implicaciones praxiológicas." *Revista de Salud Pública* 15, no. 6 (2013): 797–808.

"Morre o médico argentino Carlos Bloch." *ABRASCO* (2013). Published electronically June 14. www.abrasco.org.br/site/noticias/morre-o-medico-argentino-carlos-bloch/1050/.

Muller, Frederik. *Participación popular en programas de atención sanitaria primaria en América Latina*. Medellín: Universidad de Antioquia, Facultad Nacional de Salud Pública, 1981.

Muñoz Cortés, Víctor. *Sin dios ni patrones: historia, diversidad y conflictos del anarquismo en la región chilena*. Valparaiso: Mar y Tierra Ediciones, 2013.

Murdock, Carl J. "Physicians, the State and Public Health in Chile, 1881–1891." *Journal of Latin American Studies* 27, no. 3 (1995): 551–67.

Murillo Peña, Juan Pablo, and Gustavo Franco Paredes. "Nuestra tragedia biológica: La eugenesia peruana y su participación en el escenario internacional." In Miranda and Vallejo, *Una historia de la eugenesia*, 287–330.

Murillo Ramírez, Oscar. "América Latina y La Gran Guerra (Review)." *Historia y Sociedad* 29 (2015): 326–29.

Murray, Laura R., Jonathan Garcia, Miguel Muñoz-Laboy, and Richard G. Parker. "Strange Bedfellows: The Catholic Church and Brazilian National AIDS Program in the Response to HIV/AIDS in Brazil." *Social Science & Medicine* 72, no. 6 (2011): 945–52.

Museo Social Argentino. *Primer Congreso de la Población: 26 a 31 de Octubre de 1940*. Buenos Aires, 1941.

Navarro, Vicente. *The Politics of Health Policy: The US Reforms, 1980–1994*. Cambridge, MA: Blackwell, 1994.

———. "What Does Chile Mean: An Analysis of Events in the Health Sector before, during, and after Allende's Administration." *Milbank Memorial Fund Quarterly* 52, no. 2 (1974): 93–130.

Neely, Abigail H. *Reimagining Social Medicine from the South*. Durham, NC: Duke University Press, 2021.

Nogueira, Roberto Passos. "A segunda crítica social da saúde de Ivan Illich." *Interface-Comunicação, Saúde, Educação* 7 (2003): 185–90.

Nuccetelli, Susana. *An Introduction to Latin American Philosophy*. Cambridge: Cambridge University Press, 2020.

Nunes, Everardo Duarte. "La salud colectiva en Brasil: analizando el proceso de institucionalización." *Salud Colectiva* 12, no. 3 (2016): 347–60.

———. "Las ciencias sociales en salud en America Latina: Una historia singular." *Espacio Abierto* 6, no. 2 (1997): 215–36.

———. "O pensamento social em saúde na América Latina: revisitando Juan César García." *Cadernos de Saúde Pública* 29 (2013): 1752–62.

———. "The Path Taken by Social Sciences within Health in Latin America: Review of Scientific Production." *Revista de Saúde Pública* 40 (2006): 64–72.

———. "Salud y sociedad en América Latina: Juan César García y las primicias de una sociología de la salud." In Márquez and Rojas Ochoa, *Juan César García*, 195–212.

———. "Tendencias y perspectivas de las investigaciones en ciencias sociales en salud en América Latina: una visión general." In Márquez and Rojas Ochoa, *Juan César García*, 123–94.

Oficina Sanitaria Panamericana. "Acta Final, Décima Conferencia Sanitaria Panamericana (celebrada en Bogotá, Colombia, septiembre 4–14, 1938)." *Boletín de la Oficina Sanitaria Panamericana* 126 (1938): 1–14.

OIT (Organización Internacional del Trabajo). *Conferencia del Trabajo de los Estados de América miembros de la Organización Internacional del Trabajo: Santiago de Chile, 2 al 14 de enero de 1936, actas de las sesiones.* Ginebra: OIT, 1936.

OPS/OMS. "Aspectos teóricos de las ciencias sociales aplicadas a la medicina." *Educación Médica y Salud* 8 no. 4 (1974): 354–59.

Orrego Luco, Augusto. *La cuestión social.* Santiago: Imp. Barcelona, 1897 [1884].

Osuna, María Florencia. *La intervención social del Estado: El Ministerio de Bienestar Social entre dos dictaduras (Argentina, 1966–1983).* Rosario: Prohistoria, 2017.

Otero, Hernán. "Sueños cifrados: una arqueología de las proyecciones de población de la Argentina moderna." *Revista de Demografía Histórica* 22, no. 1 (2004): 209–39.

Pacino, Nicole L. "National Politics and Scientific Pursuits: Medical Education and the Strategic Value of Science in Postrevolutionary Bolivia." In Birn and Necochea López, *Peripheral Nerve*, 55–85.

Packard, Randall M. *A History of Global Health: Interventions into the Lives of Other Peoples.* Baltimore: Johns Hopkins University Press, 2016.

———. *The Making of a Tropical Disease: A Short History of Malaria.* Baltimore: Johns Hopkins University Press, 2007.

PAHO. "Status of National Health Planning: Provisional Agenda Item no. 13. XVI Meeting, Directing Council, PAHO." 1965. http://iris.paho.org/xmlui/handle/123456789/26146.

Paim, Jairnilson, Claudia Travassos, Celia Almeida, Ligia Bahia, and James Macinko. "The Brazilian Health System: History, Advances, and Challenges." *Lancet* 377, no. 9779 (2011): 1778–97.

Paim, Jairnilson Silva. *Desafíos para la salud colectiva en el siglo XXI.* Remedios de Escalada: Universidad Nacional de Lanús, 2021.

Paiva, Carlos Henrique Assunção, and Luiz Antonio Teixeira. "Health Reform and the Creation of the Sistema Único de Saúde: Notes on Contexts and Authors." *História, Ciências, Saúde–Manguinhos* 21, no. 1 (2014): 15–35.

Palacios, Alfredo L., and Mario R. Salomone, eds. *Alfredo L. Palacios. Legislador social e idealista militante.* Buenos Aires: Círculo de Legisladores de la Nación Argentina, 1998.

Palloni, Alberto. "Fertility and Mortality Decline in Latin America." *Annals of the American Academy of Political and Social Science* 510, no. 1 (1990): 126–44.

Palmer, Steven. *From Popular Medicine to Medical Populism: Doctors, Healers, and Public Power in Costa Rica, 1800–1940.* Durham, NC: Duke University Press, 2003.

———. *Launching Global Health: The Caribbean Odyssey of the Rockefeller Foundation.* Ann Arbor: University of Michigan Press, 2010.

Parker, Richard. "Building the Foundations for the Response to HIV/AIDS in Brazil: The Development of HIV/AIDS Policy, 1982–1996." *Divulgação em Saúde para Debate* 27 (2003): 143–83.

Partido Peronista, Consejo Superior Ejecutivo. *Manual del peronista.* Buenos Aires, 1948.

Pávez, Fabián. "Experiencias autogestionarias en salud: el legado de Gandulfo en La Hoja Sanitaria y el Policlínico de la Organización Sindical Industrial Workers of the World (1923–1942)." *Revista Médica de Chile* 137, no. 3 (2009): 426–32.

Paz Soldán, Carlos Enrique. *Demostración de asistencia y saneamiento rurales: Valle de Carabayllo, 1933*. Lima: Instituto de Medicina Social, 1933.

———. "La medicina social al servicio de la nueva época (discurso)." *La Reforma Médica (Lima, Peru)* 31(1945): 541–45.

———. *La medicina social: ensayo de sistematización*. Lima, 1916.

———. *Las bases médico-sociales de la legislación sanitaria del Perú*. 2 vols. Lima: La Reforma Médica, 1918.

Pernet, Corinne A. "Developing Nutritional Standards and Food Policy: Latin American Reformers between the ILO, the League of Nations Health Organization, and the Pan-American Sanitary Bureau." In Kott and Droux, *Globalizing Social Rights*, 249–61.

Pianetto, Ofelia. "The Historical Conjuncture: Córdoba, 1917–21." In Adelman, *Essays in Argentine Labour History*, 142–59.

Pieper Mooney, Jadwiga E. "From Cold War Pressures to State Policy to People's Health: Social Medicine and Socialized Medical Care in Chile." In Birn and Necochea López, *Peripheral Nerve*, 187–210.

———. *The Politics of Motherhood: Maternity and Women's Rights in Twentieth-Century Chile*. Pittsburgh, PA: University of Pittsburgh Press, 2009.

Pinto, Francisco, and Benjamín Viel. *Seguridad social chilena: Puntos para una reforma*. Santiago: Editorial del Pacífico, 1950.

Pires-Alves, Fernando A., and Marcos Chor Maio. "Health at the Dawn of Development: The Thought of Abraham Horwitz." *História, Ciências, Saúde–Manguinhos* 22, no. 1 (2015): 69–93.

Pires-Alves, Fernando Antonio, Carlos Henrique Assunção Paiva, and Nísia Trindade Lima. "Baixada Fluminense, in the Shadow of the 'Sphinx of Rio': Popular Movements and Health Policies in the Wake of the SUS." *Revista Ciência & Saúde Coletiva* 23, no. 6 (2018): 1849–58.

Pite, Rebekah E. *Creating a Common Table in Twentieth-Century Argentina: Doña Petrona, Women, and Food*. Chapel Hill: The University of North Carolina Press, 2013.

Plata-Stenger, Véronique. "'To Raise Awareness of Difficulties and to Assert Their Opinion': The International Labour Office and the Regionalization of International Cooperation in the 1930s." In McPherson and Wehrli, *Beyond Geopolitics*, 97–113.

Pohl-Valero, Stefan. "Alimentación, raza, productividad y desarrollo: entre problemas sociales nacionales y políticas nutricionales internacionales (Colombia, 1890–1940)." In *Aproximaciones a lo local y lo global: América Latina en la historia de la ciencia contemporánea*, edited by Gisela Mateos and Edna Suárez-Díaz, 115–54. Mexico: Centro de Estudios Filosóficos, Políticos y Sociales Vicente Lombardo Toledano, 2016.

———. "'La raza entra por la boca': Energy, Diet, and Eugenics in Colombia, 1890–1940." *Hispanic American Historical Review* 94, no. 3 (2014): 455–86.

Porter, Dorothy. "How Did Social Medicine Evolve, and Where Is It Heading?" *PLoS Med* 3, no. 10 (2006): 1667–72.

———. "Social Medicine and the New Society: Medicine and Scientific Humanism in Mid-Twentieth Century Britain." *Journal of Historical Sociology* 9, no. 2 (1996): 168–87.

Porter, Dorothy, and Roy Porter. "What Was Social Medicine? An Historiographical Essay." *Journal of Historical Sociology* 1, no. 1 (1988): 90–109.

Prainsack, Barbara, and Alena Buyx. "Solidarity in Contemporary Bioethics: Towards a New Approach." *Bioethics* 26, no. 7 (2012): 343–50.

Primer Congreso Médico Social Panamericano, Diciembre 3–10, 1946. Havana: Tamayo y Cia., 1946.

"Primer Congreso Médico Social Panamericano: Carta Médica de La Habana." *Boletín Gremial de la AMECH*, 1 no. 3 (February 1947): 7.

Quevedo, Emilio, and Claudia Cortés. "El concepto de 'sistema': de la Química y la Fisiología a la Salud Pública y las Ciencias Sociales. Bases para una investigación futura." *Ciencias de la Salud* 13, no. 4 (2015): 105–25.

Rachid, Jorge. "Perón y Carrillo hicieron de la medicina social una política de Estado." *EcoDias* (2015). Published electronically September 15. www.ecodias.com.ar/art /per%C3%B3n-y-carrillo-hicieron-de-la-medicina-social-una-pol%C3%ADtica-de-estado.

Ramacciotti, Karina Inés. "De la culpa al seguro: La Ley de Accidentes de Trabajo, Argentina (1915–1955)." *Revista Mundos do Trabalho* 3, no. 5 (2011): 266–84.

———. "Influencias internacionales sobre la gestión de los accidentes de trabajo en Argentina. Primera mitad del siglo XX." *el@ tina. Revista electrónica de estudios latinoamericanos* 12, no. 48 (2014).

———. *La política sanitaria del peronismo*. Buenos Aires: Biblos, 2009.

Ramacciotti, Karina Inés, and Federico Rayez. "Los ingenieros sanitarios en la salud pública argentina entre 1870 y 1960." *Trashumante: Revista Americana de Historia Social*, no. 11 (2018): 122–43.

Ramírez Hita, Susana. "Aspectos interculturales de la reforma del sistema de salud en Bolivia." *Revista Peruana de Medicina Experimental y Salud Pública* 31 (2014): 762–68.

Rappaport, Joanne. *Cowards Don't Make History: Orlando Fals Borda and the Origins of Participatory Action Research*. Durham, NC: Duke University Press, 2020.

Rayez, Federico. "Germinal Rodríguez: entre la higiene, el servicio social y la divulgación sanitaria." *Conceptos* 95, no. 509 (2020): 183–209.

———. "Germinal Rodríguez: salud pública, política y divulgación sanitaria en primera persona (1898–1960)." Unpublished manuscript.

Redsacol/ALAMES. "Declaración de Redsacol/ALAMES ante las amenzas de intervención militar de Los Estados Unidos en Venezuela." 2017. www.alames.org/paises/99 –declaracion-de-redsacol-alames-ante-las-amenazas-de-intervencion-militar-de-los -estados-unidos-en-venezuela.

Reggiani, Andrés H. "Depopulation, Fascism, and Eugenics in 1930s Argentina." *Hispanic American Historical Review* 90, no. 2 (2010): 283–318.

Reich, Michael R. "Restructuring Health Reform, Mexican Style." *Health Systems & Reform* 6, no. 1 (2020): e1763114.

Remen, Razel, and Lillian Holloway. "A Student Perspective on ELAM and Its Educational Program." *Social Medicine* 3, no. 2 (2008): 158–64.

Revista de Manguinhos. "Memoria (special section dedicated to Sérgio Arouca)." *Revista de Manguinhos* 1, no. 3 (2003): 30–49.

Rodriguez, Julia. *Civilizing Argentina: Science, Medicine, and the Modern State*. Chapel Hill: University of North Carolina Press, 2006.

Rodriguez B., Aurora. *El Consejo Nacional de Alimentación y su plan de alimentación popular*. Santiago: Impr. Universitaria, 1937.

Roemer, Milton I. *National Health Systems of the World. Vol. 1: The Countries.* New York: Oxford University Press, 1991.

Rojas Carvajal, Alfredo. "Aplicación de la Ley de Medicina Preventiva en la Caja de Seguro Obligatorio." *Revista Médica de Chile* 68, no. 12 (1940): 1530–43.

Rojas Ochoa, F., and M. Márquez. *ALAMES en la memoria: selección de lecturas.* Havana: Editorial Caminos, 2009.

Romero, Hernán. "Desarrollo de la medicina y la salubridad en Chile." *Revista Médica de Chile* 100 (1972): 853–903.

———. "El Colegio Médico de Chile." *Revista Médica de Chile* 91, no. 4 (1963): 237–39.

Roncali Mafezolli, Sandra. "O cenário depois do golpe." *Saúde em Debate* 1 (1976): 5–8.

Rosemblatt, Karin Alejandra. *Gendered Compromises: Political Cultures and the State in Chile, 1920–1950.* Chapel Hill: University of North Carolina Press, 2000.

———. "Por un hogar bien constituido: el estado y su política familiar en los frentes populares." In *Disciplina y desacato: Construcción de identidad en Chile, siglos XIX y XX,* edited by L. Godoy, E. Hutchison, K. Rosemblatt, and M. Zárate, 181–222. Santiago: Ediciones Sur/CEDEM, 1995.

———. *The Science and Politics of Race in Mexico and the United States, 1910–1950.* Chapel Hill: University of North Carolina Press, 2018.

Rosenberg, Charles E. "Erwin H. Ackerknecht, Social Medicine, and the History of Medicine." *Bulletin of the History of Medicine* 81, no. 3 (2007): 511–32.

———. "Holism in Twentieth-Century Medicine." In Lawrence and Weisz, *Greater Than the Parts,* 335–55.

Rosenberg, Mark B. "Social Security Policymaking in Costa Rica: A Research Report." *Latin American Research Review* 14 (1979): 116–33.

Ross, César. "Felipe Herrera: notas para la historia de su pensamiento económico, 1945–1960." *Universum (Talca)* 28 (2013): 139–67.

Rovere, Mario. "La salud en la Argentina: alianzas y conflictos en la construcción de un sistema injusto." *La Esquina del Sur* (May 2004).

Rovira, Jaime. "Chilen@s en Mozambique." *Solidaridad Internacional con Chile durante la dictadura cívico-militar* (2013). Published electronically September 14. http://solidaridadconchile.org/?p=806.

Saborío, Flory, Laura Guzman, Miguel Martínez, and Jaime Sepúlveda. "Medicina comunitaria: Un ensayo de interpretación." *Revista Centroamericana de Ciencias de Salud* 1 (1975): 53–62.

Sacchi, Mónica, Margarita Hausberger, and Adriana Pereyra. "Percepción del proceso salud-enfermedad-atención y aspectos que influyen en la baja utilización del sistema de salud, en familias pobres de la ciudad de Salta." *Salud Colectiva* 3 (2007): 271–83.

Sagan, Leonard, Albert Jonsen, and Alfonso Paredes. *Report of the Recent Mission to Chile Sponsored by the Federation of American Scientists. Doctors in Politics: Report of a Mission to Chile. Testimony Given to Human Rights in Chile Hearings before the Subcommittees on Inter-American Affairs and on International Organizations and Movements of the Committee on Foreign Affairs, House of Representatives, Ninety-Third Congress, Second Session.* Washington, DC: US Government Printing Office, 1974.

Sahlins, Marshall. "The Established Order: Do Not Fold, Spindle, or Mutilate." In Horowitz, *Rise and Fall of Project Camelot,* 71–79.

Salazar Vergara, Gabriel, and Carlos Altamirano Orrego. *Conversaciones con Carlos Altamirano: memorias críticas*. Santiago: Penguin Random House Grupo Editorial Chile, 2011.

Salvatore, Ricardo D. "Burocracias expertas y exitosas en Argentina: los casos de educación primaria y salud pública (1870–1930)." *Estudios Sociales del Estado* 2, no. 3 (2016): 22–64.

———. *Disciplinary Conquest: U.S. Scholars in South America, 1900–1945*. Durham, NC: Duke University Press, 2016.

Sánchez Delgado, Marcelo Javier, Malte Seiwerth, and Jorge Abarzúa. "Las Casas de Limpieza: antecedentes y funcionamiento en la epidemia de tifus exantemático en Chile a inicios de la década de 1930." *Historia 396* 11, no. 1 (2021): 327–60.

Sand, René. *The Advance to Social Medicine*. Translated by Rita Bradshaw. London: Staples, 1952.

———. *Medicina social y progreso nacional*. Santiago: Impresa Universitaria, 1925.

Santa Maria, Julio V. *La alimentación como problema de salubridad*. Santiago: Imprenta Universitaria, 1946.

Savala, Joshua. *Beyond Patriotic Phobias: Connections, Cooperation, and Solidarity in the Peruvian-Chilean Pacific World*. Oakland: University of California Press, 2022.

Scarzanella, Eugenia. "Los pibes en el palacio de Ginebra: las investigaciones de la Sociedad de las Naciones sobre la infancia latinoamericana (1925–1939)." *Estudios Interdisciplinarios de América Latina y el Caribe* 14, no. 2 (2003).

Schraiber, Lilia Blima, and André Mota. "The Social in Health: Trajectory and Contributions of Maria Cecilia Ferro Donnangelo." *Ciência & Saúde Coletiva* 20 (2015): 1467–73.

Schuftan, Claudio. "Una verdadera joya en los anales de la medicina social: el legado del joven Allende." *Medicina Social* 1, no. 3 (2006): 73–75.

Schuftan, Claudio, and Ravi Narayan. "People's Health Movement." In *Health Systems Policy, Finance, and Organization*, edited by Guy Carrin, 123–27. Oxford: Academic Press/Elsevier, 2009.

Selfa, Lance. "Mariátegui and Latin American Marxism." *International Socialist Review*, no. 96 (2015). https://isreview.org/issue/96/mariategui-and-latin-american-marxism.

Sen, Amartya. *Development as Freedom*. New York: Knopf, 1999.

———. "Economic Progress and Health." In *Poverty, Inequality and Health*, edited by David A Leon and Gill Walt. Oxford: Oxford University Press, 2000.

Seoane, Manuel. *Con el ojo izquierdo (mirando a Bolivia)*. Buenos Aires Imprenta Juan Perotti, 1926.

Sepúlveda Alvarez, Claudio. *De hombres y sombras, en Chile y Naciones Unidas*. Santiago: Maval Impresores, 2017.

Serra Canales, Jaime, and Gonzalo Ramírez Guier. "La experiencia del programa de salud en la comunidad 'Hospital Sin Paredes.'" *Ciencias Sociales* 40–41 (1988): 101–20.

Sigerist, Henry E. *Historia y sociología de la medicina*. Translated by Gustavo Molina Guzmán. Bogotá: Editora Guadalupe, 1974.

Silva, Patricio. "State, Politics and the Idea of Social Justice in Chile." *Development and Change* 24, no. 3 (1993): 465–86.

Singleton, Lisa. "The ILO and Social Security in Latin America, 1930–1950." In Herrera León and Herrera González, *América Latina y la Organización Internacional*, 215–43.

Smith, Benjamin T. "Towards a Typology of Rural Responses to Healthcare in Mexico, 1920–1960." *Endeavour* 37, no. 1 (2012): 39–46.

Snowden, Frank M. *The Conquest of Malaria: Italy, 1900–1962*. New Haven, CT: Yale University Press, 2006.

"Sobre un número aproximado de 10.000 médicos . . ." *Mundo Hospitalario* 179–180–181 (May–July 1958): 1–2.

Sojo, Ana. "Reformas de gestión en salud en América Latina." *Revista de la CEPAL* 74 (2001): 139–57.

Solimano, Giorgio, and Peter Hakim. "Nutrition and National Development: The Case of Chile." *International Journal of Health Services* 9, no. 3 (1979): 495–510.

Spiegel, Jerry M., Jaime Breilh, and Annalee Yassi. "Why Language Matters: Insights and Challenges in Applying a Social Determination of Health Approach in a North-South Collaborative Research Program." *Globalization and Health* 11, no. 1 (2015). https://doi.org/10.1186/s12992-015-0091-2.

Spinelli, Hugo, Juan Martín Librandi, and Juan Pablo Zábala. "Los Cuadernos Médico Sociales de Rosario y las revistas de la medicina social latinoamericana entre las décadas de 1970 y 1980." *História, Ciências, Saúde–Manguinhos* 24 (2017): 877–95.

Stehrenberger, Cécile Stephanie, and Svenja Goltermann. "Disaster Medicine: Genealogy of a Concept." *Social Science & Medicine* 120 (2014): 317–24.

Stepan, Nancy. *Eradication: Ridding the World of Diseases Forever?* Ithaca, NY: Cornell University Press, 2011.

Stepan, Nancy Leys. *"The Hour of Eugenics": Race, Gender, and Nation in Latin America*. Ithaca, NY: Cornell University Press, 1991.

Stern, Alexandra Minna. *Eugenic Nation: Faults and Frontiers of Better Breeding in Modern America*. Oakland: University of California Press, 2015.

Stonington, Scott, and Seth M. Holmes. "Social Medicine in the Twenty-First Century." *PLoS Med* 3, no. 10 (2006): e445.

Stralen, Cornelis Johannes van. "O Cebes e a defesa intransigente do direito à saúde e da democracia." *Saúde em Debate* 40, no. 108 (2016): 4–5.

Sturdy, Steve. "Biology as Social Theory: John Scott Haldane and Physiological Regulation." *British Journal for the History of Science* 21, no. 3 (1988): 315–40.

Suriano, Juan, ed. *La cuestión social en Argentina: 1870–1943*. Buenos Aires: La Colmena, 2000.

Svampa, Maristella. *Certezas, incertezas y desmesuras de un pensamiento político: conversaciones con Floreal Ferrara*. Buenos Aires: Ediciones Biblioteca Nacional, 2010.

Tabet, Livia Penna, Valney Claudino Sampaio Martins, Ana Caroline Leoncio Romano, Natan Monsores de Sá, and Volnei Garrafa. "Ivan Illich: da expropriação à desmedicalização da saúde." *Saúde em Debate* 41 (2017): 1187–98.

Tajer, Débora. "La medicina social latinoamericana en los años noventa: hechos y desafíos." In Rojas Ochoa and Márquez, *ALAMES en la memoria*, 21–37.

———. "Latin American Social Medicine: Roots, Development during the 1990s, and Current Challenges." *American Journal of Public Health* 93, no. 12 (2003): 2023–27.

Tajer, Debora, Graciela Reid, Mariana Gaba, Alejandra Lo Russo, and María Isabel Barrera. "Investigaciones sobre género y determinación psicosocial de la vulnerabilidad coronaria en varones y mujeres." *Revista Argentina de Cardiología* 81, no. 4 (2013): 344–52.

Tavares, Manuel, and Tatiana Romão. "Emerging Counterhegemonic Models in Higher Education: The Federal University of Southern Bahia (UFSB) and Its Contribution to a Renewed Geopolitics of Knowledge (Interview with Naomar De Almeida Filho)." *Encounters in Theory and History of Education* 16 (2015): 101–10.

Taylor, Rex, and Annelie Rieger. "Medicine as Social Science: Rudolf Virchow on the Typhus Epidemic in Upper Silesia." *International Journal of Health Services* 15, no. 4 (1985): 547–59.

Terán, Oscar. *Historia de las ideas en la Argentina: diez lecciones iniciales, 1810–1980*. Buenos Aires: Siglo Veintiuno Editores, 2008.

Testa, Mario. *Pensar en salud*. Buenos Aires: Organizacion Panamericana de la Salud, 1990.

Testa, Mario, and Jairnilson Silva Paim. "Memoria e historia: diálogo entre Mario Testa y Jairnilson Silva Paim." *Salud Colectiva* 6, no. 2 (2010): 211–27.

Toro-Blanco, Pablo. "La guerra santa por el bienestar de la patria: social cristianismo y política social; la campaña presidencial de Eduardo Cruz-Coke en 1946." In *Catolicismo Social chileno: desarrollo, crisis y actualidad*, edited by Fernando Berríos, Jorge Costadoat, and Diego García, 333–53. Santiago: Ediciones Universidad Alberto Hurtado, 2009.

Torres Tovar, Mauricio. "ALAMES: Organizational Expression of Social Medicine in Latin America." *Social Medicine* 2, no. 3 (2007): 125–30.

UNESCO. "Estudio de los informes de violaciones de derechos humanos en Chile, con particular referencia a la tortura y otros tratos o castigos crueles, inhumanos o degradantes (resolución 8 (XXVII) de la Subcomisión de Prevención de Discriminaciones y Protección a las Minorías y resolución 3219 (XXIX) de la Asamblea General)." Comisión de Derechos Humanos. 310. período de sesiones. Tema 7 del programa provisional, 1975.

Valdivieso, Ramón, Guillermo Adriasola, and Abraham Horwitz. "Homenaje de la Facultad de Medicina al Dr. Abraham Horwitz." *Revista Médica de Chile* 94, no. 12 (1966): 805–11.

Vargas, Juan Rafael, and Jorine Muiser. "Promoting Universal Financial Protection: A Policy Analysis of Universal Health Coverage in Costa Rica (1940–2000)." *Health Research Policy and Systems* 11, no. 1 (2013). https://doi.org/10.1186/1478-4505-11-28.

Vergara, Ángela. "De la higiene industrial a la medicina del trabajo: la salud de los trabajadores en América Latina, 1920–1970." In *Ampliando Miradas: Chile y su historia en un tiempo global*, edited by Fernando Purcell and Alfredo Riquelme. Santiago: RIL Editores–Instituto de Historia PUC, 2010.

————. "Los trabajadores chilenos y la Gran Depresión, 1930–1938." In *La Gran Depresión en América Latina*, edited by Paulo Drinot and Alan Knight, 73–108. Mexico: FCE, 2015.

————. "The Recognition of Silicosis: Labor Unions and Physicians in the Chilean Copper Industry, 1930s–1960s." *Bulletin of the History of Medicine* 79, no. 4 (2005): 723–48.

Vidal, Carlos. "Veinticinco años de *Educación Médica y Salud*." In Márquez and Rojas Ochoa, *Juan César García*, 113–20.

Vieira-da-Silva, Ligia Maria, and Patrice Pinell. "Gênese sócio-histórica da Saude Coletiva no Brasil." In Lima, Santana and Paiva, *Saúde Coletiva*, 25–48.

Viel, Benjamín. *Conferencias del Dr. Benjamín Viel*. San José: Publicaciones Caja Costarricense de Seguro Social/Imprenta Tormo Ltda., 1959.

Villarreal, Ramón. "Un hombre de estatura intelectual y moral fuera de lo común." In Márquez and Rojas Ochoa, *Juan César García*, 71–73.

Viñas, Alberto. *A la sombra de Hipócrates: episodios y relatos de un médico rural*. Buenos Aires: Editorial Metrópolis, 1936.

Wade, Peter. *Degrees of Mixture, Degrees of Freedom: Genomics, Multiculturalism, and Race in Latin America*. Durham, NC: Duke University Press, 2017.

Waitzkin, Howard. "Commentary: Salvador Allende and the Birth of Latin American Social Medicine." *International Journal of Epidemiology* 34, no. 4 (2005): 739–41.

———. *Medicine and Public Health at the End of Empire*. Boulder, CO: Paradigm, 2011.

Waitzkin, Howard, Celia Iriart, Alfredo Estrada, and Silvia Lamadrid. "Social Medicine in Latin America: Productivity and Dangers Facing the Major National Groups." *Lancet* 358, no. 9278 (2001): 315–23.

———. "Social Medicine Then and Now: Lessons from Latin America." *American Journal of Public Health* 91, no. 10 (2001): 1592–601.

Waitzkin, Howard, Rebeca Jasso-Aguilar, and Celia Iriart. "Privatization of Health Services in Less Developed Countries: An Empirical Response to the Proposals of the World Bank and Wharton School." *International Journal of Health Services* 37, no. 2 (2007): 205–27.

Wehrli, Yannick "Francisco Walker Linares: un actor del internacionalismo ginebrino en Chile (1927–1946)." In Herrera León and Herrera González, *América Latina y la Organización Internacional*, 56–85.

Weindling, Paul, ed. *International Health Organisations and Movements, 1918–1939*. Cambridge: Cambridge University Press, 1995.

———. "The League of Nations Health Organization and the Rise of Latin American Participation, 1920–40." *História, Ciências, Saúde–Manguinhos* 13, no. 3 (2006): 1–14.

———. "Social Medicine at the League of Nations Health Organisation and the International Labour Office Compared." In Weindling, *International Health Organisations*, 134–53.

Winn, Peter. "Salvador Allende: His Political Life . . . and Afterlife." *Socialism and Democracy* 19, no. 3 (2005): 129–59.

World Bank. *World Development Report 1993: Investing in Health*. Washington, DC, 1993.

Wright, Thomas C., and Rody Oñate Zúñiga. "Chilean Political Exile." *Latin American Perspectives* 34, no. 4 (2007): 31–49.

Yáñez Andrade, Juan Carlos. "Chile y la Organización Internacional del Trabajo (1919–1925): hacia una legislación social universal." *Revista de Estudios Histórico-Jurídicos*, no. 22 (2000): 317–32.

———. "La OIT y la red sudamericana de corresponsales: el caso de Moisés Poblete, 1922–1946." In Herrera León and Herrera González, *América Latina y la Organización Internacional*, 22–55.

Zabala, Juan Pablo. *La enfermedad de Chagas en la Argentina*. Bernal: Universidad Nacional de Quilmes Editorial, 2010.

Zaffaroni, Eugenio Raúl. "La mala vida o los prejuicios vestidos de ciencia." In Miranda and Vallejo, *Una historia de la eugenesia*, 123–40.

Zalaquett, Ricardo. "¡Siembra, juventud! la tierra es propicia, el momento es único: no es Neruda sino Gandulfo, el cirujano." *Revista Médica de Chile* 133, no. 3 (2005): 376–82.

Zancan, Lenira, and Álvaro Hideyoshi Matida. "Trajetórias de Joaquim Alberto Cardoso de Melo: Quincas, um berro à vida." *Ciência & Saúde Coletiva* 20 (2015): 3275–82.

Zárate Campos, María Soledad. "Alimentación y previsión biológica: la política médico-asistencial de Eduardo Cruz-Coke." In *Medicina Preventiva y Medicina Dirigida*, by Eduardo Cruz-Coke, ix–lxv. Santiago: Cámara Chilena de la Construcción, Pontífica Universidad Católica de Chile, Dibam, 2012.

Ziegler, Jean. *Betting on Famine: Why the World Still Goes Hungry*. New York: New Press, 2013.

Zimmerer, Karl S. "Ecology as Cornerstone and Chimera in Human Geography." In *Concepts in Human Geography*, edited by C. Earle, M. S. Kenzer, and K. Mathewson, 161–88. Lanham, MD: Rowman and Littlefield, 1996.

Zimmermann, Eduardo A. "Intellectuals, Universities and the Social Question." In Adelman, *Essays in Argentine Labour History*, 199–216.

———. *Los liberales reformistas: la cuestión social en la Argentina 1890–1916*. Buenos Aires: Editorial Sudamericana Universidad de San Andrés, 1995.

Zylberman, Patrick. "Fewer Parallels than Antitheses: René Sand and Andrija Stampar on Social Medicine, 1919–1955." *Social History of Medicine* 17, no. 1 (2004): 77–92.

Index

Abad Gómez, Héctor, 161

abortion, 30, 38, 39, 70, 77–78, 82, 83, 107

ABRASCO, 14, 153, 173, 180–83, 198, 204, 210, 213. *See also* saúde coletiva

Aguirre Cerda, Pedro, 85, 90

ALAMES, 4, 14, 18, 147, 165, 175, 178–79, 189, 190, 192–97, 198, 199, 204, 207, 208, 210, 212–16

alcoholism: eugenics and, 38, 43; nutrition and, 84; as social disease, 29, 31, 52, 87; as vice, 27, 42

Alessandri, Arturo, 71, 85

Allende, Salvador, 4, 72; advocacy for national health service, 90, 137; Colegio Médico and, 143; eugenics and, 36, 39; gender ideology of, 89, 104; as minister of health, 79, 86–92; overthrow in 1973 coup, 147, 150, 157–63, 215; political philosophy of, 43, 63, 64, 65, 70, 81, 88, 219; as president of Chile, 18, 129, 133, 136, 143–44, 153, 155–57; social medicine and, 10, 36, 64, 68–72, 86–92, 222; as student activist, 74, 76, 151; Vanguardia Médica and, 67, 75–77, 81, 85, 91

Alliance for Progress, 57, 126, 130–35, 140, 146, 161

Alma Ata conference, 161, 187, 206, 210. *See also* primary health care (PHC) model

Almeida Filho, Naomar, 139, 174, 199, 200, 203–4

American Medical Association, 62, 140

American Popular Revolutionary Alliance (APRA). *See* Apristas

American Public Health Association (APHA), 158, 161, 162

anarchism: in Argentina, 105–9, 121, 141; in Chile, 40–44, 71; gender ideology of, 40, 42, 69, 105–9; sexuality and, 40, 42, 69,

105–9; social medicine and, 20, 21, 40–44, 69, 96, 105–9

anarcho-feminism, 30, 39, 43, 107. *See also* anarchism; feminism

anticommunism, 124, 136, 145. *See also* Cold War geopolitics; medical McCarthyism

Apristas, 63–64, 67, 88

Aráoz Alfaro, Gregorio, 28, 39, 52, 98, 99, 101, 102

Argentina: authoritarianism in, 164–68; doctors' strike in, 142; eugenics in, 29, 36, 97–98, 101–3, 105, 107, 110; health system in, 17, 100–101, 106–9, 112–21, 142–43, 213; hygiene movement in, 96–98, 101–3, 105, 113; immigrants in, 97, 98, 99, 100; labor unions in, 95, 96, 100, 105, 106, 108, 114–20, 141–43; medical labor organizing in, 61, 101, 106–8, 118–21, 141, 142, 166, 217; mutual-aid societies in, 99–100, 101, 108, 113; neoliberal reforms of health sector in, 189–91; populism in, 94–95, 106, 109–17; rural medicine in, 34–35

Argentine Association for Biotypology, Eugenics, and Social Medicine, 36, 102–03. *See also* Argentina: eugenics in; eugenics; social medicine: eugenics and

Argentine Department of Labor, 24, 30, 103

Argentine Ministry of Health, 109, 110–16, 119

Arouca, Sergio, 1–2, 139, 154, 169, 170, 171–73, 176, 177, 182, 183, 199, 219, 223, 245n124

Baixada Fluminense, 181–82

Bambarén, Carlos, 29, 36

Bard, Leopoldo, 29, 31, 98–99, 105, 119

Basaglia, Franco, 169

9 781469 674452